NEW CHROMOSOMAL AND
MALFORMATION SYNDROMES

Birth Defects: Original Article Series
THE NATIONAL FOUNDATION
March of Dimes

VOL. XI, NO. 5
1975

NEW CHROMOSOMAL AND MALFORMATION SYNDROMES

Editor
DANIEL BERGSMA, M.D.

Associate Editors
David L. Rimoin, M.D., Ph.D.
David W. Smith, M.D.
Robert S. Sparkes, M.D.

Assistant Editors
Sue Conde Greene
Jaakko Leisti, M.D.
Jonathan Zonana, M.D.

The 1974 Birth Defects Conference held at Newport Beach, California, sponsored by The Harbor General Hospital Campus of the UCLA School of Medicine and The National Foundation-March of Dimes.

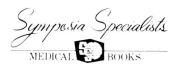

 STRATTON INTERCONTINENTAL MEDICAL BOOK CORPORATION

381 Park Avenue South, New York, New York 10016

To enhance medical communication in the birth defects field, The National Foundation publishes the *Birth Defects Atlas and Compendium,* an *Original Article Series, Syndrome Identification,* a *Reprint Series* and provides a series of films and related brochures.

Further information can be obtained from:

Daniel Bergsma, M.D.
Vice President for Professional Education and
    Director, Professional Education Department
The National Foundation-March of Dimes
1275 Mamaroneck Avenue
White Plains, New York 10605

Published by

Symposia Specialists

MIAMI, FLORIDA, 33161

Printed in the U.S.A.

Library of Congress
Catalog Card Number 75-16885

ISBN 0-88372-032-9

Received for publication October 21, 1974.

THE NATIONAL FOUNDATION is dedicated to the long-range goal of preventing birth defects. Our interim goal is to search for ways to ameliorate those birth defects which cannot be prevented.

As a part of our efforts to achieve these goals, we sponsor, or participate in, a variety of scientific meetings and symposia where all questions relating to birth defects are freely discussed. Through our professional educational program we speed the dissemination of information by publishing the proceedings of these meetings and symposia. Now and then, in the course of these discussions, individual participants may express personal viewpoints which go beyond the purely scientific in nature and into controversial matters; abortion for example. It should be noted, therefore, that personal viewpoints about such matters will not be censored but obviously this does not constitute an endorsement of them by The National Foundation.

Contents

Malformation Syndromes

Internipple Distance and Hand Measurements in Various Syndromes

Marilyn Preus, M.S., Murray Feingold, M.D.
and F. Clarke Fraser, Ph.D., M.D.

One of the difficulties encountered in syndrome diagnosis is the lack of specific measurements that allow the clinician to describe facial abnormalities and other physical features. In a study reported elsewhere,[1] 2403 normal patients were measured for various physical parameters including low-set ears; ear length; inner and outer canthal distance; interpupillary distance; internipple distance (IND); and hand, palm and finger lengths. By utilizing these normal measurements we attempted to determine if the above parameters were abnormal in various syndromes. For example, is the IND in Turner syndrome increased as we have always believed? We measured the chest circumference and the IND and then determined the ratio. For example, if the chest circumference was 60 cm and the IND 15 cm, the IND would be 25% of the total chest circumference. By utilizing Figure 1 the percentile can then be determined. Collins[2]

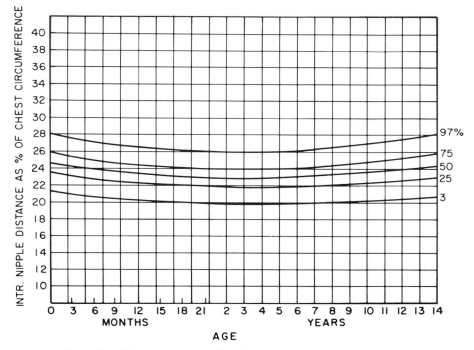

Fig. 1. The IND as a percentage of the chest circumference in normal children.

Table 1. Percentile of the IND as Percentage of Chest Circumference in Turner Patients

Age	Newborn	5 mos	2-5 yrs	8-10 yrs	11-12 yrs	14 yrs
Percentile	90	80	50	65	35	15
	90	70	75	70	40	20
	90		85	78	70	20
			97	78	85	25
			97	97		45
						50

Summary of Results

1) None of the 25 patients had an IND greater than the 97th percentile.
2) Sixteen of 25 patients had an IND greater than the 65th percentile (14 of whom were 10 years of age and younger).
3) None of 6 patients who were 14 years of age had an IND greater than the 50th percentile and 4 had an IND less than the 25th percentile.

recently reported that the IND was not increased in Turner syndrome but appeared increased because the acromial ends of the clavicles were positioned at a higher level than normal causing the shoulder width to be decreased. This resulted in an apparent increase in the IND which she described as an "illusion" secondary to the decreased shoulder width. Collins measured the IND and the chest width at the nipple level and then calculated an IND/chest width percentage ratio. No difference was found in patients with Turner syndrome and the normal controls.

We have studied a total of 25 patients with Turner syndrome — 18 with an XO karyotype and the remainder with an isochromosome X or mosaicism. These groups were first studied separately and then combined because the findings in both groups were similar. The results of this study are shown in Table 1.

None of the patients had an IND that was greater than the 97th percentile. However, as a child grows older the IND appears to decrease relative to normal. The patients 10 years of age and younger were on the average at the 81st percentile, those 11-12 years at the 41st percentile and those 14 years of age at the 29th percentile. Before any definite conclusions can be made, a greater number of patients with Turner syndrome need to be examined. At the present time it appears that as the child with Turner syndrome becomes older, the IND decreases relative to normal and this measurement is therefore most useful in the younger patient.

The same measurements performed on 17 patients with Noonan syndrome were within normal limits.

Measurements of total hand size, palm and finger length were also obtained. The palm length (Fig. 2-B) was obtained by measuring the distance from the distal flexion at the wrist to the proximal flexion crease of the middle finger. The middle finger length (Fig. 2-A) was obtained by measuring the distance from the proximal flexion crease of the middle finger to the tip of the middle finger. The length of the middle finger

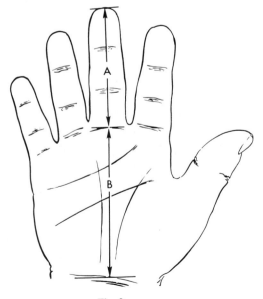

Fig. 2.

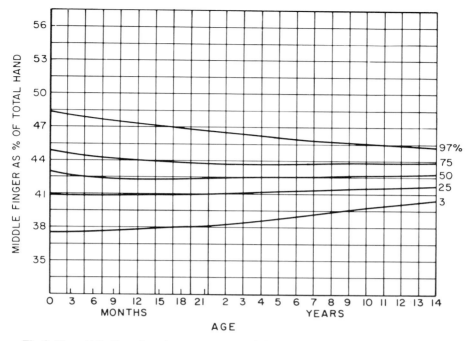

Fig. 3. The middle finger length as a percentage of the total hand length in normal children.

as a percentage of the total hand size was then determined. Figure 3 shows that when the finger size is 42-43% of the total hand size it is in the 50th percentile range. A marked increase in this percentage would indicate arachnodactyly which is associated with a variety of malformation syndromes including Marfan syndrome, which is often difficult to diagnose during infancy. The hands of 3 newborn infants who were suspected of having Marfan syndrome were measured. Two of the 3 have subsequently been proved to have this syndrome. The hand size of these 2 patients was in the 75th percentile or greater. Their middle finger size as a percentage of total hand size was in the 97th percentile in one infant and greater than the 97th percentile in another. Therefore, these preliminary findings suggest that this type of measurement may be helpful in making the diagnosis of Marfan syndrome in the newborn period.

Hand measurements of 22 patients with de Lange syndrome were also studied. The middle finger, as a percentage of the total hand size, was less than the 3rd percentile in 11 of the 22 patients, less than the 25th percentile in 17 of the 22 patients and less than the 40th percentile in 21 of the 22 patients. From our initial study it appears that in patients with de Lange syndrome who do not have major hand malformations, the hands, particularly the fingers, are short.

All of the patients with achondroplasia who were studied had a hand size less than the 3rd percentile with a proportionate decrease in the finger length. Eight patients with Treacher Collins syndrome had normal hand lengths.

Much work needs to be done in determining the measurements of various physical parameters in patients with syndromes. These measurements need to be standardized so that investigators will be measuring the same parameters and utilizing similar methods. A workshop is planned in the near future to consider standardization of such measurements.

References

1. Feingold, M. and Bossert, W. H.: *Normal Values for Selected Physical Parameters: An Aid to Syndrome Delineation.* In Bergsma, D. (ed.): Birth Defects:

Orig. Art. Ser., vol X, no. 13. White Plains:The National Foundation-March of Dimes, 1974.

2. Collins, E.: The illusion of widely spaced nipples in the Noonan and Turner syndromes. *J. Pediatr.* *83*:557-561, 1973.

Discussion

Moderator: Dr. Feingold, where will the data on your normal standards be published?

Dr. Feingold: The data will be published in The National Foundation's Original Articles Series.

Dr. Luzzatti: I am afraid I missed the number of normal children you measured. I would like to know how they were divided among the 20 age groups that you have there? How many per group did you have?

Dr. Feingold: We measured a total number of 2400. However, within each parameter, it varied tremendously.

Dr. Luzzatti: Do you feel that your figures are reliable for each age group?

Dr. Feingold: Yes, within the limits of sampling error. We still need more data for some age groups and some parameters.

Dr. Luzzatti: You are probably aware that the late Helen Pryor, in the late 1960s, studied 20,000 children in the Bay Area, from newborn to adult age group, and studied 19 different anthropometric measurements, for which we have means and standard deviations. I wonder if it would be worthwhile comparing your data with her data?

Dr. Feingold: We have done that. Dr. Pryor's original work was in 1935 (Lucas, W. P. and Pryor, H. B.: Range and standard deviations of certain physical measurements in healthy children. *J. Pediatr.* *6*:533-545, 1935). We measured many more different parameters than she did. However, we both measured interpupillary distances and obtained different results. One reason was that the formula used by Dr. Pryor to obtain the interpupillary distance did not take into consideration that the interpupillary distance is more dependent upon the inner canthal distance than the outer canthal distance.

The KBG Syndrome– A Syndrome of Short Stature, Characteristic Facies, Mental Retardation, Macrodontia and Skeletal Anomalies*

Jürgen Herrmann, M.D., Philip D. Pallister, M.D.,
William Tiddy, D.D.S. and John M. Opitz, M.D.

A "new" malformation/retardation syndrome is described in 7 patients from 3 unrelated families. Affected individuals presented with mild mental retardation, shortness of stature, characteristic facial appearance, macrodontia and multiple other anomalies primarily of the skeleton. Using the patients' initials, the condition has been designated the KBG syndrome. It is caused by an autosomal dominant mutant gene.

Case Reports

Case 1

The propositus *R.K.* was born at term 10/24/60, with a weight of 2700 gm and a length of 47 cm. He did not walk until 2 to 3 years of age. His performance in kindergarten and first grade was inadequate. Psychologic testing at 8 years showed an IQ of about 60.

Family history showed lack of information about the father. He was reportedly well, about 26 years old at the time the patient was born and 170 cm tall. The mother's age was 32 at that time. *R.K.* represents her only pregnancy. She was 163 cm tall, had no physical illnesses, but was admitted to a state mental institution at 40 years of age. Her mother and sister have been patients in the same institution. There is no family history of congenital abnormalities.

R.K. was evaluated at the Boulder River School and Hospital (BRSH) in Boulder, Montana, at 8 years of age (Figs. 1 and 2). Measurements for height (116 cm),

*Paper No. 1662 from the University of Wisconsin Genetics Laboratory. These studies were supported by NIH grants GM 15422 and 5 KO4 HD 18982. Previously presented in part at the 7th Annual Genetics Seminar, Boulder River School and Hospital on July 3, 1973 (Studies of Malformation Syndromes of Man XXXIV).

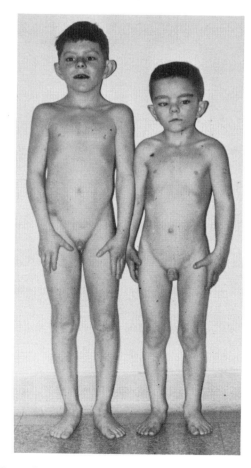

Fig. 1. *Case 1* (left) at 8 years of age. Note shortness of stature, pectus excavatum, cryptorchidism and facial appearance. *Case 2* (right) at 7 years of age. Note the similar general appearance to *Case 1*.

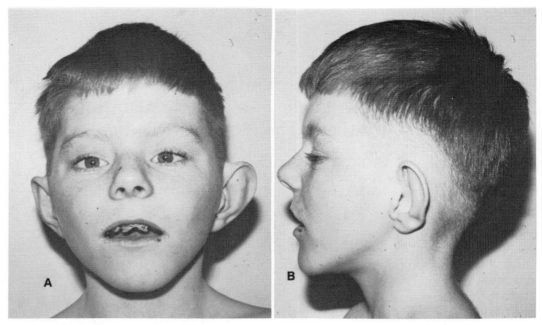

Fig. 2. A) *Case 1.* Note round face, redundant eyebrows, telecanthus, left internal strabismus and widely arched maxilla. B) Note brachycephaly, high bridge of nose, anteverted nostrils, relative micrognathia and abnormal auricles.

weight (20.4 kg) and head circumference (49.2 cm) were, respectively, below the 3rd, at the 3rd and at the 2nd percentile for age. The inner and outer canthal distances were 32 mm and 85 mm, respectively. The skull was turribrachycephalic and the face was broad. The left side was slightly more prominent than the right. The eyebrows were rather bushy, broad and widely arched. He had mild synophrys, slight mongoloid slanting of the palpebral fissures, bilateral epicanthic folds and left internal strabismus. The bridge of his nose was high but the nose was short and there was marked anteversion of the nostrils. The maxilla and palate were broad and there was maxillary overbite since the arch of the mandible was narrow. The uvula deviated to the left. There was posterior angulation and abnormal differentiation of the auricles. The helix was hypoplastic and unrolled; the anthelix was prominent; and the tragus was "rigid" bilaterally. The left helix showed anteflexion. The AP diameter of the thoracic cage was increased; the sternum was short; and there was a mild pectus excavatum. The lower portions of the scapulas were prominent. There was a double pilonidal dimple. The penis was small with a secondary meatal stenosis. There was bilateral cryptorchidism. Both feet showed a varus deformity and 25% cutaneous syndactyly of toes 2-3. The 5th fingers were short, had a short middle phalanx and mild clinodactyly. A simian crease was present bilaterally. Dermatoglyphic examination showed on the right *t, t', t''*, hypothenar ulnar loop, third interdigital distal loop and on fingers 1-5: U,PU,

W,W,U; and on the left *t''*, third interdigital distal loop and on fingers 1-5: U,PU,PU,W,PU. An open field was present in the right and a small whorl in the left hallucal area.

Dental examination showed the maxilla to be widely arched and the alveolar ridge to be short. Crowding of the unerupted permanent teeth was seen on roentgenogram. Both permanent upper central incisors and the permanent left upper lateral incisors were enlarged (Fig. 3). The right upper lateral incisor had not erupted. The right upper central incisor measured 15.5 mm in width, 11 mm in height and was also of increased thickness. It

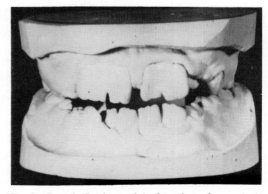

Fig. 3. *Case 1.* **Study** model of teeth to demonstrate macrodontia.

had 5 mamelons and was separated by a cleft with a depth of 3 mm into a mesial portion with 2 mamelons and a distal portion with 3 mamelons. The left upper central incisor measured 13.6 mm in width and was similar in height and thickness to the right upper incisor. A cleft of 2.5 mm separated 2 mesial and 3 distal mamelons which were closer together than on the right. According to Moyers,[1] 80% of central incisors measure between 7.7 and 9.2 mm in width, and 80% of lateral incisors measure 5.8 to 7.4 mm in width. A height of 11 mm is apparently within normal limits. We are not aware of any standards for tooth thickness. The lower (permanent) incisors also were enlarged, measuring 6.5 mm (right central), 7 mm (left central), 8 mm (right lateral) and 8 mm (left lateral). The width of 80% of lower central incisors ranges from 4.8 to 5.8 mm, and of 80% of lower lateral incisors from 5.3 to 6.3 mm.[1] The lower incisors all had 3 mamelons. The deciduous teeth were of apparently normal size. The color of the teeth was within normal limits. The enamel was smooth and without hypoplastic pitting. Roentgenograms of the enlarged teeth showed a single root and thinning of the enamel at the mesial and distal surfaces. The mandibular incisors were malpositioned due to a narrow mandible.

Laboratory examinations, including urinalysis, CBC, VDRL, urine chromatography and peripheral lymphocyte karyotyping, were within normal limits. The EEG was abnormal; it showed 5/second high volt-age rhythmic slowing, particularly in the frontal and occipital areas. Slowing was not aggravated by hyperventilation but was possibly decreased by stroboscopic photic stimulation.

Roentgenographic examination (Fig. 4) confirmed brachycephaly and macrodontia of the upper central incisors, and showed the presence of 7 cervical, 11 thoracic, 5 lumbar, 6 sacral and 3 coccygeal vertebras. There was one rudimentary pair of cervical ribs and 11 pairs of thoracic ribs. The bodies of C3 and C4 appeared to be fused. There was anterior notching and irregularity of the upper and lower plates in the thoracic and lumbar spine. The intervertebral distances were irregular. The iliac bones were hypoplastic and the femoral necks were short. The tubular bones of the hands and feet were short. The carpal bone age was 8 years at a chronologic age of 11 4/12 years. An IVP was normal.

Case 2

Cases 2, 3, 4, and 5 are members of the *B Family* (Fig. 5). The propositus (*Case 2*), his 2 younger brothers (*Cases 3, 4*) and their mother (*Case 5*) are described in detail. The mother is 1 of 7 sibs, 2 of which reportedly had "large front teeth." No further details of family history are available.

The propositus, *E.B. (III-10)*, was born 3/3/65, at term after an uncomplicated pregnancy. Delivery was

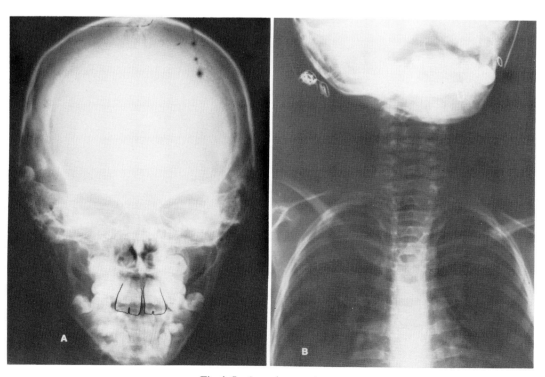

Fig. 4. See legend on next page.

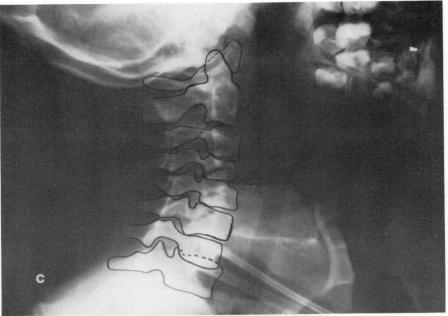

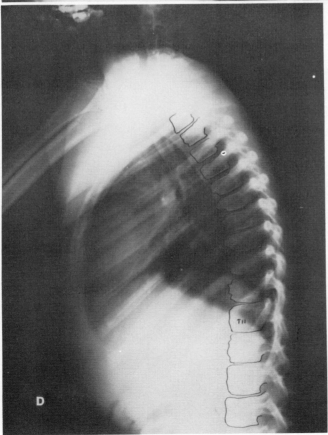

Fig. 4. *Case 1*, roentgenograms at 8 years of age. A) Skull with increased biparietal diameter and macrodontia. B and C) AP and lateral views of the cervical spine segmentation defects. D) Thoracic spine with irregular upper and lower vertebral plates, and anterior tonguing and notching of vertebral bodies. E) Pelvis with irregular intervertebral spaces, small iliac wings and short femoral necks. F) Hands with short tubular bones.

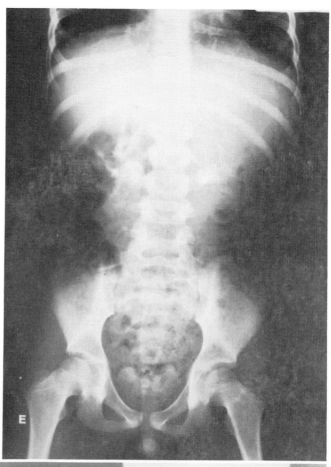

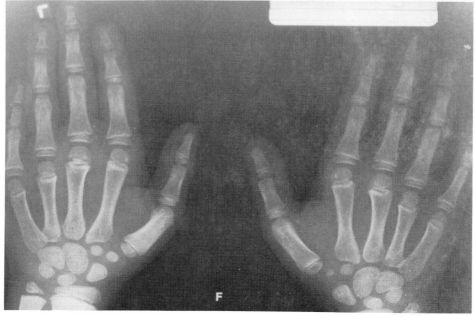

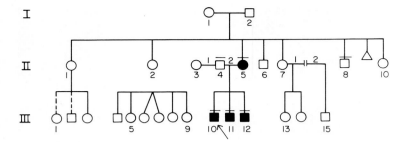

Fig. 5. Pedigree of the *B Family*.

aided by instruments which reportedly caused "his head to be bruised and to have marks showing for 6 months." Birthweight was 3810 gm and length 52 cm. Psychomotor development was delayed. At 4 years of age *E.B.* was treated with Ritalin for hyperactivity. At 7 years of age he was found to have an IQ of 40, to be frustrated easily, and to have a mild speech defect with expulsion of air before speaking a word. *E.B.* was evaluated at the BRSH at 7 years of age for a limping gait and mental retardation (Fig. 1). Height was 11.8 cm (below the 3rd%), weight 20.2 kg (25th%), head circumference 52.9 cm (60th%), inner canthal distance 35 mm (95th%) and outer canthal distance 86 mm. The skull showed prominence of parietal eminences, flat occiput, mild frontal bossing and a slightly prominent, and in part,

open metopic suture (Fig. 6). The posterior hairline was low. The anterior hairline showed a cowlick pattern on the left. The eyebrows were widely arched and very broad. Laterally they extended onto the upper eyelids and medially they joined across a relatively high bridge of the nose. The face was round. There was moderate telecanthus and right internal strabismus. The bridge of the nose was wide; the tip of the nose was broad; and nostrils were anteverted. The lips were thin and the upper lip was shaped like a hunter's bow. The maxillary arch was of normal width, but the mandible was narrowly arched. The mandible was short and had a central symphyseal depression and 2 inferior lateral prominences similar to the spurs in the Brachman-de Lange syndrome.

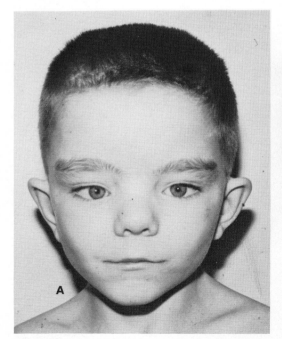

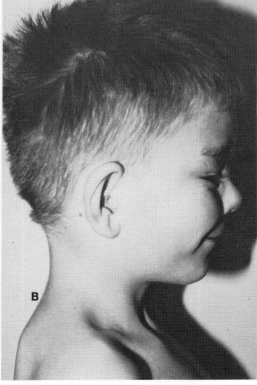

Fig. 6. *Case 2.* A) Note telecanthus, redundant eyebrows, internal strabismus, upper lip thin and shaped like hunter's bow and round face. B) Note brachycephaly, anteverted nostrils, micrognathia and abnormal auricles.

Dental examination showed a delay of about 18 months in the eruption of the permanent teeth. The length of the alveolar ridges was normal. Radiographically, the width of the unerupted permanent upper central incisors was increased. It was not possible to adequately evaluate the enamel of the permanent teeth. Dark coloration of the deciduous teeth presumably was due to tetracycline therapy.

The auricles showed moderate anteflexion and an accessory fold of the lobules. Mild tightness of the trapezius muscles suggested webbing of the neck and sloping shoulders. The lower portions of the scapulas were prominent. A sacral dimple was over 1 cm long. There was 25% cutaneous syndactyly between toes 2 and 3 bilaterally. The hands were short and broad. There was slight cutaneous syndactyly between the index and the middle fingers bilaterally. The 5th fingers were short and clinodactylous. The palmar flexion creases were hypoplastic. Dermatoglyphic examination showed bilaterally a *t* and absence of the *c* triradius, an ulnar loop on each thumb, middle and 5th finger, a whorl on both 4th fingers, a radial loop on the right index and a tented arch on the left index. A distal loop was present in each hallucal area. The right hip was subluxated. There was bilateral tendon adductor and iliopsoas tightness secondary to hip dysplasia. Deep tendon reflexes were present with summation; muscle tone and proprioception were normal.

Laboratory examination was normal. An EEG showed convulsive activity with high voltage paroxysmal slowing which was widespread and not completely rhythmic. A considerable amount of normal sigma wave activity was seen during sleep. From time to time there was an unusually sharp wave discharge, indicating that the patient might develop grand mal seizures.

Roentgenographic examination showed an increased biparietal diameter of the skull, delayed closure of cranial sutures and apparent "Catlin spot" defects. There was a complete left and a rudimentary right cervical rib. The lateral view showed tonguing and rounded edges of multiple vertebral bodies. There was spina bifida occulta L4 through S1. The iliac bones were small (Fig. 7). There was marked dysplasia of the femoral heads and necks, and secondarily, of the acetabula. The hands and feet showed shortness of the tubular bones and a bone age between 5 to 6 years at a chronologic age of 7 years.

Innominate osteotomies were done on the right on 6/7/72 and on the left on 3/21/73. Subsequently *E.B.* has returned home and to school with a markedly improved, painless gait.

Case 3

V.B. (born 3/30/67; *III-11*) is a younger brother of *Case 2*. He was examined at 4 11/12 years. Height was 100 cm (slightly below 3rd%) weight 16.3 kg (25th%), head circumference 49.2 cm (25th%), inner canthal distance 30 mm (80th%), and outer canthal distance 74 mm. *V.B.* was still talking "baby talk" and an undefined speech problem was present. The posterior hairline was slightly low, and there was mild synophrys. The face was normal. There was a long and deep sacral dimple, bilateral 30% cutaneous syndactyly of toes 2-3, shortness and clinodactyly of the 5th fingers, a simian crease on the right, and an absent proximal flexion crease of the 5th finger. The left hand and foot showed evidence of surgically treated postaxial hexadactyly. The *d* triradius of the right hand was laterally displaced. Dermatoglyphic examination showed on the right *t'*, proximally located hypothenar ulnar loop, third interdigital distal loop, and on the fingertips ulnar loops except for a radial loop on the index. The left hand showed a *t''*, a third interdigital distal loop and ulnar loops on the fingertips except for a large radial loop on the index.

Dental examination showed complete deciduous dentition for age; the teeth appeared normal. Roentgenograms suggested that the (unerupted) permanent upper central incisors were of increased width and that each had 4 or more mamelons. The permanent right upper lateral incisor was apparently absent.

Roentgenographic examination showed wormian bones, increased biparietal diameter, anterior tonguing of thoracic and lumbar vertebral bodies, shortness of femoral necks, slight flaring of tibial and femoral metaphyses, shortness of tubular bones in the hands and feet. The carpal bone age was 2 6/12 at a chronologic age of 4 11/12 years.

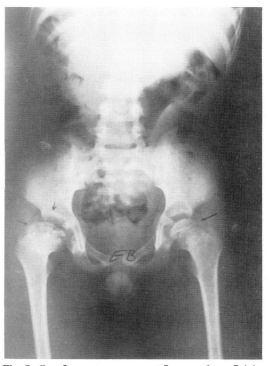

Fig. 7. *Case 2*, roentgenograms at 7 years of age. Pelvis with small iliac wings and bilateral hip dysplasia.

Case 4

J.B. (born 7/1/70; *III-12*) is the youngest brother of *Case 2*. He was examined at 19 months. He measured in height 78 cm (3rd%), weight 11.6 kg (50th%), head circumference 46.7 cm (20th%), inner canthal distance 32 mm (95th%) and outer canthal distance 74 mm. He had not walked until 16 months and only used 3 to 4 words at 20 months. The anterior fontanel was open. The face was round. There was slight mongoloid slanting of the palpebral fissures. The uvula was bifid. The deciduous upper central incisors had erupted and were large, the lateral upper incisors were just erupting. The deciduous right upper lateral incisor was small; the left one was malpositioned and large. The 2 lower central incisors were the only other teeth present. Radiographically the unerupted upper central incisors appeared wide. There was shortness, clinodactyly and hypoplasia of the proximal flexion crease of the 5th fingers. Dermatoglyphically he had bilateral hypothenar ulnar loops, vestigial third interdigital loops and ulnar loops on all fingertips except for the indices which had low ridge-count radial loops (or tented arches). The hallucal pattern on the right was a fibular loop and that on the left, a whorl. The right elbow showed an additional flexion crease. Neurologic examination was normal.

Roentgenographic examination showed open cranial sutures and wormian bones at the lambdoid suture. The parietal bones appeared thin. The neural arches of C2-7 were open. There were bilateral hypoplastic cervical ribs. Anterior tonguing was noted in the thoracic vertebras. There was mild flaring of the femoral and tibial metaphyses. The tibias were short. The tubular bones in the hands and feet were short. The carpal bone age was 9 months at a chronologic age of 19 months.

Case 5

N.B. (born November 1942; *II-5*) is the mother of *Cases 2, 3, and 4*. She was examined at 29 years of age. Her height was 149 cm and weight was 85.5 kg. The biparietal diameter was increased and the face was round. There was mild telecanthus. The face was normal. The bridge of the nose was high and the nose was short. There was slight anteversion of nostrils. The mandible was of normal height and length but it was narrow-ly arched. The dermatoglyphics show a *t″*, third interdigital distal loop and simian crease bilaterally, and ulnar loops on all fingertips except for a medial loop on the right index and a low arch on the left index.

Dental examination showed absence of the upper right third molar and left lateral incisor, and in the mandible, of the left and right first molar, and left and right lateral incisors. Some of these teeth had been surgically removed. Both upper central incisors were unusually wide and probably had 4 mamelons. Hypoplastic pitting of the enamel was noticed on the maxillary right first molar, right cuspid, right lateral incisor and right and left central incisors. The lower central incisors showed a "sand-blasted" effect. Roentgenograms showed hypoplastic cervical ribs bilaterally, increased thoracic kyphosis, slight shortness of femoral neck and shortness of tubular bones in both hands.

Case 6

R.G. (born 3/28/64; *III-23* in Fig. 8) is the propositus of the *G Family*. Pregnancy was complicated by an upper respiratory infection at 5 months; it was treated with penicillin and an unknown cough medicine. Delivery was at term and uncomplicated. Birthweight was about 4.5 kg; length is unknown, but the patient was said to be "short." Psychomotor development: sat at 6 to 7 months, walked at 2½ years and spoke words at about 3 years of age. *R.G.* suffered an accidental skull fracture at 5½ months. Hearing loss was noticed at 4 to 5 years. At 6½ years of age, an audiogram showed complete hearing loss on the right. He had a markedly nasal speech and his soft palate did not move well. Psychologic testing suggested an IQ of 62. Height measurements at 6, 7 and 8 years were all below the 3rd percentile. The corresponding weight values were at the 5th percentile.

R.G. was evaluated at the BRSH at 8½ years of age (Fig. 9). Height was 116 cm (below 3rd%), weight 24.8 kg (45th%), head circumference 51.8 cm (40th%), inner canthal distance 31 mm (80th%) and outer canthal distance 87 mm. The skull showed biparietal prominence and slight brachycephaly.

The hair was coarse and extended laterally onto the forehead. The eyebrows were broad and laterally

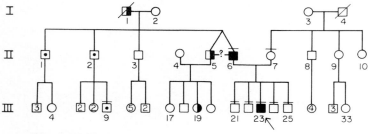

= AFFECTED

= REPORTEDLY AFFECTED

= SEIZURE DISORDER

Fig. 8. Pedigree of the *G Family*.

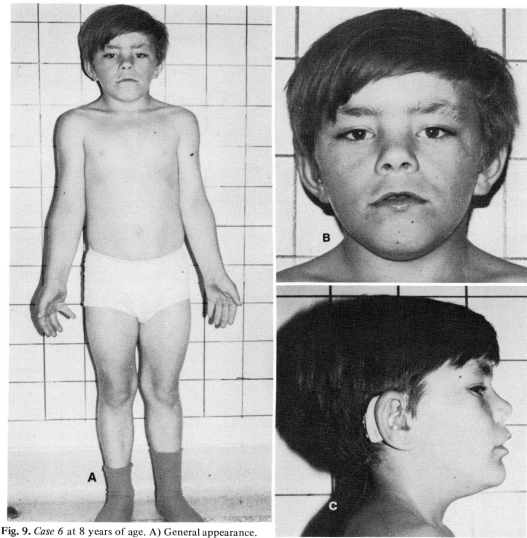

Fig. 9. *Case 6* at 8 years of age. A) General appearance. B) Note round face, telecanthus, wide eyebrows, long nasolabial distance and upper lip shaped like hunter's bow. C) Note anteverted nostrils, abnormal auricles and hearing aid in place.

extended almost to the upper lid. The face was normal, but the left side of the face appeared slightly smaller than the right. There was minimal mongoloid slanting of the palpebral fissures. The bridge of the nose was broad and there was anteversion of the nostrils. The nasolabial distance was increased and the philtrum was not well indicated. He had a relatively large mouth; the upper lip was thin and bow-shaped. The lower lip had a small midline fissure. The auricles showed tightly curled helices and prominence of the anthelices. On the left there were 2 to 3 small pretragal eminences. The xiphisternum was prominent. The nipples were located almost on the

anterior axillary lines. The umbilicus was prominent. There was some shoulder rigidity. The hands were wide and broad. A long (? accidental) scar from the base of the right thumb across the palm and the thenar area was noted. There appeared to be wasting of this area, suggesting nerve damage. There was a single palmar crease bilaterally; the finger flexion creases were normal; but the middle phalanx of the 5th fingers was short. A paronychia of the thumb was healing and index and middle fingers had overgrowth of cuticles. There was some leukoplasia of fingernails 3, 4 and 5. The nails of both 5th fingers were hyperconvex. There was a right hypothenar ulnar loop with a *t* and a secondary *t'*, a third interdigital distal loop, a small fourth interdigital whorl but no *c* triradius. On the left there was a *t*. There were low ridge-count ulnar loops on all fingertips except

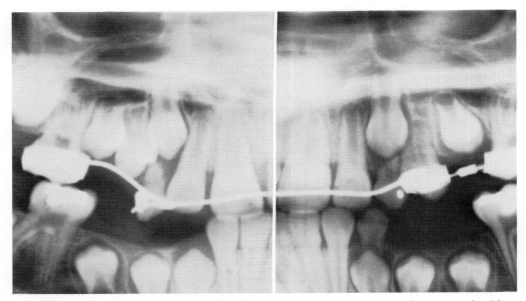

Fig. 10. *Case 6.* Panorex film demonstrates macrodontia and crowding of unerupted permanent dentition.

for a tented arch on the left thumb and a radial loop on the left index finger. The right hallucal area showed a tibial loop; the left, a distal loop. There was slight varus deformity of both knees. Both 5th toenails were hypoplastic. The feet were broad and wide. There was a mild flat foot deformity.

Dental examination showed a wide maxillary arch and shortness of the alveolar ridge. Roentgenograms (Fig. 10) indicated crowding of the unerupted permanent teeth. Both upper central incisors measured 11.3 mm in width; they appeared to have 4 mamelons. The upper lateral incisors also were of increased width. The right one measured 8.2 mm and the left one 8.3 mm. The lower incisors were not enlarged. There was no evidence of enamel hypoplasia.

Skull films showed an increased bitemporal diameter. Roentgenographically no asymmetry of facial bones or of the calvarium was present. There was slight irregularity of the upper and lower vertebral plates and there was anterior tonguing. Lumbar lordosis was decreased. Carpal bone age was about 4 years at a chronologic age of 8½ years.

Case 7

G.G. (born 6/14/34; *II-6*) is the father of the propositus. He is of Norwegian and American Indian ancestry. Height was 173 cm. He had a rectangular and massive face with a wide mouth. There was moderate telecanthus. The upper lip was shaped like a hunter's bow. All teeth had been pulled because of progressive decay and abscesses by age 31. Reportedly the upper central incisors had been unusually wide and the lower central incisors never erupted. On examination the neck

was short and the hands were large and broad and showed "spoon" nails. There was a single transverse palmar crease on the right and a high total fingertip ridge-count. Roentgenograms showed thickening of the calvarium with increased calcification of the sutures, a cervical rib bilaterally, short femoral necks, block (fused) vertebras D12-L2, and deformed and partially collapsed vertebral bodies L3-L5 (Fig. 11). These findings correspond to a history of "hip problems" and chronic back pain particularly during his early teenage years. He had no history of seizures.

Family history suggests that other members possibly are also affected. *Case 7* has 3 older unaffected brothers and a (? identical) twin brother who is reported to have "large front teeth," oligodontia, cutaneous syndactyly of toes 2-3 and a history of "hip problems"; he refused to be examined. His 4 children include a daughter who is reported to have a hearing deficit and wide upper central incisors, but not to be mentally retarded. The paternal grandfather of the propositus had an undefined hip problem. Four brothers of the propositus were examined and found to be unaffected. An autosomal dominant seizure disorder on the paternal side is segregating apparently independently of the KBG syndrome.

Discussion

The clinical findings of 7 patients with the KBG syndrome are summarized in Table 1. The most consistent features are mental retardation (5/7), shortness of stature (6/7), telecanthus

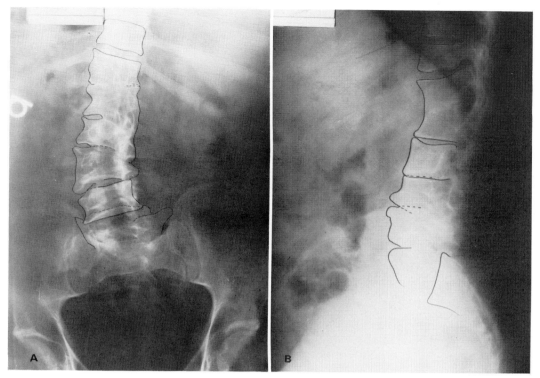

Fig. 11. *Case 7* at 38 years of age. Lower spine and pelvis. A) AP and B) lateral views. Note the block vertebras D12-L2, deformed and partially collapsed vertebral bodies L3-L5 and short femoral necks.

(7/7), wide biparietal diameter (7/7), brachycephaly (5/7), widely arched maxilla with short alveolar ridge (6/7), macrodontia (7/7), oligodontia (3/7), hand abnormalities (6/7), syndactyly of toes 2-3 (4/7), radiographic costovertebral abnormalities (7/7), and delayed bone age (5/5). The anomalies of the teeth and the skeleton are most striking. The incisors have 4 to 5 mamelons (instead of the usual 3) and appear enlarged in width, height and thickness. At times other teeth are also enlarged. Macrodontia may be associated with enamel hypoplasia and there may be malpositioning of teeth.

The skeletal abnormalities include brachycephaly, biparietal prominence, and an increased incidence of wormian bones and cervical ribs. The most consistent vertebral anomalies were anterior notching, hypoplasia of the upper and lower plates, open neural arches and block vertebral formation. *Case 2* presented with severe dysplasia of the femoral heads and necks. Mild

metaphyseal flaring was seen in several instances. The bone age was delayed in all cases.

Affected individuals have a similar facial appearance. The face is round, the eyebrows are wide and synophrys may be present. There is telecanthus and the bridge of the nose is often high, but the nose is short and the nostrils are anteverted. The philtrum is often long and the upper lip thin and shaped like a hunter's bow. Mandibular spurs similar to those in the Brachman-de Lange syndrome may be felt on palpation. The hands frequently are broad, the fingers short. A distal axial triradius and cutaneous syndactyly between toes 2-3 were present on several occasions.

The KBG syndrome is apparently caused by an autosomal dominant gene; genetic heterogeneity cannot be excluded at this time. Male-to-male transmission is demonstrated in the *G Family*. The significance of the 6 male:1 female preponderance is undetermined, but could repre-

Table 1. Clinical Manifestations of the KBG Syndrome

Case	1	2	3	4	5	6	7
General features							
Sex	m	m	m	m	f	m	m
Age (years)	8	7	5	2	29	8	38
Height (percentile)	<3	<3	<3	3	<3	<3	50
Weight (percentile)	3	25	25	50	>97	45	
Head circumference (percentile)	2	60	25	20		40	
Mental retardation (IQ)	60	40	+	+	-	62	-
Abnormal EEG	+	+					
Speech defect	-	+	+	-	-	+	-
Craniofacial features							
Biparietal prominence	+	+	+	+	+	+	+
Brachycephaly	+	+	-	-	+	+	+
Round face	+	+	+	+	+	+	+
Telecanthus (mm)	32	35	30	32	+	31	+
Wide eyebrows	+	+	+	-	-	+	-
Short alveolar ridges	+	-	+	+	+	+	+
Dental features							
Macrodontia	+	+	+	+	+	+	+
Oligodontia	-	-	+	-	+	-	+
Malposition	+	-	-	+	-	+	
Enamel hypoplasia	-	-	-	-	+	-	
Skeletal features							
Cervical ribs	+	+	-	+	+	-	+
Abnormal vertebras	+	+	+	+	+	+	+
Short femoral neck	+	+	+	+	+	-	+
Short tubular bones in hands	+	+	+	+	+	+	-
Delayed bone age	+	+	+	+		+	
Palmar and digital features							
Syndactyly of toes 2-3	+	+	+	-	-	-	+
Distal axial triradius	+	-	+	+	+	+	-
Simian crease	+	-	+	-	+	+	+

Additional features

Case 1: cryptorchidism, pectus excavatus, abnormal auricles, internal strabismus
Case 2: severe hip dysplasia, internal strabismus, mandibular spur, abnormal auricles
Case 3: postaxial hexadactyly left hand and foot (surgically removed)
Case 4: bifid uvula
Case 6: hearing deficit, facial asymmetry, abnormal auricles
Case 7: all teeth removed by age 31; history of "hip problems"

sent biased ascertainment. The range of expressivity of the KBG syndrome cannot be determined from these few patients.

Reference

1. Moyers, R.E.: *Handbook of Orthodontics.* Chicago: The Year Book Publication, Inc., 1958.

Leukonychia Totalis, Multiple Sebaceous Cysts and Renal Calculi: A Syndrome*

Robert J. Gorlin, D.D.S., M.S., Lawrence L. Bushkell, M.D.
and Guy Jensen, D.D.S.

Hereditary leukonychia was first described by Lawrence in 1893.[1] His patient was a healthy middle-aged man with leukonychia striata whose 5-year-old son had a similar pattern. Since then, many cases of hereditary leukonychia in healthy individuals have been reported. A minority has had association with defects of various organ systems such as autosomal dominant inheritance of total leukonychia, keratosis palmaris et plantaris, knuckle pads and mixed deafness.[2,3]

The observation of a syndrome including leukonychia totalis, multiple sebaceous cysts and renal calculi in several generations prompts this report.

Case Reports

Case 1

IV-19, the propositus (Fig. 1), was a 27-year-old white male with leukonychia totalis of all fingernails and toenails (Fig. 2). The terminal portion of all nails was translucent and koilonychia was present on both index fingers (Fig. 3). Numerous sebaceous cysts had been removed from the scalp, thorax and thigh. Intravenous pyelography demonstrated a cluster of small calculi, each measuring about 2 mm in diameter, overlying the lower pole of the left kidney. The dye studies suggested that the calculi were located within a calyceal diverticulum with a normal collecting system. A 3-hour glucose tolerance test showed glycosuria.

*This study was supported in part by the USPHS Program Grant in Oral Pathology DE-1770 and Research Training Grant in Dermatology 5-TO1-AM05560.

Case 2

III-14 a 65-year-old male, the father of *IV-19* and the brother of *III-9*, had leukonychia of all nails with only the terminal portions being translucent. His index fingers exhibited koilonychia. He had had numerous sebaceous cysts removed from various areas of his skin, and had cysts of the occipital region, crown, buttocks and anterior chest, ranging in size from 1 to 4 cm. Renal calculi were found during hospitalization for acute pancreatitis when the patient was 50 years of age. Glycosuria was ascertained at that time, but more recent studies showed no sugar in the urine.

Case 3

III-9, a 78-year-old male, had leukonychia totalis of fingers and toes. There was koilonychia of the middle finger, index finger and thumb of one hand. He stated that other fingernails had been deformed earlier in life but had "rounded out" with age. He had no history of renal calculi or other renal disease. Numerous sebaceous

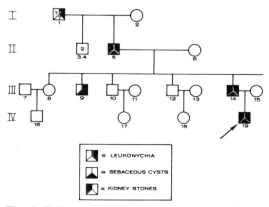

Fig. 1. Pedigree showing variable expression of syndrome. Inadequate information available on *I-1*.

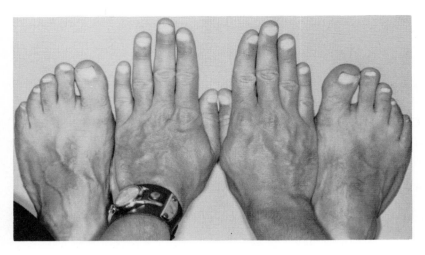

Fig. 2. Leukonychia totalis of all fingernails and toenails.

cysts of the skin had been removed. Cysts were present in the scalp, in the right biceps area and in the left popliteal area. Except for benign prostatic hypertrophy, the patient has been healthy.

Case 4

II-5 died in 1910 at 58 years of age. History, obtained from his sons, *III-14* and *III-9*, indicated that he had leukonychia totalis, numerous sebaceous cysts, renal calculi and gall bladder disease. Cause of death was unknown. No information regarding glycosuria was known.

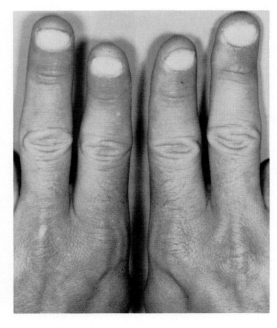

Fig. 3. Koilonychia of index fingers.

Case 5

I-1, the great-grandfather of the propositus, *IV-19*, was known to have had total leukonychia. No further information was available.

Discussion

The classification of leukonychia became more precise when, in 1896, Unna[4] described 3 types: leukonychia totalis, leukonychia striata and leukonychia punctata. A fourth type, leukonychia partialis, was added by Parkes-Weber[5] in 1918. In leukonychia totalis, the entire nail, from its origin to the free margin, is white. Leukonychia partialis indicates that only the distal portion is involved. In practice, photographs and case descriptions of these 2 forms so overlap that they are often discussed as leukonychia totalis. Leukonychia striata indicates either a single broad transverse band or multiple thin bands; the bands may or may not traverse the nail completely. Leukonychia punctata is the term applied to the ubiquitous tiny white spots in fingernails and toenails.

Albright and Wheeler[6] classified leukonychia according to etiology. They subdivided the hereditary and congenital forms into total, partial, or striate; acquired forms into total, partial, striate or punctate. Acquired leukonychia totalis has been reported with hepatic cirrhosis, leprosy, typhoid fever, ulcerative colitis, nail biting, trichinosis and following emetine therapy.

The only pedigree similar to that described in the present report was published by Bauer[7] in

1920. He described 5 generations of a family in which 19 individuals (10 men, 9 women) exhibited leukonychia totalis. Seventeen of the 19 affected family members also had multiple sebaceous cysts. No mention was made of renal calculi. Autosomal dominant inheritance was postulated.

Summary

We have presented a family of 4 generations demonstrating total leukonychia. Multiple sebaceous cysts and renal calculi are associated features of the syndrome. Inheritance is autosomal dominant. We cannot determine whether renal glycosuria is a component of this syndrome.

References

1. Lawrence, H.: Leukopathia unguium. *Aust. Med. J. 15*:483, 1893.
2. Schwann, V. J.: Keratosis palmaris et plantaris cum surditate congenita et leuconychia totali unguium. *Dermatologica 126*:335-353, 1963.
3. Bart, R. S. and Pumphrey, R. E.: Knuckle pads, leukonychia and deafness: A dominantly inherited syndrome. *N. Engl. J. Med. 276*:202-207, 1967.
4. Unna, P. G.: Histopathology of Diseases of the Skin. New York:MacMillan, 1896, pp. 1049-51.
5. Parkes-Weber, F.: Some pathologic conditions of the nails. *Int. Clin. 1*:108-130, 1918.
6. Albright, S. D. and Wheeler, C. E.: Leukonychia. *Arch. Dermatol. 90*:392-399, 1964.
7. Bauer, A. W.: Beiträge zur klinischen Konstitutionspathologie. V. Heredofamiliäre Leukonychie und multiple Athermbilderung der Kopfhaut. *Z. Ang. Anat. 5*:47-58, 1920.

Alopecia Totalis, Nail Dysplasia and Amelogenesis Imperfecta*

Robert J. Gorlin, D.D.S., M.S. and Jaroslav Červenka, M.D.

The disorder described in the following case presentation is probably a new one.

Case Report

D.T., a 26-year-old girl, was first seen in June 1973 for chromosome analysis. She had been examined at the age of 19 years by a gynecologist because of absent menses. At that time she stated that every few months she developed lower abdominal pain that lasted for a few hours and then relented.

Physical examination showed that she had alopecia totalis and bilateral ptosis of the upper eyelids. There was no evidence of breast tissue and the nipples were small and infantile (Fig. 1). There was complete absence of the labia majora and minora and no subcutaneous fat in the pubic area. The clitoris was present and hypertrophic. There was complete absence of the vestibule of the vagina and no vaginal opening could be demonstrated.

A surgical procedure was performed and agenesis of the distal one third of the vagina with a rigid imperforate hymen was demonstrated. This was opened and a

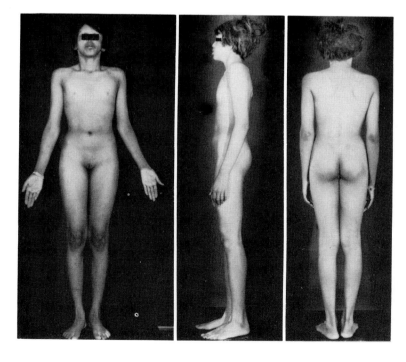

Fig. 1. Patient at 16 years of age. She is wearing a wig due to alopecia totalis. She has no breast development and absent menses. Subsequent chromosome study showed her to be an XO/XX Turner syndrome mosaic.

*This study was made possible by USPHS Program Grant in Oral Pathology DE-1770.

normal vagina was noted in normal position. Upon introduction of a speculum, a hypoplastic cervix was observed. Z-plasty was performed to enlarge the vaginal opening and the patient was placed on estrogen-progesterone combination. Subsequently she had a mild degree of menstrual flow.

Buccal smear studies done at that time showed a deficiency of Barr bodies but no karyotypes were carried out. She was referred to a psychiatrist for evaluation. He indicated that she had a schizoid personality. She was "largely a stranger from society and people by virtue of her atypical physical and psychosexual development and her low intellectual caliber." Her IQ measured 86. She did, however, have feminine identification.

At the time we saw her on 6/15/73, it was noted that she had deficient fingernails and toenails (Fig. 2) and that she was wearing dentures. She stated that she had "had bad teeth which were all extracted." Radiographs obtained from her dentist showed amelogenesis imperfecta of both the deciduous and permanent dentition (Fig. 3). Karyotypes of 30 mitoses from peripheral blood cells showed that 40% were 45,XO and 60% were 46,XX. Her height was 167 cm. Sweat tests performed with O-phthalaldialdehyde and sweat pore counts were normal.

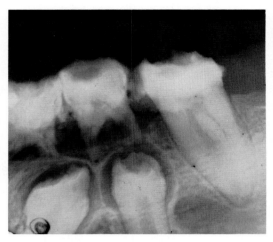

Fig. 3. Amelogenesis imperfecta of both primary and secondary dentitions.

Discussion

We are not familiar with a syndrome in which alopecia totalis, nail dysplasia and amelogenesis imperfecta are combined. In so-called hidrotic ectodermal dysplasia (Clouston type) there are alopecia totalis, nail dysplasia and normal sweating but the enamel is normal. The XO/XX Turner mosaicism is compatible with the lack of breast development, hypoplastic genitalia and normal height but cannot explain the other findings.

Summary

A patient with Turner XO/XX mosaicism is presented who also exhibits alopecia totalis, nail dysplasia and amelogenesis imperfecta. This combination has not been previously reported. What relationship the clinical manifestations have to the chromosome status is also unknown.

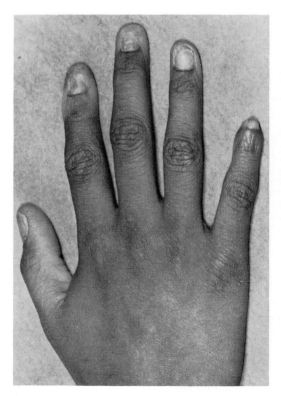

Fig. 2. Dysplasia of several fingernails. Similar alterations were present on the other hand and both feet.

Study of a Family with a New Progeroid Syndrome

Oliverio Welsh, M.D.

Two forms of systemic progeria have been described. The first usually begins in children from 6 to 12 months of age and phenotypically it is fully developed before puberty. The first cases were reported by Hutchinson in 1886[1] and Gilford in 1904.[2] By 1972, a total of 61 cases had been reported.[3,4] The first case in Mexico was presented by Rotberg in 1964.[5] The other form of progeria usually starts at puberty or later. In 1904 Werner described the first 4 cases.[6] Since then 127 cases have been reported in the world literature.[7-11]

The purpose of the present paper is to report the findings of a family with atypical progeria. The patients are 2 males and 2 females in a family of 14 (Fig. 1). There was no history of consanguinity, nor is there knowledge of similar cases or other abnormalities among their relatives. All of the pregnancies and deliveries were normal.

Case Reports

Case 1 was a 26-year-old single Mexican male (*II-7*). He began his somatic changes at age 6, with a somatic

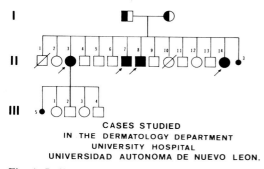

CASES STUDIED
IN THE DERMATOLOGY DEPARTMENT
UNIVERSITY HOSPITAL
UNIVERSIDAD AUTONOMA DE NUEVO LEON.

Fig. 1. Pedigree of the reported family with atypical progeria.

growth delay, sclerodermoid skin, changes and deformities on his chest, hands and feet, as well as micrognathia.

On recent examination the findings were: height 140 cm; weight 27.5 kg; baldness of the frontoparieto-occipital region, with only a few large hairs and without greying; prominent scalp veins; bird-like facies with hypodevelopment of facial bones and marked micrognathia; proptosis; beaked nose; small mouth; crowded teeth; high-pitched voice; and adherent ear lobes (Fig. 2). Audition was within normal limits. The larynx was apparently normal; there were no cataracts. There was sparse body hair on upper lip, chin and axillas, but of

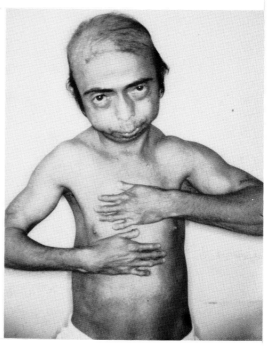

Fig. 2. *Case 1.* Partial alopecia, bird-like facies, proptosis, beaked nose, micrognathia, absence of clavicles, mottled hyperpigmentation of the skin of thorax and abdomen.

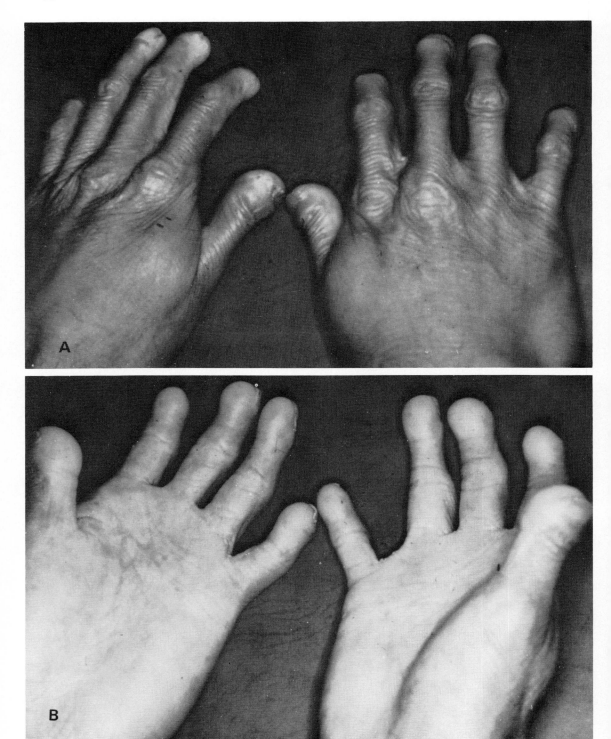

Fig. 3. *Case 1.* A and B) Sclerodermoid skin changes, short fingers and dystrophic fingernails.

normal quantity and distribution in the pubic area. The skin of the neck, chest and abdomen revealed a mottled brownish hyperpigmentation and, due to the poor development of the subcutaneous tissue, it seemed fixed onto the muscles. The thorax was bell-shaped because of the absence of both clavicles. The biacromial diameter was 25 cm and the thoracic perimeter measured at the fourth intercostal space was 64 cm. BP was 120/60 and pulse was regular, 80/min. The abdomen was prominent without visceromegaly. The genitalia were normal.

There were sclerodermoid skin changes on the hands and feet. The fingers were short and with interphalangeal prominent joints. Several fingernails and toenails were dystrophic or absent and there were callouses in both plantar regions (Figs. 3 and 4).

The laboratory findings, including FSH and LH, were below normal. The phosphorus was 6 mg%, alkaline phosphatase 150 mU/ml (normal 30-80 mU/ml). The glucose tolerance test showed a borderline pattern. Two karyotypes were not conclusive.

Two skin biopsies taken from the chest showed moderate homogenization of the dermis and mild elastosis (Fig. 5). The resting ECG was normal. The treadmill effort test with telemetry was incomplete due to the development of pain in his callouses.

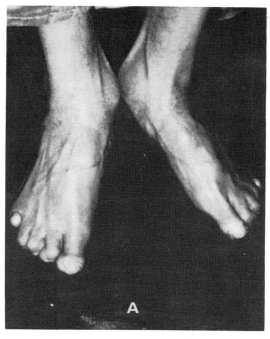

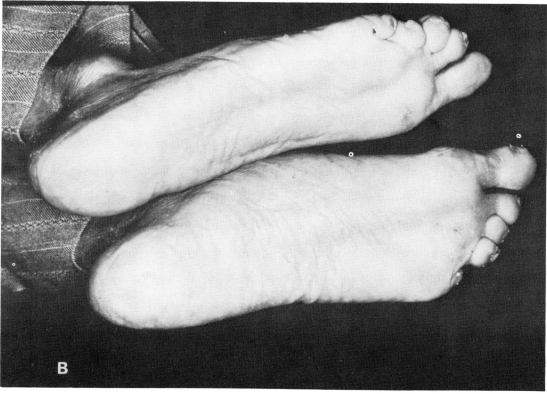

Fig. 4. *Case 1.* A and B) Dystrophic toenails and callouses.

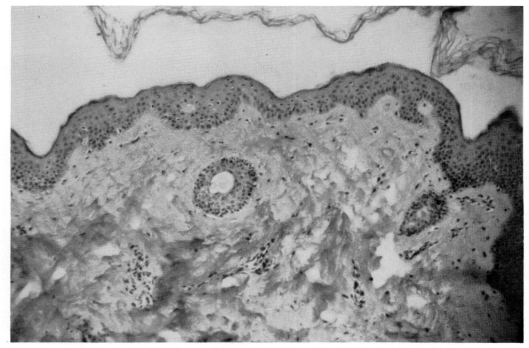

Fig. 5. *Case 1.* Skin biopsy showing mild collagen homogenization, (H and E, × 48).

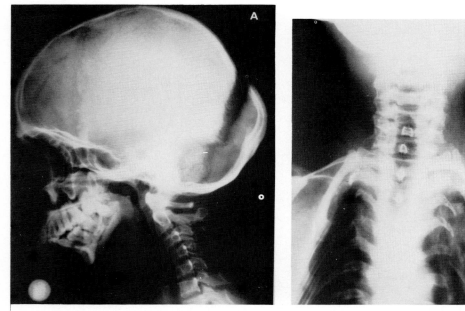

Fig. 6. *Case 1.* A) The lateral skull roentgenogram reveals widening of the sutures, mainly the parietooccipital; hypoplasia of the facial bones; crowded teeth; and micrognathia. B) PA chest roentgenogram shows a bell-shaped thorax, absence of both clavicles and of posterior segment of upper ribs collapsing the thoracic wall.

X-ray studies showed the following changes: widening of the fontanel and sutures with reabsorption of their borders and increase in the number of wormian bones; micrognathia, hypoplasia of the facial bones and crowded teeth (Fig. 6A); bell-shaped thorax, absence of both clavicles, bone reabsorption of the posterior segment of the upper ribs and partial collapse of the thoracic cage (Fig. 6B); coxa valga (Fig. 7); small calcifications over the trochanter major and right acetabulum; and acroosteolysis, more accentuated in feet than in hands (Fig. 8).

Case 2 (II-14) was a 14-year-old single Mexican female, a 4th grade student, and the youngest in the family. She began her somatic changes at age 6. Her somatic growth stopped at 10½ years of age; menarche at age 12. The clinical findings were similar to her brother (*Case 1*) with the following variants: height 126 cm; no alopecia; pseudopterygium in the left eye, absence of hair in the left axilla, and normal pubic hair with gynecoid distribution; biacromial diameter 26 cm; chest perimeter 28 cm; absence of the distal third of both clavicles (Fig. 9). Breast development responded to that of a 10-year-old girl. Fingernails were normal and there was anonychia of the right toenail (Fig. 10).

The laboratory studies, including FSH and LH, were normal with the exception of a diabetic type of glucose tolerance test. The skin biopsy showed changes similar to *Case 1*. The ECG revealed changes compatible with right ventricular hypertrophy. The treadmill effort test with telemetry was normal.

With the exception of reabsorption of the distal two thirds of the clavicles, mild heart hypertrophy and absence of soft tissue calcifications, the radiologic

changes were similar to those of *Case 1*, although less pronounced (Figs. 11-13).

Case 3 (II-3) was a 37-year-old married female, gravida 10, para 5, ab 5; one child died at 4 months of age of an unknown cause, and the 4 living children are in apparently good health. She was the third in a family of 14. She began her somatic changes at the age of 6 years. Clinical data were similar to the former cases (her 2 sibs) with the following variants: height 138 cm, weight 35 kg; ocular proptosis was less pronounced (Fig. 14). Almost complete destruction of fingernails and distal phalanges in both hands was found (Fig. 15). Her breast development was normal. The radiologic studies revealed changes similar to the former cases but the acroosteolysis was more prominent in her hands; there was a complete absence of both clavicles and less pronounced changes in the skull (Figs. 16-18). The laboratory tests were within normal limits, except for a borderline

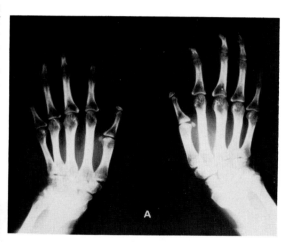

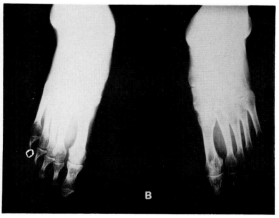

Fig. 7. *Case 1*. Coxa valga.

Fig. 8. *Case 1*. Marked acroosteolysis on both A) hands and B) feet.

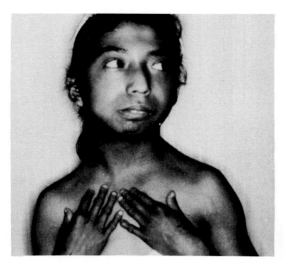

Fig. 9. *Case 2.* Patient with changes similar to her brother (*Case 1*) but to a lesser degree.

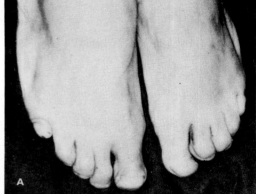

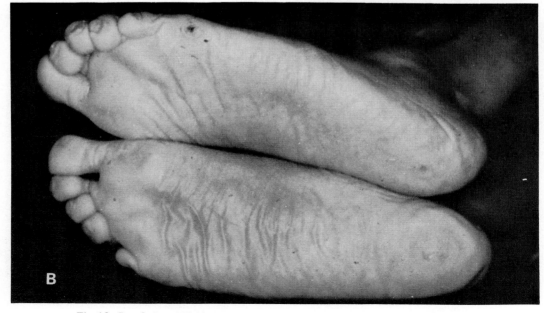

Fig. 10. *Case 2.* A and B) Note anonychia of the 5th toe and the presence of callouses.

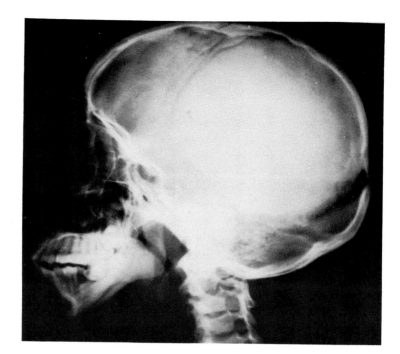

Fig. 11. *Case 2.* A lateral view of skull roentgenogram revealing widening of the sutures, hypoplasia of the facial bones, micrognathia and crowded teeth, but to lesser degree than her brother (*Case 1*).

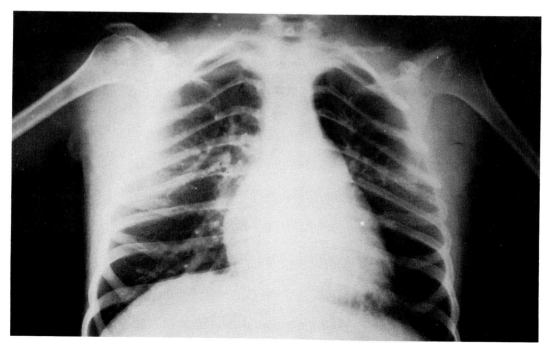

Fig. 12. *Case 2.* Bell-shaped thorax, the absence of the distal two thirds of the clavicles and the reabsorption of the posterior-superior region of the upper ribs. There is mild cardiac enlargement.

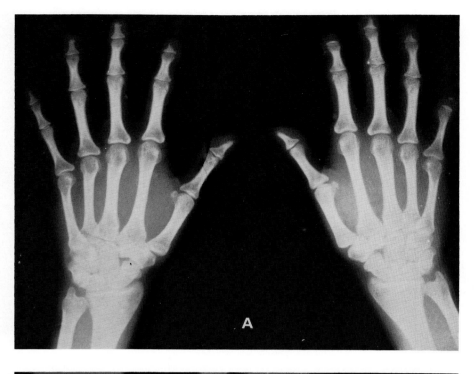

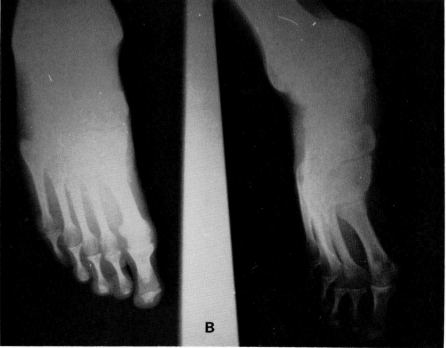

Fig. 13. *Case 2.* A and B) The hands and feet show acroosteolysis, but to a lesser degree than *Case 1.*

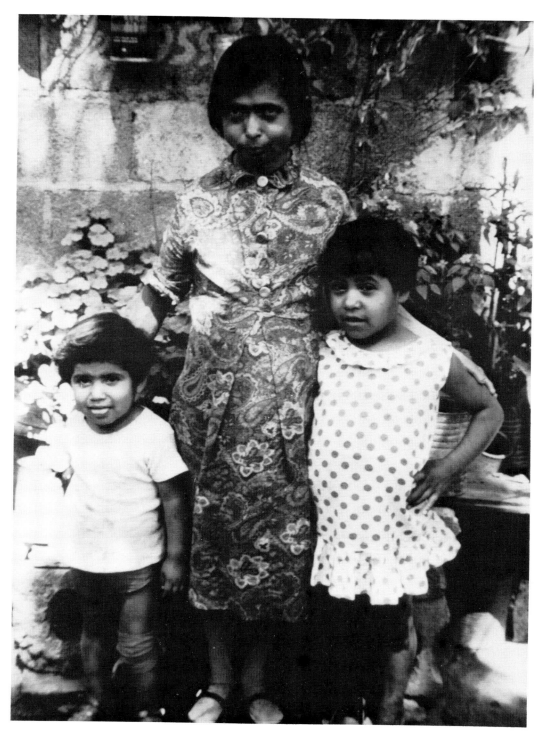

Fig. 14. *Case 3.* Patient with similar facies, bell-shaped thorax and skin changes similar to her 2 sibs (*Cases 1 and 2*); *Case 3* is shown with 2 of her 4 children.

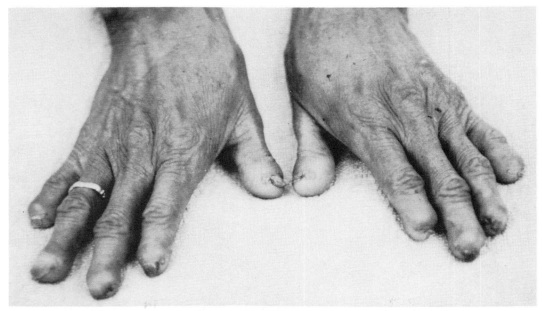

Fig. 15. *Case 3.* Sclerodermoid changes, short fingers, bulging of the finger joints and dystrophic fingernails.

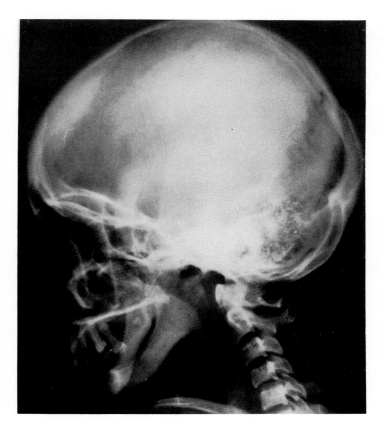

Fig. 16. *Case 3.* The skull roentgenogram (lateral view) shows hypoplasia of the facial bones, micrognathia and absence of several teeth.

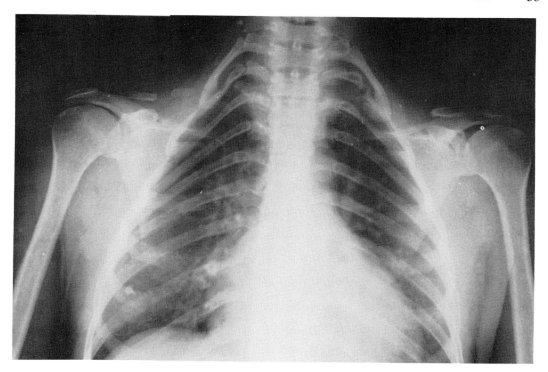

Fig. 17. *Case 3.* PA chest roentgenogram shows a bell-shaped thorax; absence of the left clavicle and a small segment of the right; and reabsorption of the posterior segment of the upper ribs.

glucose tolerance test, abnormal phospholipids and mild anemia. The karyotype and ECG were normal.

Case 4 (II-8) was a single 21-year-old Mexican male. He began his somatic changes at age 7. His clinical course was closely similar to his sibs (*Cases 1-3*) with the following differences: height 150 cm, weight 40 kg, and biacromial diameter 30 cm. The alopecia and micrognathia were less pronounced, and there was absence of only the distal two thirds of both clavicles. We have been unable to obtain the cooperation of this patient for ECG, biopsy and laboratory tests, or clinical photographs.

In the first 3 cases complete laboratory studies including CBC, urinalysis, chemistry profile, lipid profile, glucose tolerance test, VDRL, and when indicated (*Case 1 and 2*), FSH and LH were obtained. Only the abnormal values were reported in each case. The rest of the above-mentioned studies were normal. Three attempts to obtain a karyotype in each of the first 2 cases have been unsuccessful to date, but they will be attempted periodically. Growth hormone and humoral or cellular immunity were not determined.

Discussion

The clinical picture most generally found in the Werner syndrome is as follows[6-13]: 1) arrest of somatic growth at puberty; 2) appearance of cataracts between the second and fourth decades; 3) bird-like facies; 4) greying and baldness between the second and fourth decades; 5) sclerodermoid changes with bulging of the interphalangeal joints; 6) muscular atrophy and hypoplasia of the subcutaneous tissues of the limbs appearing between the first and fifth decades; 7) beaked nose, discrete micrognathia; atrophy of the skin with sclerodermoid changes, and hyperpigmented or hypopigmented mottling; skin ulcers on pressure sites of lower limbs and painful callouses; premature arteriosclerosis and death caused by myocardial infarction or cerebral vascular accident and 8) appearance of moderate diabetes mellitus in 44.4% of the cases.

The following symptoms and laboratory data[14-18] may or may not be present: pseudo-exophthalmos; floppy ears; scanty or absent hair on the upper lip, chin, axillas and pubis; dystrophic fingernails and toenails; calcifications of soft tissues and arteries; or hypogonadism. Occasionally there is a family history of consanguinity and familial incidence.

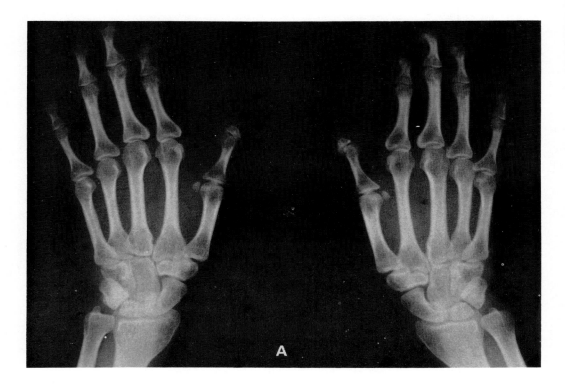

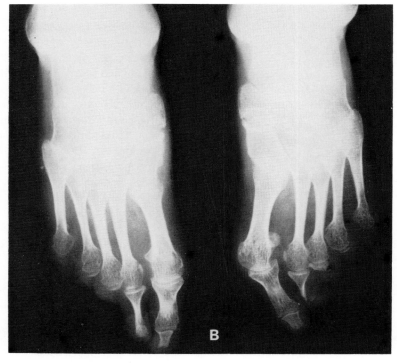

Fig. 18. *Case 3.* A and B) Severe acroosteolysis of hands and feet.

Neoplasias were present in 10% of the cases. The culture of fibroblasts was difficult. This syndrome is inherited by an autosomal recessive gene with a normal karyotype,[16,17] although Ferramosca et al had reported a diploidism XXYY.[18]

The Hutchinson-Gilford progeria syndrome is differentiated from the Werner syndrome by the following[19]: earlier onset of symptoms (generally from 6 to 12 months of age); total or almost total alopecia, with prominent veins and absence or scarcity of eyebrows and eyelashes; open skull sutures with increased wormian bones and marked micrognathia; crowded teeth; bell-shaped thorax and severe narrowing of the posterior segment of the ribs; absence or partial reabsorption of clavicles; and acroosteolysis in hands and feet. Generally, there are no cataracts, hyperkeratosis, calcinosis or skin ulcers. Diabetes mellitus is rare.

Analysis of the data in our cases showed that they do not fit into any of the 2 classic forms of progeria. Some of the clinical and laboratory findings corresponded to the Werner syndrome, while others corresponded more to the Hutchinson-Gilford syndrome. We believe that these cases have enough findings of their own to be considered as a new progeroid syndrome, which could be classified as an intermediate or juvenile form of progeria.

Summary

From a family of 14 sibs, we described 2 males and 2 females with a new progeroid syndrome. The clinical characteristics of this syndrome are as follows: complete arrest of somatic growth by age 11; initiation of somatic changes at age 6 or 7 years; partial alopecia in the males, without greying of the hair; skeletal changes of skull and facies giving a bird-like appearance; micrognathia; total or partial absence of both clavicles; bell-shaped thorax with severe acroosteolysis; and coxa valga. In one case there was presence of soft tissue calcifications. Marked hypoplasia of the subcutaneous tissue and mottled hyperpigmentation of the skin, with sclerodermoid changes of hands and feet, and dystrophic nails were prominent features. Two of the patients (*Cases 1 and 3*) had a borderline glucose tolerance test. *Case 2* showed a diabetic curve and *Case 4* was not investigated.

We believe that these cases have enough clinical and radiographic findings to be considered a new progeroid syndrome, autosomal recessive, and different from the classically described Werner and Hutchinson-Gilford syndromes.

Comment

These patients were reported as atypical cases of progeria at The First International Symposium of Pediatric Dermatology held in Mexico City in October 1973.

References

1. Hutchinson, J.: Congenital absence of hair and mammary glands, with atrophic condition of the skin and its appendages in a boy whose mother had been almost wholly bald from alopecia areata from the age of six. *Trans. R. Med. Chir. Soc. Lond.* 69:473-477, 1886.
2. Gilford, H.: Progeria, a form of senilism. *Practitioner 73*:188, 1904.
3. Fleischmajer, R. and Nedwich, A.: Progeria (Hutchinson-Gilford). *Arch. Dermatol. 107*:253-258, 1973.
4. DeBusk, F. L.: The Hutchinson-Gilford progeria syndrome. *J. Pediatr. 80*:697-724, 1972.
5. Rotberg, T. et al: Progeria. Reporte de un caso con estudio histoquímico comparativo. Revisión bibliográfica. *Arch. Inst. Cardiol. Mex. 34*:242, 1964.
6. Werner, C. W. O.: Über Katarakt in Vebindung mit Sclerodermie. *Inaugeral Dissertation Kiel*, Schmidt Klauning, 1904. Cited by Jacobson, H. G. (ref. 14).
7. Oppenheimer, B. S. and Kugel, V. H.: Werner's syndrome a heredofamilial disorder with scleroderma, bilateral juvenile cataract, precocious graying of hair, and endocrine stigmatization. *Trans. Assoc. Am. Physicians 49*:358, 1934.
8. Thannhauser, S. J.: Werner's syndrome (progeria of the adult) and Rothmund's syndrome; two types of closely related, heredofamiliar atrophic dermatoses with juvenile cataracts and endocrine features; A critical study with five new cases. *Ann. Intern. Med. 23*:559-629, 1945.
9. Petrohelos, M. A.: Werner's syndrome: A survey of three cases, with review of the literature. *Am. J. Ophthalmol. 56*:941-953, 1963.
10. Epstein, C. J. et al: Werner's syndrome: A review of its symptomatology, natural history, pathologic features, genetics, and relationship to the natural aging process. *Medicine (Baltimore) 45*:177, 1966.

11. Fleischmajer, R. and Nedwich, A.: Werner's syndrome. *Am. J. Med. 54*:111-118, 1973.
12. Irwin, G. W. and Ward, P. E.: Werner's syndrome, with a report of two cases. *Am. J. Med. 15*:266-271, 1965.
13. Riley, T. R. et al: Werner's syndrome. *Ann. Intern. Med. 63*:285-294, 1965.
14. Jacobson, H. G. et al: Werner's syndrome: A clinical roentgen entity. *Radiology 74*:373-385, 1960.
15. Schott, J. and Dann, S.: Werner's syndrome. A report of two cases. *N. Engl. J. Med. 240*:641-645, 1949.
16. Cohen, L. K. et al: Werner's syndrome. *Cutis 12*:76-80, 1973.
17. Stecker, E. and Gardner, H. A.: Werner's syndrome. *Lancet 2*:1317, 1970.
18. Ferramosca, B. and Basiello, O.: Su un caso singolare di dismortia corporea con-diploidia XXYY. *Folia Endocrinol. 25(2)*:161-173, 1972.
19. Danowski, T. S.: Progeria in children and adults with the Hutchinson-Gilford and Werner syndromes. In *Clinical Endocrinology*. Baltimore: Williams & Wilkins Co., 1962, vol. I, pp. 244-255.

Discussion

Dr. McKusick: I think that there are 2 cases of this condition reported in the proceedings of earlier Birth Defects Conferences, as mandibuloacrodysplasia, the MAD syndrome. One was an Italian boy, whom we saw in Baltimore some years ago. The second was a patient of Dr. Young, formerly of Rochester, New York, whom he had followed for many years. These were both sporadic cases. The identity is very striking. Your contribution of information on the genetics is very valuable.

Dr. DeBusk: I would certainly agree that this is a very distinct phenotypic expression of something. It is not the Hutchinson-Gilford, and it is certainly not Werner. In some of the older literature, there are some people with oligophrenia, premature senility and bad bones; some of them look sort of like this. I cannot offhand recall the references.

Dr. Welsh: These patients do not have mental retardation. I did not present the picture of *Case 4*, because up until today he has refused permission to be photographed.

The 3-M Syndrome:
A Heritable Low Birthweight Dwarfism

J. Daniel Miller, M.D., Victor A. McKusick, M.D., Paul Malvaux, M.D.,
Samia Temtamy, M.D., Ph.D. and Carlos Salinas, D.D.S.

Four dwarfed children, each of whom had low birthweight at term, from 2 unrelated families had similar dysmorphic features. Comparison of clinical findings showed that they all had a syndrome which could be distinguished from other dwarfed conditions. The main features of the 3-M syndrome (M is the first letter of 3 of the authors' last names) include low birthweight, proportionate dwarfism, hatchet-shaped craniofacial configuration, a short broad neck with prominent trapezius muscles, deformed sternum, transverse grooves of the anterior chest, winged scapulas, and abnormalities of the mouth and teeth. The occurrence of the same syndrome in sibs, the offspring of normal parents who in one of the 2 families were consanguineous, suggests autosomal recessive inheritance.

Case Reports

The pedigrees of the 2 families are shown in Figure 1. *Family P* is from Sicily and presently lives in the United States. *Family W* lives in Belgium and the ancestors came from that country.

Family P

Case 1. R.P. (JHH 1536994), a 12-year-old white male, was the product of a full-term uncomplicated pregnancy. The mother, age 27, and the father, age 32 at the time of the birth of *R.P.*, were first cousins. Other family members were of normal stature. Previously there had been one normal pregnancy resulting in a normal female child. Fetal activity and maternal weight gain during pregnancy were normal. The birthweight was 2159 gm and the birth length was 38 cm. The placenta was grossly normal. In 1969 evaluation at another hospital resulted in the diagnosis of Russell

dwarfism. There had been no clinical response to a 6-month trial of growth hormone (2 mg every other day). On examination at age 12 years he was prepubertal. His height was 109 cm and head circumference was 51 cm with a U/L segment ratio of 1.09. Due to dolichocephaly and pointed facial features, the craniofacial configuration appeared hatchet-shaped (Figs. 2 and 3). The facial appearance was triangular with flattened malar region and relative prominence of the lower part of the face. His father had somewhat similar facies. The subject's thorax was short with mild pectus carinatum and anterior transverse grooves above both costal margins (Fig. 4). The neck was short and the shoulders were high-set and square. The scapulas were prominent and

The P Family

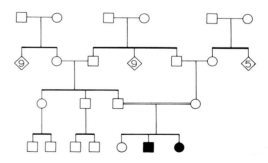

The W Family

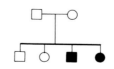

■ ● Affected, The 3—M Syndrome.

Fig. 1. Pedigrees of 2 families affected with the 3-M syndrome.

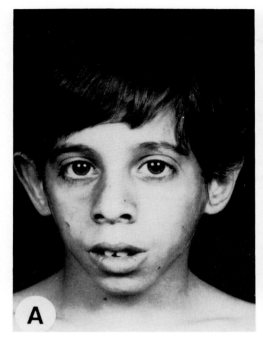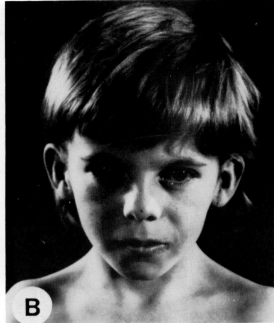

Fig. 2. Facial appearance of A) *Case 1* and B) *Case 3*. Note similarities: triangular shape of face, flattened malar regions, prominent ears and pinched mouth and chin.

slightly winged. There was mild diastasis recti. His intelligence was normal. An arginine-insulin-tolerance test showed a partial but incomplete response of growth hormone (6.2 ng/ml). Laboratory tests including chromosome analysis by Giemsa banding method, biochemical analysis of collagen from skin biopsy, and assay of LH, FSH and T_4 were normal.

Case 2. L.P. (JHH 1533994), the 11-year-old sister of *Case 1* was also the product of a full-term pregnancy during which the mother did not need to wear maternity clothes until the seventh month. At birth, the weight was 1864 gm, the length was 39 cm and the placenta was grossly normal. Evaluation in 1969 led to the diagnosis of Russell dwarfism. Growth hormone (2 mg every other day) given over a 6-month period had no beneficial effects. On examination at age 11, her height was 108 cm, her head circumference was 51 cm and the U/L segment ratio was 1.00. Her appearance was strikingly similar to that of her brother including the same facial appearance, and minor musculoskeletal abnormalities of the upper part of the body. There was an early breast development noted at age 11. Her intelligence was normal. All laboratory tests which included those done on her brother were normal. The growth hormone assay peaked at 21.2 ng/ml after insulin stimulation.

Family W

Case 3. D.W., a 7 3/4-year-old white male, was the product of a 40-week normal gestation. The mother, age

31, and the father, age 33 at the time of the birth of *D.W.*, were not known to be related. There had been 2 previous pregnancies resulting in a normal boy and a normal girl. The placenta was small. At birth the weight was 2100 gm and the length was 41 cm. At 6 weeks of age pyloric stenosis was surgically corrected. On examination at age 7 3/4 the height was 98 cm, the head circumference 53.5 cm and the U/L segment ratio 1.17. The face appeared similar to that of *R.P.* and *L.P.* being triangular, with the upper part of the face relatively broad with flat malar regions and the lower part pointed with a prominent mouth (Figs. 2 and 3). There was pectus carinatum and pectus excavatum with anterior chest grooves above both costal margins (Fig. 4). The neck was short with prominent trapezius muscle and winged scapulas (Fig. 5). Intelligence was normal. Tests including assay of growth hormone after arginine-insulin-tolerance test, LH, FSH, T_4 and chromosome analysis were normal.

Case 4. M.W., the 4½-year-old sister of *Case 3*, was also the product of a full-term uncomplicated pregnancy. At birth the length was 40 cm, the weight 1810 gm and the placenta normal. On examination at age 4½ her height was 83 cm, her head circumference was 50 cm and her U/L segment ratio was 1.18. Her face was triangular but the malar areas were not flattened (Fig. 6). Musculoskeletal abnormalities of the upper part of the body were similar to those of the above described 3 cases. The intelligence was normal. Chromosome analysis was normal. Endocrine assays were not performed.

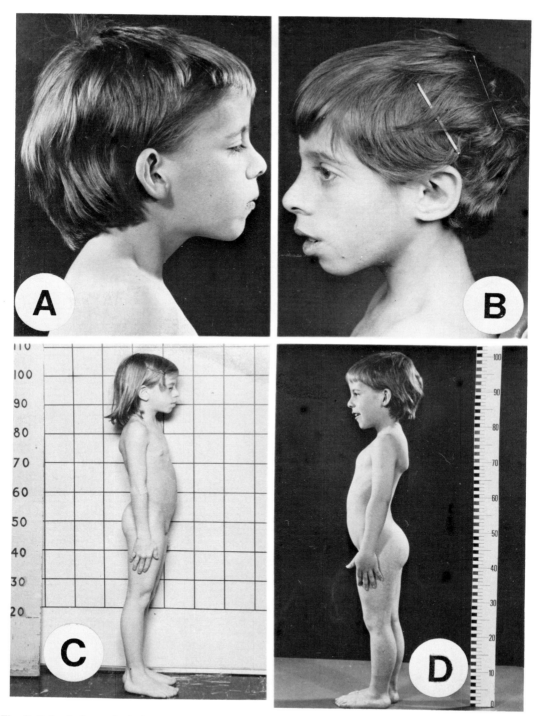

Fig. 3. Lateral views of A) *Case 3*, B) *Case 1*, C) *Case 2* and D) *Case 3* showing hatchet-shaped craniofacial configuration and prominent scapulas.

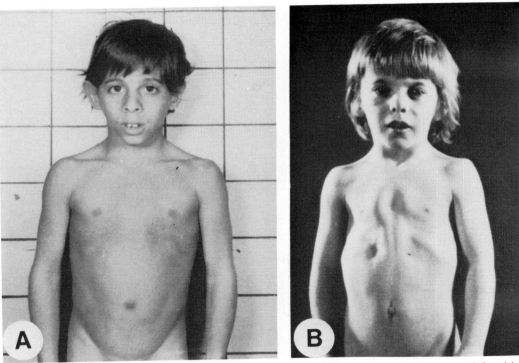

Fig. 4. Frontal views of A) *Case 1* and B) *Case 3* showing short neck, prominent trapezius, pectus deformities, transverse grooves above both costal margins, and diastasis recti.

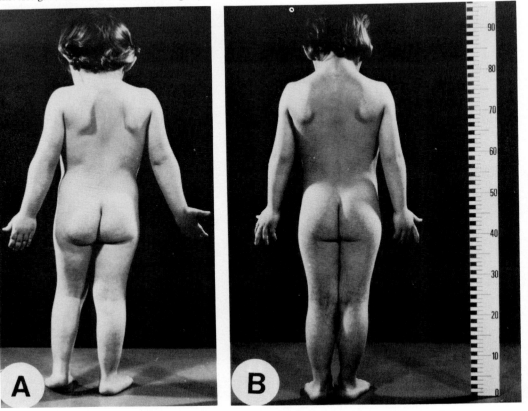

Fig. 5. Posterior view of A) *Case 4* and B) *Case 3* showing prominence of the scapulas.

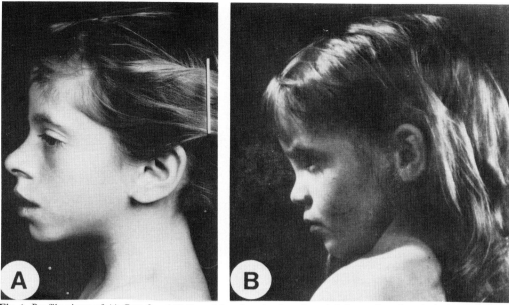

Fig. 6. Profile views of A) *Case 2* and B) *Case 4* showing short neck, pointed mouth and posteriorly rotated ears.

Discussion

The pattern of dysmorphic features in the 4 cases described is distinctive (Table 1). Despite clinical similarities to other dwarfisms with low birthweight, the 3-M syndrome can be differentiated from them.

Differentiation between the 3-M syndrome and the Russell-Silver syndrome, the diagnosis originally made for *Cases 1 and 2*, is important. Two of the major manifestations of the Russell-Silver syndrome, body asymmetry and altered patterns of sexual development,[1-3] are not features of the 3-M syndrome.

The 3-M syndrome also can be distinguished from the symmetric variant of the Russell-Silver syndrome[4] by the lack of craniofacial dispropor-

Table 1. Summary of Main Clinical Features in 3-M Syndrome

	Case 1	Case 2	Case 3	Case 4
Low birthweight	+	+	+	+
Proportionate dwarfism	+	+	+	+
Lack of body asymmetry	+	+	+	+
Hatchet-shaped craniofacial configuration	+	+	+	-
Triangular face shape	+	+	+	+
Frontal bossing	+	+	+	+
Flattened malar region	+	+	+	-
Pointed or pinched mouth and chin	+	+	+	-
Prominent ears	+	+	+	+
Short neck with prominent trapezius	+	+	+	+
High square shoulders	+	+	+	+
Short thorax	+	+	+	+
Pectus deformity (carinatum or excavatum)	+	+	+	+
Transverse grooves of anterior chest	+	+	+	+
Diastasis recti	+	-	+	-
Winging of scapulas	+	+	+	+
Short 5th finger	+	+	+	-
Normal sexual development	+	+	+	+
Hyperextensible joints	+	+	+	+

Table 2. Summary of Orodental Findings in 3-M Syndrome

	Case 1	Case 2	Case 3	Case 4
Normal philtrum	+	+	+	+
Absence of downturned (inverted V) corners of mouth	+	+	+	+
V-shaped dental arch	+	+	+	+
Anterior crowding of teeth	+	+	+	-
Numerous dental caries	+	+	+	-
Malocclusion	+	+	·+	+
Congenitally absent lower 2nd molar	-	-	+	-

tion, pseudohydrocephalus and delayed closure of the anterior fontanel present in the latter syndrome. The head is dolichocephalic and craniofacial configuration is hatchet-shaped in the 3-M syndrome (Figs. 2 and 3). The face in the 3-M syndrome is triangular with malar flattening and relative prominence of the mouth and chin (Figs. 2 and 3). The lips are patulous and the ears are prominent. The short neck with prominent trapezius, sternal abnormalities, winged scapulas, anterior chest grooves and diastasis recti (Figs. 3 and 4) seen in the 4 cases that we studied are not features of the Russell-Silver syndrome. Other clinical findings reported in the Russell-Silver syndrome are turned down corners of the mouth, café-au-lait spots, syndactyly of 2nd and 3rd toes, delayed motor milestones, excessive sweating and clinodactyly of the 5th finger.[5] These are not features of the 3-M syndrome.

The facies in the 3-M syndrome resembles that seen in Bloom syndrome, an autosomal recessive dwarfism with low birthweight.[6] The absence of telangiectatic lesions and chromosomal breaks, which are features of Bloom syndrome, allows for differentiation between these 2 disorders.

The orodental abnormalities in the 3-M syndrome (Table 2) may be related to the shape of the maxilla. Because of the V-shape of the dental arch, the teeth are crowded anteriorly and malocclusion occurs. Crowding of the teeth and the absence of molars noted in our Case 3 also have been reported in the Russell-Silver syndrome.[5,7] There is a high prevalence of dental caries in both sexes and in both deciduous and permanent dentition. The pinching of facial features may be progressive as this feature is less obvious in photographs of our patients at an earlier age. This observation may explain the absence of pinched facies in Case 4 at age 4½.

The dermatoglyphic findings in the 3-M syndrome are recorded in Table 3 in accordance with the format of Cummins and Midlo.[8] Low total ridge count, transitional simian crease and proximal axial triradius may be features of the syndrome, but because of the small number of patients studied no conclusions about the dermatoglyphic findings can be made.

Radiographic findings in the 3-M syndrome (Table 4) are nonspecific. The bones are slender and the diaphyses in particular are narrowed (Fig. 7). The pelvic bones, especially the pubis

Table 3. Dermatoglyphic Findings in 3-M Syndrome

Patient		1	Fingers 2	3	4	5	TRC	Palms	atd angles	a-b ridge-count	transition simian crease
R.P.	left	W	UL	UL	UL	UL	143	9.7.5′.3.t.dL.0.0.0.L	40	54	-
	right	W	RL	UL	UL	UL		9.7.5″.3.t.dL.0.0.0.L	42	51	+
L.P.	left	UL	RL	RL	UL	UL	99	9.7.5′.3.t′.V.0.0.0.L	45	54	-
	right	W	RL	UL	W	UL		9.7.5′.3.t.RA.0.0.0.L	42	51	+
D.W.	left	UL	UL	UL	UL	UL	91	9.7.5″.3.t.0.0.0.0.L	42	-	+
	right	UL	UL	A	RL	UL		9.0.5″.3.t.0.0.0.0.0	42	-	+
M.W.	left	UL	A	UL	A	A	39	11.X.7.3.t′.0.0.0.0.0	47	-	+
	right	UL	A	A	UL	UL		11.0.7.3.t.0.0.0.0.0	43	-	+

Table 4. Radiographic Findings in 3-M Syndrome

	Case 1	Case 2	Case 3	Case 4
Slender bones with thin diaphyses	+	+	+	+
Relatively small pelvis	+	+	+	+
Moderate flaring of iliac wings	+	+	+	+
Small ischium and pubis	+	+	+	+
Small obturator foramen	+	+	+	+
Osteoporotic appearance	−	−	+	+
Pseudoepiphyses	+ (2nd metacarpal)	+ (2nd metacarpal)	−	−
Retarded bone age	+ (BA = 10 CA = 12¼)	+ (BA = 8 5/6 CA = 11)	+ (BA 4 1/5 CA 7 1/3)	+ (BA 2 3/4 CA 4½)
Narrowed intraorbital distance	+	+	−	−

BA = Bone age
CA = Chronologic age

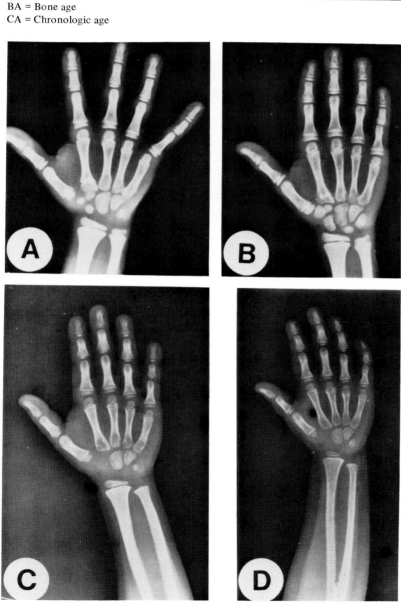

Fig. 7. Radiographs of the hands: A) *Case 1*, B) *Case 2*, C) *Case 3* and D) *Case 4*. Note slender bones and pseudo-epiphyses of 2nd meta-carpal in A and B.

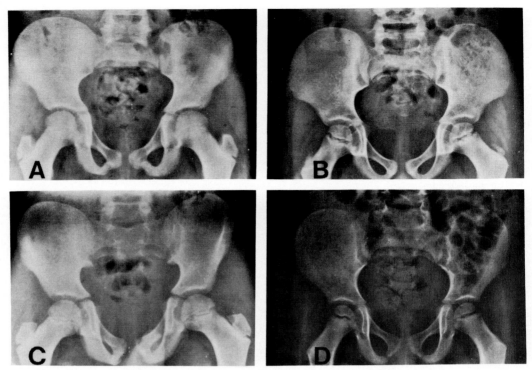

Fig. 8. Radiographs of pelvis: A) *Case 2*, B) *Case 3*, C) *Case 1* and D) *Case 4*. Note flaring of iliac wings and small ischium, pubis and obturator foramina.

and the ischium, are small. The iliac wings are flared and the obturator foramina are small (Fig. 8). The bone age is slightly delayed. Pseudo-epiphyses and osteoporosis are occasional findings. The father and both affected children in the *P Family* had narrow interorbital distance. This may be a family trait and not a feature of the 3-M syndrome as these distances were normal in *Cases 3 and 4*.

There is some evidence for autosomal recessive inheritance of the 3-M syndrome. A brother and a sister were affected in both families that we studied and in one of them the parents were first cousins. In neither family is there an affected individual in more than one generation.

Previously reported cases of the Russell-Silver syndrome have, for the most part, been sporadic. Smith[9] has suggested that sporadic cases of Russell-Silver syndrome may represent new dominant mutations. Rimoin's report of Silver syndrome in monozygotic twins[10] does not define the etiology of this disorder. There has

been one report of asymmetric Russell-Silver syndrome in sibs.[11]

It is possible that in the past other cases of the 3-M syndrome have been diagnosed as Russell-Silver syndrome without asymmetry. In the report by Fuleihan et al[12] 3 sibs from a consanguineous marriage were described as having the Russell-Silver syndrome without asymmetry. From the published photographs of these children sternal abnormalities and chest grooves appear to be present and the facial appearance of the oldest affected child is similar to that in our cases.

The 3-M syndrome is an autosomal recessive proportionate dwarfism characterized by low birthweight, a hatchet-shaped craniofacial configuration, pinched facies, minor musculoskeletal abnormalities of the neck and thoracic wall and normal growth hormone levels. For proper management, prognosis and genetic counseling, differentiation from other types of low birthweight dwarfism, particularly from Russell-

Silver dwarfism and from Bloom syndrome, is important.

References

1. Silver, H. K., Kiyasu, W., George, J. and Deamer, W. C.: Syndrome of congenital hemihypertrophy, shortness of stature, and elevated urinary gonadotrophins. *Pediatrics 12:*368, 1953.
2. Russell, A.: A syndrome of "intra-uterine" dwarfism recognizable at birth with craniofacial dysostosis, disproportionately short arms, and other anomalies (5 examples). *Proc. R. Soc. Med. 47:*1040, 1954.
3. Silver, H. K.: Asymmetry, short stature, and variations in sexual development. A syndrome of congenital malformations. *Am. J. Dis. Child. 107:*495, 1964.
4. Gareis, F. J., Smith, D. W. and Summitt, R. L.: The Russell-Silver syndrome without asymmetry. *J. Pediatr. 79:*775, 1971.
5. Taussig, L. M., Braunstein, G. D., White, B. J. and Christiansen, R. L.: Silver-Russell dwarfism and cystic fibrosis in a twin. *Am. J. Dis. Child. 125:*495, 1973.
6. German, J.: Bloom's syndrome: I. Genetical and clinical observations in the first 27 patients. *Am. J. Hum. Genet. 21:*196, 1969.
7. Szalay, G. C.: Pseudohydrocephalus in dwarfs: The Russell dwarf. *J. Pediatr. 63:*622, 1963.
8. Cummins, H. and Midlo, C.: *Finger Prints, Palms and Soles. An introduction to Dermatoglyphics.* New York:Dover Publications, Inc., 1961.
9. Smith, D. W.: *Recognizable Patterns of Human Malformation.* Philadelphia:W. B. Saunders Co., 1970, p. 66.
10. Rimoin, D. L.: The Silver syndrome in twins. In Bergsma, D. (ed.): Part II. *Malformation Syndromes,* Birth defects: Orig. Art. Ser., vol. V, no. 2. White Plains:The National Foundation-March of Dimes, 1969, pp. 183-187.
11. Callaghan, K. A.: Asymmetrical dwarfism, or Silver's syndrome in two male siblings. *Med. J. Aust. 2:*789, 1970.
12. Fuleihan, D. S., DerKaloustian, V. M. and Najjar, S. S.: The Russell-Silver syndrome: Report on two siblings. *J. Pediatr. 78:*654, 1971.

A Newly Recognized Inherited Syndrome of Dwarfism, Craniosynostosis, Retinitis Pigmentosa and Multiple Congenital Malformations*

Salvador Armendares, M.D., Florencio Antillón, M.D., Victoria del Castillo, M.D. and Miguel Jiménez, M.D.

Three male sibs with growth deficiency have a previously unrecognized pattern of craniofacial and limb anomalies. Two were fully studied, whereas the third was evaluated from medical records. The family pedigree is shown in Figure 1 and characteristics of the syndrome are summarized in Table 1 and illustrated in Figures 2-5. A brief report has been published about this disorder, without photographs.[1]

Case Reports

Case 1 (Figs. 2A and B), a Mexican mestizo male, was the term product of the fifth normal pregnancy and delivery to a 31-year-old mother and 33-year-old father. Birthweight was 2.8 kg.

At 7 1/12 years, his length was 93 cm (height age, 2 7/12 years); weight was 12 kg (3rd% for height age) and his head circumference was 45 cm (below the 3rd%). The upper segment was 50.5 cm with U/L ratio of 1.18 (below the 3rd%), corresponding to a 25-

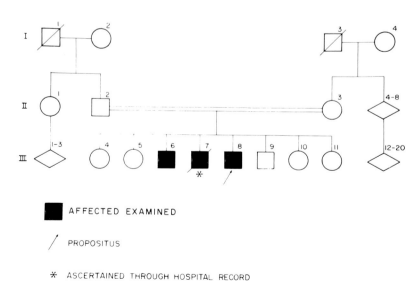

Fig. 1. Pedigree. Parents were born in a small isolated village in the State of Colima (México), where inbreeding is known to be high. They assure that they are consanguineous but we were unable to establish the precise degree of relationship.

AFFECTED EXAMINED

/ PROPOSITUS

* ASCERTAINED THROUGH HOSPITAL RECORD

*This work was partially supported by a grant from The Ford Foundation.

Table 1. Characteristics of the Syndrome*

	Abnormality	Patient 1	Patient 2	Patient 3
Growth	Growth deficiency, apparently postnatal	+	+	+
Craniofacies	Microcephaly and cranial asymmetry	+	+	+
	Craniosynostosis	+	+	+
	Small face	+	+	+
	Scant eyebrows	+	+	?
	Short obtuse nose	+	+	+
	Micrognathia	+	+	+
	High palate	+	+	+
	Ptosis of the eyelids	±	+	+
	Epicanthic folds	±	+	?
	Telecanthus	+	+	?
	Antimongoloid slant eyes	-	+	?
	Atypical retinitis pigmentosa	+	+	?
	Prominent or malformed auricles	+	+	+
Limbs	Short 5th fingers with clinodactyly and hypoplasia of middle phalanx	+	+	+
	Wide 4th interdigital space	+	+	?
	Hypoplastic thenar and hypothenar regions	+	+	?
	Simian creases, partial-to-complete	+	+	?
Other	Retarded bone age	+	+	?

' + = present; ± = mild degree; ? = not stated in the hospital record.
*From *J. Pediatr.* vol. 85, no. 6, p. 872, 1974, with permission.

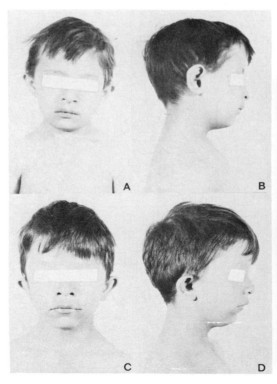

Fig. 2. A and B) *Case 1.* C and D) *Case 2.*   **Fig. 3.** Hands of A) *Case 1* and B) *Case 2.*

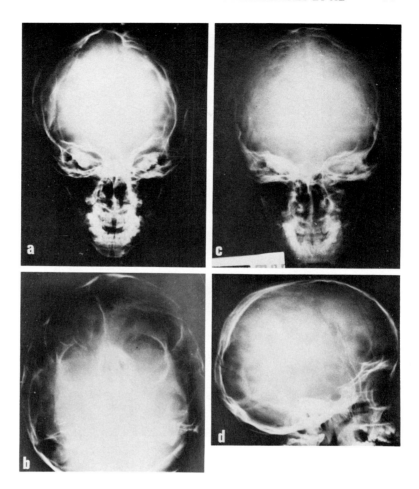

Fig. 4. Roentgenograms of the skull of A and B) *Case 1* and C and D) *Case 2.*

month-old boy. The penis was normal, but testes and scrotum were hypoplastic. The IQ was 100 (Wisc and Bender).

Roentgenograms of the skull (Figs. 4A and B) disclosed premature synostosis of the right coronal suture and the sagittal suture, plagiocephaly, hypoplasia of the paranasal sinuses and prominent convulsional markings. Bone age was 5 years.

Case 2 (Figs. 2C and D) was the product of a normal 40-week pregnancy. Birthweight was 3.2 kg.

At 10 years of age his height was 112.5 cm (height age, 5 10/12 years), weight was 19 kg (which was 1 kg below that expected for length) and head circumference was 48 cm (below the 3rd%). The upper segment was 61.1 cm with a U/L ratio of 1.18 (below the 3rd%) corresponding to a 25-month-old boy. The penis, testes and scrotum were normal. The IQ was 92 (Wisc and Bender).

Roentgenograms of the skull (Figs. 4C and D) showed complete synostosis of the coronal and sagittal sutures, and hypoplasia of the paranasal sinuses. Bone age corresponded to a 7-year-old boy.

Case 3 died at the age of 5 months with the following diagnosis: malnutrition, acute enteritis (*Shigella flexneri, E. coli* 055 and 0119), craniosynostosis and anemia.

He was the term product of the fourth uneventful pregnancy. Birthweight was 3.1 kg. Asymmetry of the cranium was noticed by the parents from birth. He was able to hold his head at 3 months of age. At 4 months of age, his height was 56.5 cm (height age of less than 2 months), weight was 3.2 kg (below the 3rd% for height age) and head circumference was 36 cm (below the 3rd%). Cranial asymmetry with left frontal and lateral prominence was present. The anterior fontanel was small, measuring less than 0.5 cm.

Roentgenographic studies of the cranium revealed premature synostosis of the sutures and prominent convulsional markings.

Specific Studies – Abnormal

Ophthalmology. Ophthalmologic examination was performed in *Cases 1 and 2*, their sibs and both par-

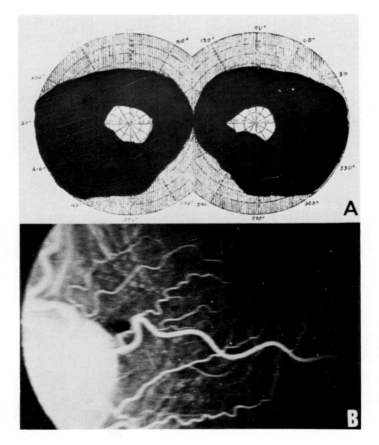

Fig. 5. A) Constriction of the visual fields of *Case 1*. B) Fluorescein angiography of the fundus of *Case 2*. Due to the pigment dispersion, the choroid fluorescence is clearly seen through the retina.

ents. All were normal except *Cases 1 and 2*. Both presented in common the following abnormalities: marked diminution of visual acuity, irregular dispersion of the pigment of the retina (Fig. 5B) more accentuated at the periphery and less marked at the posterior pole, constriction of the visual fields (Fig. 5A) and narrowing of the retinal arteries. Electroretinogram disclosed diminution of the b-wave. *Case 1* also had bilateral pallor of the optic disks.

Specific Studies – Normal

The following studies showed no abnormality: hemogram, urinalysis, PBI, fasting growth hormone levels, chromosome karyotypes, EEG and complete dermatoglyphics.

Discussion

Since birthweights were essentially normal when compared to both the normal sibs and to normal Mexican newborns, the growth defect in these 3 affected brothers was not evident at birth. No data of birth lengths are available, unfortunately. These would be indispensable to assure that the growth retardation was essentially postnatal.

The 3 patients had microcephaly. Mental development was normal, however, at least in *Cases 1 and 2*. The most likely consequence of variable craniosynostosis was cranial asymmetry.

In *Cases 1 and 2*, the retinopathy observed is difficult to classify. It bears resemblance to the atypical peripheral pigmentary retinopathy with little pigment (retinitis pigmentosa sine pigmento) of the tapetoretinal degenerations classification (Duke-Elder 1967).[2]

Since the abnormal phenotype is present in 3 sibs with presumed parental consanguinity and there are no phenotypic manifestations in the parents or other first-degree relatives, the pedigree analysis shows a pattern compatible with an autosomal recessive inheritance. It could be explained by chance alone that all 3 patients are males; however, an X-linked recessive mutant cannot be ruled out at the present time. Since the patients derive from a relatively inbred population, one would have to consider consanguinity as a coincidence in this case.

Acknowledgments

The authors are greatly indebted to Professor David W. Smith and Dr. Kenneth Jones from the Department of Pediatrics, School of Medicine, University of Washington for their most valuable advice with the manuscript. We also thank Miss Luz Elena Hernández de Alba for her secretarial assistance.

References

1. Armendares, S., Antillón, F., del Castillo, V. and Jiménez, M.: A newly recognized inherited syndrome of dwarfism, craniosynostosis, retinitis pigmentosa and multiple congenital malformations. *J. Pediatr. 85*:872, 1974.
2. Duke-Elder, S.: *Diseases of the Retina*, System of Ophthalmology. London:Kimpton, 1967, vol. X, p. 574.

Familial Frontometaphyseal Dysplasia—
Evidence for Dominant Inheritance

Lester Weiss, M.D., William A. Reynolds, M.D. and Romuald T. Szymanowski, M.D.

Frontometaphyseal dysplasia was first described as a distinct clinical entity by Gorlin and Cohen in 1969.[1] The abnormalities described were marked overgrowth of the supraorbital ridges, absence of the frontal sinuses, defective modeling of the metaphyses of the long bones, flared ilia, antegonal notching of the mandibles, conductive deafness and hirsutism. In 1972, Holt and his associates reported 2 additional cases of frontometaphyseal dysplasia, emphasizing new or previously minimized abnormalities in the hands, feet, spine and ribs.[2] The purpose of this paper is to describe a 10-year-old black male with frontometaphyseal dysplasia whose mother has many of the clinical and radiographic features of the same syndrome, and to suggest dominant inheritance.

Case Report

The proband was admitted to Henry Ford Hospital for external auditory canalplasty and middle ear exploration. His hearing loss was first noted when he was 2 years old. He was referred because of his unusual facial features. The prominent supraorbital ridges were first noted when he was one year old. He was of normal intelligence. There was height-span disproportion. His hands and feet were large. The distal phalanges of the thumbs were broad. The coronal, lambdoidal and metopic sutures were prominent to palpation. There was marked prominence of the supraorbital ridges. There was hypoplasia of the maxilla and an antimongoloid slant to the palpebral fissures, with a wide-eyed appearance. He had a pointed chin, broad bridge of the nose, stenosis of the ear canals and an anterior polar cataract in the left eye. He had malaligned malformed teeth with dysplastic enamel and retained deciduous and absent permanent teeth. The clavicles were prominent and the scapulas winged. He had generalized muscular underdevelopment, with limitation of extension of the elbows, knees and 5th fingers.

His mother was 31 years old. She had an unaffected male child. She had prominent supraorbital ridges, marked scoliosis, conductive hearing loss and limited extension of the 5th finger. The maternal grandmother and grandfather were unaffected.

The radiographs of the skull and facial bones of the proband showed marked thickening of the supraorbital ridges, thickening and sclerosis of the mastoid, perisutural sclerosis, internal hyperostosis, absent frontal sinuses, prominent occipital condyles, hypoplasia of the maxilla and antegonal notching of the mandible. The thoracic and lumbar vertebras were flattened; the posterior portions of the ribs had irregular margins, some displaying a coat-hanger configuration. There was moderate pectus excavatum. The clavicles were thickened medially. The scapulas were also thickened. The pelvis showed some iliac flaring and there was midpelvic constriction. There was slight widening of the metaphyses of the humeri. The diaphyses of the humeri were also widened. All of the metacarpals and most of the phalanges were elongated and wide. The distal phalanges of the thumb were short and broad. Similar abnormalities were present in the feet.

The mother's skull radiographs showed hyperostosis of the supraorbital ridges, internal hyperostosis, mastoid sclerosis, hypoplasia of the frontal sinuses, prominent occipital condyles and increased mandibular angle. There was severe thoracic scoliosis. The ilia were only mildly flared. The appendicular skeleton showed only minor abnormalities. The middle phalanges of the 5th finger of each hand were slightly widened. The metatarsals of both feet appeared elongated.

55

Discussion

The proband demonstrates the full range of abnormalities previously described for frontometaphyseal dysplasia. The variation in expression possible is demonstrated by the less severe manifestations in the mother. Her conductive hearing loss is mild enough so that she does not wear a hearing aid. The supraorbital hyperostosis is not as striking as it was in the child. She does have contractures of the 5th fingers bilaterally but does not have hypoplastic musculature. Her radiographs show abnormalities of the skull, thoracic scoliosis and flared ilia, but she does not have the midpelvic constriction or the striking abnormalities in the ribs and tubular bones. All previously reported cases have been sporadic. The occurrence of frontometaphyseal dysplasia in a mother and son strongly suggests that this condition is genetic and inherited as a mendelian dominant.

References

1. Gorlin, R. J. and Cohen, M. M.: Frontometaphyseal dysplasia — A new syndrome. *Am. J. Dis. Child. 118*:487-494, 1969.
2. Holt, J. F., Thompson, G. R. and Arenberg, I. K.: Frontometaphyseal dysplasia. *Radiol. Clin. North Am. 10*:225-243, 1972.

Discussion

Dr. Gorlin: It certainly is a beautiful example and we are indebted to you for finding out what the heredity is in this disorder. Dave Danks reported another case, as you probably know, and found metachromasia in the fibroblasts. I was wondering if you were planning to pursue this line of inquiry?

Dr. Weiss: We looked for and did not find metachromasia in peripheral blood lymphocytes and in the Rebuck skin window.

Dr. Rimoin: I would like to point out that we have a family with dominant inheritance of just the frontal part of frontal dysplasia. The interesting thing is that one of them has a very enlarged frontal sinus, and the other one has hyperostosis of the frontal area. They have nothing else but this frontal change, although they look identical. (See Case Reports, Case G.)

Dr. Poznanski: I think that this is a fascinating addition, from the point of view of the hand radiograph, where the pattern of elongation is so typical. The very long proximal phalanges are very typical. Dr. Weiss was nice enough to send us his case, and we measured it. It fits beautifully with the pattern profiles of our cases, as well as the case we received from a doctor in Paris, France, and another case as well.

Dr. Weiss: Interestingly enough, the mother did not fit that pattern.

Dr. Poznanski: That is right, but the mother had much milder skeletal changes generally. The mother's pattern did not fit well. The boy's fit beautifully.

A Syndrome of Systemic Hyalinosis, Short-Limb Dwarfism and Possible Thymic Dysplasia

Omar S. Alfi, M.D., Eva T. Heuser, M.D., Benjamin H. Landing, M.D.,
Ricki E. Robinson, M.D., Spencer Nadler, M.D. and George N. Donnell, M.D.

The term systemic hyalinosis seems to represent a nonspecific finding present in a category of disorders including mesenchymal dysplasia of Puretic,[1,2] systemic hyalinosis of Ishikawa-Hori,[3] fibromatosis hyalinica multiplex juvenilis,[4] Winchester syndrome[5,6] and possibly others.

The present report describes a disorder falling within this general category of disorders showing systemic hyalinosis, affecting 2 female sibs and compatible with autosomal recessive inheritance.

Case Reports

The proband and her sib are Mexican sisters born to second cousin parents. There have been 4 pregnancies, the first resulted in a stillborn male and the second, a 5-year-old healthy female; the proband and her sib were the third and fourth offspring, respectively.

Case 1

G.R., born 1/6/71, was the product of a full-term, normal pregnancy and delivery; birthweight was 2.78 kg. At 6 days of age, she was noted to have decreased movements of limbs, cried continuously and appeared in pain when touched. By 2 months, she had developed flexion contractures in both upper and lower limbs. She also developed thick skin with periodic peeling and redness in the skin crease areas. On examination she was below the 3rd percentile for weight and height, had a relatively large head, short neck and marked flexion contractures in both upper and lower limbs. The skin was generally thickened, with erythematous areas in the skin creases. There was no facial dysmorphology. Examination of the eyes showed normal corneas and fundi.

There were no cardiac murmurs and the lungs were clear. Examination of the abdomen was within normal limits. Skeletal radiographs revealed generalized demineralization. The results of extensive laboratory investigation were within normal, except for one alkaline phosphatase that was elevated on one occasion, but normal on repeat; a serum ANA that was positive 1:16 on one occasion and negative on repeat, and a slightly elevated IgM. Urine showed no mucopolysaccharides.

Over the next 12 months the contractures increased and involved the wrists, elbows, hips, knees and ankles. She developed spade-like hands with relatively short, swollen, sausage-like fingers (Fig. 1). Her skin remained

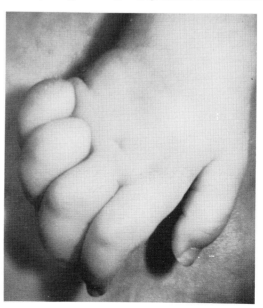

Fig. 1. Hand of *Case 1*, the proband.

thickened and developed a violatious discoloration over the neck and ears. A nodule was noted on her lip and several small nodules were seen on the external ears (Fig. 2). She developed gum hypertrophy. She was taken to Mexico from age 3 months to age 12 months, during which time she was tried on steroids without improvement. She developed episodes of pneumonia and gastroenteritis. At 14 months, she had a severe episode of diarrhea with dehydration and septisemia, and expired after a brief terminal illness.

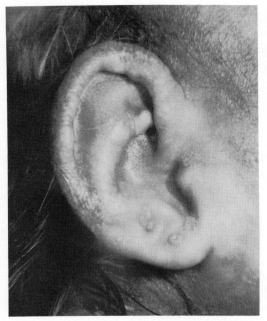

Fig. 2. *Case 1.* Note nodules on external ear.

Case 2

F.R., born 9/22/73, presented at 5 weeks of age with a similar history and findings. She was the product of a normal pregnancy and delivery. Birthweight was 2.61 kg. During the first week of life her parents noted that she, too, would not move her upper limbs and seemed to cry in pain if touched. She was referred for evaluation at 5 weeks of age (Fig. 3). At that time, height and weight were at the 10th percentile and head circumference was at the 50th percentile, giving an appearance of relative macrocephaly, with a short neck. Her upper limbs were shortened. She was very irritable and cried when touched. Her skin was generally thickened, but no skin or lip nodules were noted at that age. She had hyperpigmented areas over the metacarpophalangeal joints bilaterally and a violatious discoloration of the eyelids. No contractures were noted. Examination of the eyes, ears, nose and throat, lungs and heart were within normal limits. Skeletal radiographs confirmed the short upper limbs and revealed demineralization of the long bones. Laboratory investigations included quantitative immunoglobulins, latex flocculation, ANA test, erythrocyte sedimentation rate, alkaline phosphatase and urine mucopolysaccharides, all of which showed normal findings. Chromosome analysis of the peripheral blood was 46,XX. Steroid treatment for 3 weeks did not alter the symptomatology.

Pathologic Findings of Case 1

Autopsy confirmed the short-limbed dwarfism, short neck, macrocranium, sausage-like fingers, nodules of lip, gum hypertrophy, conjunctivitis and skin changes noted on physical examination. Microscopically, much of the cutaneous induration of the thorax and neck was found to be due to a severe acute cellulitis, with visible microorganisms consistent with streptococci present in

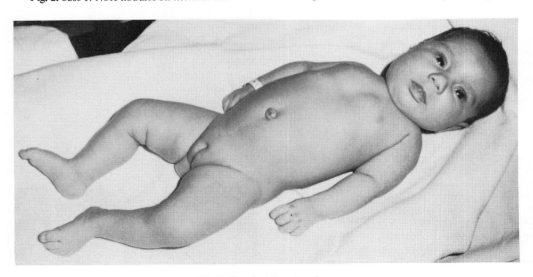

Fig. 3. *Case 2* at 5 weeks of age.

the inflamed tissues. The nodular lesions of the lip and the erythematous scaling lesions of the ear could not be sampled. Other evidence of infection was a well-developed, histologically active, nonspecific enteritis. Striking systemic findings apparently unrelated to these infectious processes were also present. They consisted of a marked hyalinosis of the stroma of villi in the small intestine, lobules of the thymus and in the walls of parathyroid sinusoids. A lesser degree of hyalinosis was seen in the central regions of the adrenal glands. Hyalinosis also involved muscles of the anterior chest wall, lymph nodes from a variety of sites and the soft tissues about the lateral ends of the clavicles. These, at autopsy, were encased in voluminous, edematous, firm, but easily cut, tissue which proved to be fibrohyaline microscopically.

In the thymus, the hyalinosis appeared to replace the normal epithelial core of the lobules, with (apparently resulting) total absence of Hassall corpuscles (Fig. 4). In the kidneys there was extensive calcification in distal convoluted tubules. (This is interesting in view of the history of an earlier episode of aminoaciduria, and possible but unproved renal tubular acidosis.) The parathyroid glands, besides the hyalinosis, consisted of a marked preponderance of clear cells. Various medium-ized arteries showed patches of medial calcinosis.

Random cuts of mesenteric and coronary artery showed focal intimal sclerosis. Such carotid artery branches as were sampled showed no abnormalities, but the brain contained a large area of very old left-sided encephalomalacia.

The lungs showed nonspecific pneumonitis and acute bronchitis. There were no germinal centers in an otherwise normal spleen. The liver showed portal triaditis and some foci of bile ductular proliferation. The pancreas was normal. The long bones were not sampled. Ribs and vertebras showed osteoporosis, with thin cortices and normal but not too active conversion. Sections of skin were all from the thorax and were affected by the cellulitis. However, there was a band of hyalinosis in the papillary layer of the dermis, underlying the epidermal basement membrane. No deeper dermal or subcutaneous hyalinosis was present.

Electron Microscopy

Electron microscopy from skin biopsy of both patients and of cultured skin fibroblasts from the younger sib was performed. There was distention of cisternas and hyperplasia of rough endoplasmic reticulum (Figs. 5 and 6). Mitochondria varied from apparent

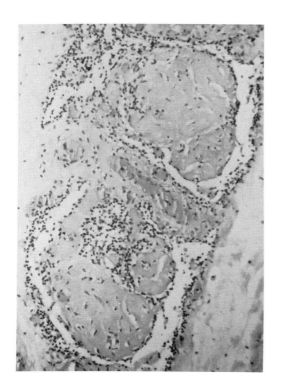

Fig. 4. *Case 1.* Section of thymus showing hyaline deposits and absence of Hassall corpuscles.

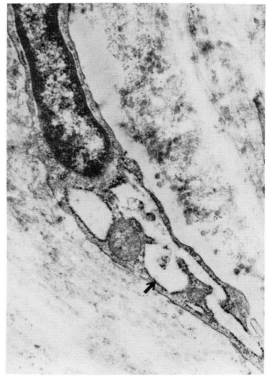

Fig. 5. Dermal fibroblast showing markedly distended and hyperplastic endoplasmic reticumum ($\times$ 18,000).

Table 1. Comparison of the Main Features in the Two Patients with Those in Puretic/Ishikawa and Winchester Syndromes

	Puretic/Ishikawa	Winchester	Case 1	Case 2
Mode of Inheritance	Aut. rec.	Aut. rec.	Aut. rec.	Aut. rec.
Mentality	N	N	N	N
Craniofacial Appearance:				
Relative macrocephaly	+	?	+	+
Coarse facies	+	+	+	+
Corneal opacity		+	-	-
Gum hypertrophy	+	+	+	-
Skin and Subcutaneous Tissue:				
Thick skin	+	+	+	+
Skin nodules	+	+	+	+
Pigmentary changes	+	+	+	+
Swollen fingers	+	+	+	+
Musculoskeletal Changes:				
Short stature	+	+	+	+
Short neck	+	+	+	+
Muscle and/or joint pains	+	+	+	+
Contractures	+	+	+	+
Osteoporosis	+	+	+	+
Osteolysis	+	+	-	-
Immunologic Response:				
Recurrent infections	+	+	+	+
Thymic dysplasia			+	
High IgM	-	+	+	?
Skin Microscopic Changes	+	+	+	+
EM Cultured Fibroblasts	+	+	+	+
MPS in Urine	-	-	-	-

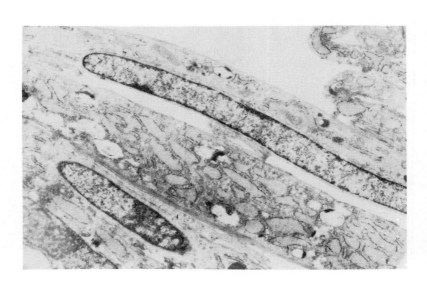

Fig. 6. Fibroblasts in tissue culture showing endoplasmic reticulum changes similar to Figure 5 (× 9,000).

normal appearance to markedly swollen and vacuolated organelles. Occasional laminated bodies, similar to myelin figures, were noted in the cytoplasm. There was no prominence of the nuclear limiting zonules similar to that reported by Hollister et al[6] in the Winchester syndrome.

Discussion

This reported disorder of systemic hyalinosis, short-limb dwarfism and possible thymic dysplasia shares many of the clinical features reported in Puretic syndrome[1,2] and Winchester syndrome[5,6] (Table 1). However, there were some differences — the osteolysis described in the Puretic and Winchester syndromes was not significant in the present probands and the corneal opacity in the Winchester syndrome was not present either in the Puretic syndrome or in our patients.

The EM picture in the present disorder is of interest. We are not aware of any EM studies in patients with Puretic syndrome. The EM of skin fibroblasts in the Winchester syndrome[6] is somewhat similar to that of our patients in regard to distention of endoplasmic reticulum and the presence of mitochondrial changes. However, there was greater distention of the endoplasmic reticulum and far less mitochondrial changes in our patients than in those with Winchester syndrome. Also there was no prominence of the nuclear limiting zonule as reported in the Winchester syndrome.

Because of their microscopic picture, this disorder, the Puretic syndrome and the Winchester syndrome may all be considered as connective tissue disorders. Further studies of function of the immune system in disorders with systemic hyalinosis, and of the association of skeletal dysplasia and dwarfism with immunologic deficiency, are needed.

References

1. Puretic, S. et al: A unique form of mesenchymal dysplasia. *Brit. J. Dermatol. 74*:8, 1962.
2. Puretic, S. and Puretic, B.: Mesenchymal dysplasia of Puretic. In Bergsma, D. (ed.): *Birth Defects: Atlas and Compendium*. Baltimore:Williams & Wilkins Co. for the National Foundation-March of Dimes, 1973, p. 608.
3. Ishikawa, H. and Hori, Y.: Systematisierte Hyalinose im Zusammenhang mit Epidermolysis bullosa polydystrophica und Hyalinosis cutis et mucosae. *Arch. Klin. Exp. Dermatol. 281*:30, 1963.
4. Drescher, E. et al: Juvenile fibromatosis in siblings (fibromatosis hyalinica multiplex juvenilis). *J. Pediatr. Surg. 2*:427, 1967.
5. Winchester, P. et al: A new acid mucopolysaccharidosis with skeletal deformities stimulating rheumatoid arthritis. *Am. J. Roentgenol. Radium Ther. Nucl. Med. 106*:121, 1969.
6. Hollister, D. et al: The Winchester syndrome: A nonlysosomal connective tissue disease. *J. Pediatr. 84*:701, 1974.

Discussion

Moderator: Dr. Robinson, do you feel that these are separable entities, these 3 that you showed, the Winchester and the 2 others?

Dr. Robinson: We feel that they all have the systemic hyalinosis and fit into a class. Now, whether or not they are separate entities is another question.

Dr. Rimoin: I really fail to see the similarity. The EM changes are quite different. What is hyalinosis? The osteolysis was really quite different. The eye changes were quite different.

Dr. Robinson: I believe that in the Winchester syndrome you found a hyperplastic, distended, endoplastic reticulum?

Dr. Rimoin: Yes, that was in the description. There was some. It was the mitochondria that were consistently abnormal, plus more changes around the nuclear membrane.

Moderator: Southern Californians, from USC and from UCLA, always act this way when they get on the field of battle!

Dr. Rimoin: They are nonlysosomal connective tissue diseases, but I do not know that there is any closer relationship than that. I think that they are quite clearly distinguishable.

Dr. Robinson: We felt that the hyalinosis was actually collagen deposition. We found that the light microscopic findings in both of our cases were similar in that respect.

Dr. Rimoin: The interesting thing is that the light microscopic changes in our cases were quite dissimilar in the same family, dependent upon age. I think that it is hard to make any comparison because they are really quite nonspecific changes.

Dr. Robinson: In the Puretic syndrome, the light microscopic findings show the swirls of collagen that were in the deep dermis, as you found, I think, in your cases.

Dr. Rimoin: Yes, that is right, but I would not try to make a big point of it. I think that it is clear that they are different diseases. Whether you want to class them together and call them hyalinosis, into which we could put another 20 to 30 diseases, all having abnormal collagen or increased deposition, is a matter of how broad one wants to make the categories. But to claim any close etiologic link, I just do not think that the evidence is there as yet. I think that the biochemists are going to have to tell us eventually.

Dr. Alfi: I think that the EM pictures of the Winchester syndrome published by Drs. Rimoin,

Hollister et al are very similar to the ones that Dr. Robinson just presented, regarding the dilatation of the endoplasmic reticulum, which could be within the normal or a bit beyond the normal limit, in both situations. Mitochondrial abnormality is closely similar in both. The additional part of nuclear membrane abnormality described in the Winchester is possibly seen in some of the normal fibroblast preparations, too, and the definition or the demarcation between what is normal and what is abnormal there is not very sharp. But the similarity in the EM is very striking between both of them. Clinically, however, there are some differences; the corneal opacity is definitely not seen in the 2 cases reported, while it is mentioned in the Winchester syndrome, in most of the cases. Susceptibility to infection is also another difference.

Familial Multiforme Ventricular Extrasystoles with Short Stature, Hyperpigmentation and Microcephaly—A New Syndrome

Florence Char, M.D., John E. Douglas, M.D. and
William T. Dungan, M.D.

The familial occurrence of multiforme ventricular extrasystoles has been well-documented.[1-3] Previous reports of such arrhythmias did not mention associated somatic abnormalities.

The purpose of this communication is to report a previously undescribed syndrome in a mother and son (Fig. 1) with multiforme ventricular extrasystoles who also presented with short stature, hyperpigmentation, microcephaly, peculiar dermatoglyphics and borderline intelligence.

Case Reports

Case 1

This 10-year-old white male (Fig. 2) was referred for evaluation because of a fainting episode while climbing into a truck.

The patient, born to an 18-year-old woman and her 27-year-old husband, was the product of a full-term uncomplicated pregnancy. The birthweight was 3.6 kg. He was considered to be in good health except for slow growth and poor school work, having had to repeat the second grade. He had no history of exercise intolerance, previous fainting episodes or seizures.

The family history was negative for consanguinity. His father was 190.5 cm tall. His 147 cm mother distinctly resembled the patient and will be described. There were no sibs and no family history of similarly affected individuals.

Examination showed a well-proportioned prepubertal male whose height was 125 cm and who weighed 25 kg. The head circumference was 49 cm. The facies appeared infantile. The interpupillary distance was 5.7 cm. The fundi were normal. There was mild esotropia. The hearing was grossly normal. The mandible appeared small. The 1st mandible molars were missing bilaterally. The pulse rate was 90-100/minute and was irregular. BP was 90/60 mm Hg. No significant heart murmurs were noted. There was no organomegaly. The genitalia appeared normal with both testes descended. There were large areas of hyperpigmentation on the right chest with midline delineation, right shoulder, neck and arm. There was no abnormal hair over the pigmentated areas. The limbs were normal. There was no hypermobility of the joints. There was a simian line on the left, increased Atd angle and peculiar hypothenar pattern. Neurologic exam was normal. He was somewhat dull and general behavior was immature for age.

ECG showed multiforme ventricular extrasystoles with runs of ventricular tachycardia and variable bigeminal and trigeminal rhythm. The Q-T interval was normal.

Full skeletal survey revealed normal bony structures. The bone age was approximately 8 years. Cardiac series showed normal heart size and lung

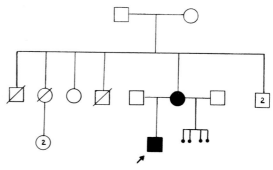

Fig. 1. Pedigree.

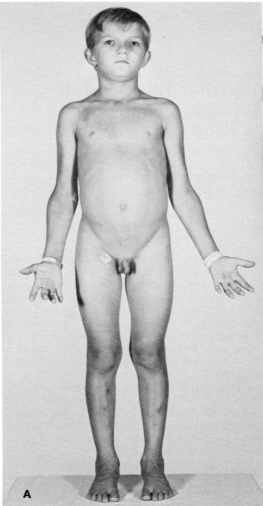

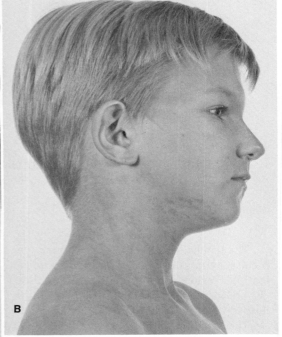

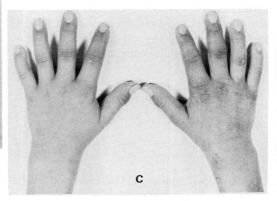

Fig. 2. A-C) *Case 1* showing infantile facies and hyperpigmentation on neck, chest and dorsum of hands.

fields. IVP was normal. Dental films showed missing 1st mandibular molars, and absence of 3rd molar tooth buds.

Laboratory findings revealed normal urinalysis, CBC, serum electrolytes, SGOT and T_4.

EEG, audiogram and chromosome studies were normal. Psychometric evaluation revealed borderline intellectual ability, functioning at approximately 80% of his age in years.

Dermatoglyphics revealed on the left: a simian crease – Atd angle 66°, whorls in interdigital areas 3 and 4; digital patterns – double loop in L_1, whorls in L_2-L_5. Revealed on the right were normal flexion creases – Atd angle 63°, arch pattern in hypothenar area; digital patterns – double loop in R_1, whorls in R_2-R_5. Total ridge count 156.

Case 2

This patient (Fig. 3), the 28-year-old mother of the propositus, fainted while visiting him during his hospitalization.

The patient was well until she was 20 years of age when she first experienced cardiac irregularity associated with substernal pain. Since then she has had 8-10 similar episodes, some of which were accompanied by syncopal episodes. Cardiac arrhythmia was documented at several hospitals as being multifocal ventricular extrasystoles. Further evaluation for the ventricu-

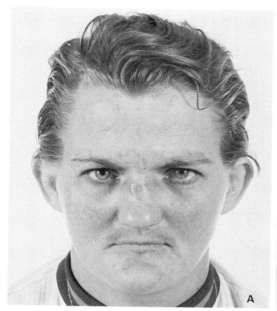
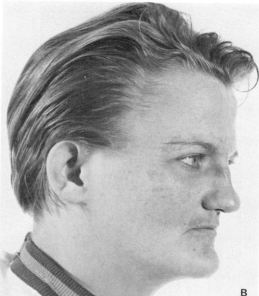
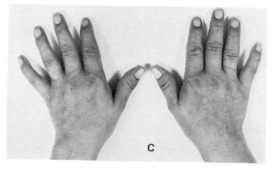

lar tachyarrhythmia was recommended; however, the patient had refused. She had normal exercise tolerance and led an active live.

The patient was the fifth of 7 sibs. Her parents were 28 years of age at the time of her birth. Her father was 178 cm tall and her mother was 170 cm tall. A brother died at one day of age, cause unknown, and a second brother died of pneumonia at age 3 years. A diabetic sister died accidently of gun shot wounds. Two living brothers and one sister were in good health. There was no family history of cardiac arrhythmia, hyperpigmentation or short stature.

Her menses began at 15 years. She had 4 other pregnancies which all ended in miscarriage at approximately 4-5 months. She fractured her nose in an automobile accident. A hysterectomy was performed at age 26 years for menorrhagia. She lost all her teeth by age 22; some "fell out" and others were extracted because "they were loose."

Examination showed an edentulous female who measured 147 cm in height and weighed 55 kg. Head circumference was 50 cm. Pulse rate was irregular and varied from 50-90/minute. BP was 116/70 mm Hg. There were several areas of hyperpigmentation over her cheeks, left forearm and dorsum of the right hand. The interpapillary distance was 5.8 cm. The fundi were normal. There were no significant heart murmurs. Limbs were normal except for peculiar dermatoglyphics. Heurologic examination showed no abnormal reflexes. General behavior was immature.

ECG showed ventricular premature contractions similar to *Case 1* (Fig. 4 and 5).

Skull series, chest roentgenograms and EEG were normal.

Fig. 3. A-C) *Case 2* showing hyperpigmentation on face and hands.

Dermatoglyphics revealed on the left: a simian crease — Atd angle 57°, whorl in hypothenar area; digital pattern — ulnar loop in L_1, L_4, L_5, radial loop in L_2 and L_3. Revealed on the right were normal flexion crease — Atd angle 68°, double loop in hypothenar area; digital pattern — double loop in R_1, radial loop in R_2, ulnar loop in R_3, R_4 and R_5. Total ridge count 93.

Cardiovascular Studies

Cardiac catheterization studies were done only on the propositus, *Case 1*. Data obtained from the right heart catheterization showed normal intracardiac pressures and no evidence of a shunt.

Portable electrocardiographic monitoring of the Holter type was performed during his hospital stay, and although he had short runs of ventricular tachycardia, this caused no symptoms. The presumption

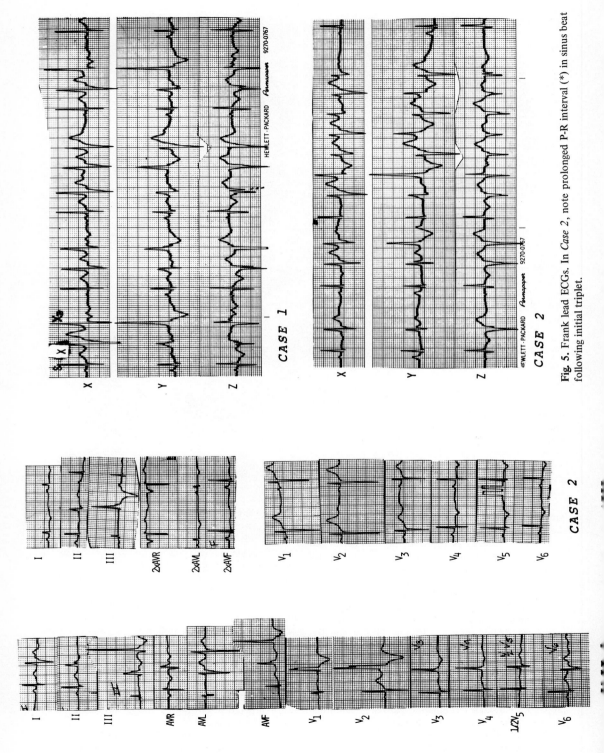

Fig. 5. Frank lead ECGs. In *Case 2*, note prolonged P-R interval (*) in sinus beat following initial triplet.

was, however, that his syncopal episode was due to an episode of ventricular tachycardia.

Conventional orthogonal 12 lead ECGs and Frank lead ECGs were obtained and tape recorded for subsequent analysis. Examples of this patient's and his mother's 12 lead ECGs are shown in Figure 4. Their X,Y,Z ECGs during paroxysms of arrhythmias are shown in Figure 5. The similarities are obvious. The basic cardiac rhythm was characterized by triplet or couplet beats. The first beat was apparently of normal sinus origin (S) with a normal QRS configuration. The second beat (X_A) had a QRS configuration resembling right bundle branch block, with possible left posterior fascicular block. The third beat of the triplet (X_B) was also ectopic occurring with a slightly shorter, less distorted QRS complex. Though the typical sequence of beats was S-X_A-X_B, occasionally X_B preceded X_A.

Vector display of beats S, X_A, X_B for *Case 1* are shown in Figure 6.

Intracardiac recording and pacing studies were performed using conventional techniques to obtain high right atrial and His bundle electrograms. His bundle records demonstrated that both beats X_A and X_B arose below the His bundle (Fig. 7). Three to 15 beat salvos of these infra-Hisian beats occurred frequently at rest and consisted predominantly of beats resembling X_A and X_B though intermediate forms emerged during the latter beats of longer salvos (Fig. 5).

During isoproterenol infusion the S-X coupling interval decreased from 0.42 seconds to 0.38 seconds and salvos became more frequent and persistent. During these salvos, it was possible to detect atrial activity independent of the ventricular arrhythmia.

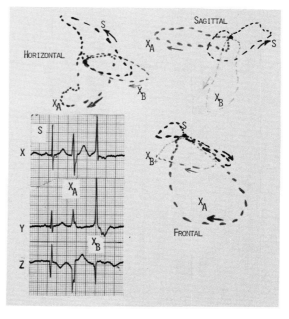

Fig. 6. Frank vectorcardiogram of *Case 1.*

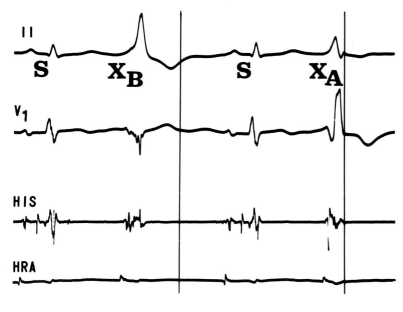

Fig. 7. ECG and His bundle electrogram at rest. Note His spikes with the S beats and no His spike before the X beats.

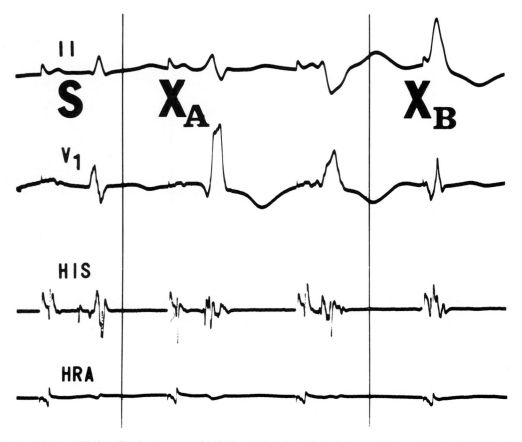

Fig. 8. ECG and His bundle electrogram with high atrial pacing. Note despite atrial and His bundle capture, the arrhythmia persists.

At atrial pacing rates of 150, he demonstrated Mobitz I block. The ventricular arrhythmia (S-$X_A X_B$) persisted despite capture of the atria via His bundle catheter pacing (Fig. 8). Ventricular pacing, at between 100 and 140/minute abolished the arrhythmia.

After propranolol, the S to X_A coupling interval increased to 0.47 seconds and the frequency and duration of ventricular salvos decreased. In addition, ectopic beats were frequently associated with discernible retrograde P waves.

These results suggest the mechanism of our patients' arrhythmias depends on multiple alternating reentrant pathways occurring below the His bundle, possibly promoted by depolarization wave dispersion secondary to adrenergic influence and partially suppressed with beta adrenergic blockade.

Course. Both patients were placed on propranolol therapy. Both demonstrated persistence of multiforme ventricular extrasystoles, though in less frequency. During the 12-month follow-up period, *Case 1* had one

syncopal episode, apparently brought on by stress and excitement while carrying a pail of water to fill a boiling car radiator. *Case 2* refused to continue on her medications after about a one-month period and has denied symptoms.

Evaluation of Other Members in the Family. The maternal grandparents and a maternal uncle were available for evaluation. None of these individuals demonstrated similar findings of the 2 cases presented. ECGs of these individuals were all normal.

Discussion

The association of skin manifestations and arrhythmia has been well-described in the multiple lentigines syndrome or LEOPARD syndrome.[4,5] Lentigines is a cardinal feature of that syndrome. Our cases presented skin lesions consisting of patchy areas of brown macular hyperpigmentation, distinctly different from lentigines. Presence of dental abnormalities and premature loss of teeth may be speculative. Ventricular ectopic beats, mild microcephaly, hypertelorism, short stature and peculiar dermatoglyphics present in both mother and son suggest the mode of inheritance as being autosomal dominant with high penetrance and variable expressivity.

Summary

A previously undescribed syndrome with ventricular extrasystoles and presumed cardiac syncopy, hyperpigmentation, short stature and microcephaly in a mother and son was presented. Physiologic and pharmacologic studies suggest that the mechanism of the ventricular arrhythmia depends on multiple reentrant pathways occurring below the bundle of His.

Acknowledgments

The authors wish to express their appreciation to Dr. J. Bissett for his assistance in the His bundle studies and Dr. Roosevelt Brown for dental evaluation.

References

1. Berg, K. J.: Multifocal ventricular extrasystoles with Adams-Stokes syndrome in siblings. *Am. Heart J. 60*:965-970, 1960.
2. Kuhn, E., Wold, D. and Stieler, M.: Familial polytopic and polymorphic extrasystoles. *Jap. Heart J. 5*:81-84, 1964.
3. Gualt, J. H., Cantwell, J., Lev, M. and Braunwald, E.: Fatal familial cardiac arrhythmias. *Am. J. Cardiol. 29*:548-553, 1972.
4. Smith, R. F., Pulicicchio, L. U. and Holmes, A. V.: Generalized lentigo: Electrocardiographic abnormalities, conduction disorders and arrhythmias in these cases. *Am. J. Cardiol. 25*:501, 1970.
5. Gorlin, R. J., Anderson, R. C. and Blau, M.: Multiple lentigines syndrome. *Am. J. Dis. Child. 117*:652, 1969.

Skeletal Dysplasia, Occipital Horns, Diarrhea and Obstructive Uropathy– A New Hereditary Syndrome

Stephen G. Lazoff, M.D., James J. Rybak, M.D.,
Bruce R. Parker, M.D. and Luigi Luzzatti, M.D.

A previously undescribed complex of clinical and roentgenographic abnormalities including a unique bone dysplasia, chronic diarrhea and urinary tract obstruction has been identified in 3 members of a family seen recently at the Stanford University Medical Center. The proband was an 11-year-old boy who presented to the Birth Defects Center with a chief complaint of lifelong diarrhea. At age 2 he was noted to have an unusual facial appearance and prominent elbows similar to those of 3 male relatives of his mother. The proband underwent repair of bilateral bladder diverticula and surgical repair of bladder neck obstruction at age 5. Exhaustive psychologic testing at age 7, because of poor school performance, demonstrated poor learning capability with a borderline IQ and problems in coordination. At the age of 9 he underwent open reduction of a dislocated right radial head.

Physical examination revealed an alert, cooperative 11-year-old boy whose appearance was distinctive because of a high forehead and narrow face. Height and weight were at the 50th percentile for age and anthropometric measurements were within normal limits. His hands were broad with short fingers. His elbows were prominent and he had a genu valgum deformity. Dermatoglyphics revealed all 10 fingers to have ulnar loop patterns. The remainder of the physical examination was normal.

Radiographic findings included the unique appearance of "occipital horns." These are bony projections extending inferiorly from the occiput; they are parasagittal in location and bilaterally symmetric (Fig. 1). Radiographic examination of the wrists revealed capitate-hamate fusion and a slight increase of the radioulnar angle (Fig. 2). Mild platyspondyly with diffuse demineralization of the vertebral bodies was present in the thoracolumbar spine (Fig. 3). The interpediculate distances were normal. The acetabular roofs were flattened

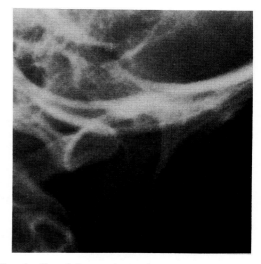

Fig. 1. Coned-down view of the occipital bone showing bilaterally symmetric bony protuberances ("occipital horns").

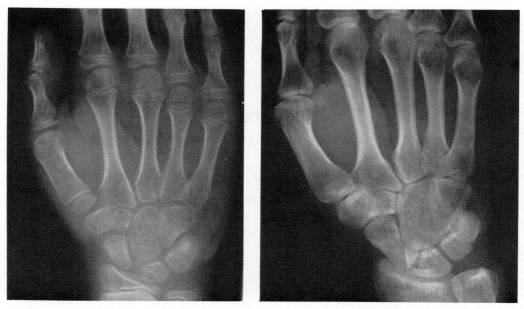

Fig. 2. Left: Proband's hand and wrist showing capitate-hamate fusion and slight increase in radioulnar angle. Right: Similar findings in the wrist of the proband's uncle.

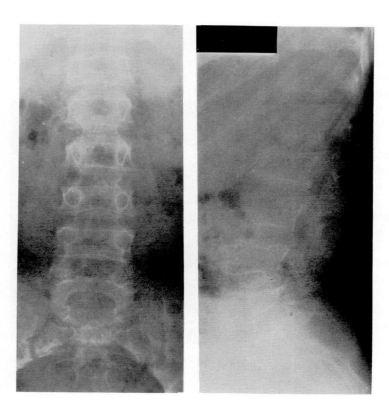

Fig. 3. AP and lateral views of the proband's lumbar spine demonstrating marked osteoporosis and mild platyspondyly.

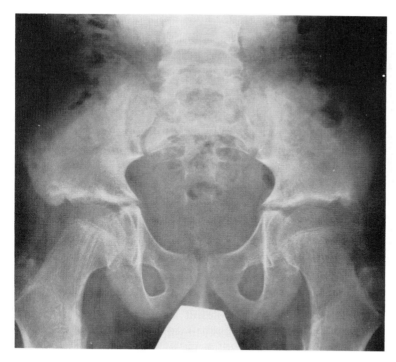

Fig. 4. AP view of the proband's pelvis. Marked flattening of the acetabular angle and bilateral coxa valga in association with diffuse osteoporosis.

bilaterally and coxa valga was present (Fig. 4). The cortical margins of the long bones were undulating with alternate widening and narrowing of the cortical width. The long bones were not shortened.

Laboratory studies were all within normal limits including evaluation of the serum, calcium, phosphorus, alkaline phosphatase and electrolytes. Urinary mucopolysaccharides were within normal range. The karyotype was normal.

The patient's GI complaints were evaluated by means of barium enema, upper GI series with a small bowel follow-through, 3-day fecal fat excretion, d-xylose absorption, sweat chloride determination, and a small bowel biopsy. All of these studies were within normal limits.

IVP and voiding cystoureterogram demonstrated normal upper tracts with a markedly irregular bladder and multiple diverticula. These changes were felt to be consistent with previous bladder surgery. Urinalysis, urine culture, BUN and creatinine were within normal limits.

No recent psychometric testing had been performed, but the patient was in a class for educationally handicapped children at an appropriate grade level.

Three members of the proband's mother's family have physical resemblance to the patient in terms of facial features and prominent elbows (Fig. 5). One uncle (III-5) suffered from lifelong diarrhea. He was 183 cm in height, weighed 59 kg and had 20 bowel movements per day. Barium enema, upper GI series with small intestinal follow-through and intestinal biopsy were all within normal limits. Radiographic examination of his skeletal system revealed changes similar to those seen in the proband. Another uncle (III-6) has had multiple surgical procedures for lower urinary tract obstruction since childhood and has had an ileal loop diversion. He had frequent watery stools. Radiographic examination of the skeleton was similar to that of the proband and of the other uncle.

Both of these apparently affected uncles have low-normal intelligence and did not complete high school, in comparison to their sibs who were all college graduates.

The proband's mother, his sister and his other maternal uncles have normal intelligence, normal GI and GU tract functions, and no abnormalities of the skeletal system by radiographic evaluation.

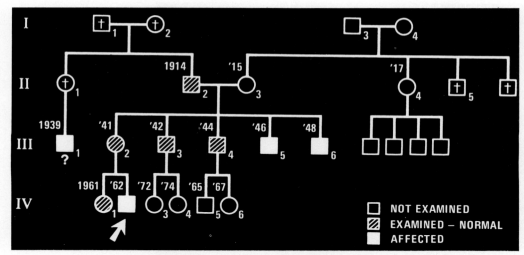

Fig. 5. Family pedigree. The proband is identified by the arrow.

A maternal cousin (*III-1*) has a facial appearance and prominent elbows similar to the proband. He lived at a distance from the Stanford University Medical Center and refused to see a physician or to have radiographs performed.

The pattern of inheritance is not yet certain. If the cousin (*III-1*) is not affected, the inheritance would appear to be an X-linked recessive pattern. If he is affected, however, this may represent an autosomal dominant with variable penetrance.

Further characterization of this syndrome and the inheritance pattern will depend upon the accumulation of more data from members of this family and from patients found by other investigators.

Dominantly Inherited Ulnar Drift

Roger E. Stevenson, M.D., Charles I. Scott, Jr., M.D.
and Michael Epstein, M.D.

In 1972, Sallis and Beighton[1] described a large South African kindred with ulnar deviation of phalanges, flexion contractures of interphalangeal joints, soft tissue webbing between the thumb and palm, vertical talus with "rocker bottom" feet and short stature. Other cases of this dominantly transmitted syndrome, termed digitotalar dysmorphism by the authors, have not been reported. Members of a similarly large kindred with the same hand features but lacking vertical talus and short stature form the basis for this report. Although conclusive evidence that the 2 syndromes arise from different dominant mutations cannot be given, the designation "congenital ulnar drift with webbing and flexion contractures of the fingers" better characterizes the entity herein reported.

Case Reports

M.S. was examined at age 73 years (Fig. 1, *I-2*). She denied visual or auditory impairment and her facial features appeared normal. The fingers of each hand deviated towards the ulna, a deformity which became more pronounced when supination was attempted. Flexion contractures limited both 5th fingers at the proximal interphalangeal (PIP) joint. The toes tended to deviate laterally with prominence of the distal and medial aspects of the 1st metatarsal bone. These skeletal features had been present since birth, had not progressed and produced little functional impairment.

V.B. was examined at age 40 years (Fig. 1, *II-4*). Her facial features, hearing and vision were normal. The fingers were positioned in marked ulnar deviation with flexion contractures of the 5th fingers (Fig. 2). Her skeletal anomalies had not been progressive and had produced only mild impairment of hand function.

M.W. was examined at age 38 years (Fig. 1, *II-9*). She had normal vision and hearing. She had epilepsy, with

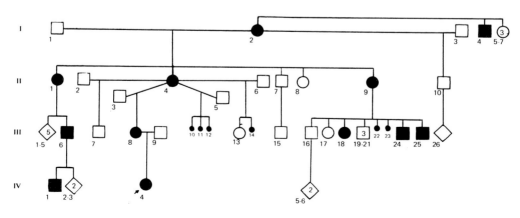

Fig. 1. Pedigree of a kindred with dominantly inherited ulnar drift.

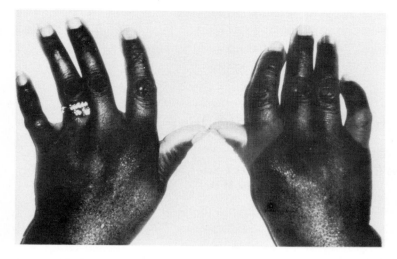

Fig. 2. Hands of *V.B.* *(II-4)* demonstrating ulnar drift of hand and fingers with flexion contractures of 5th fingers.

the onset of seizures in the second decade of life. There was ulnar drift of both hands. No contractures were present but the IP joint of the left 5th finger was flexed and the PIP joints of the left 4th and 5th fingers hyperextended. The toes of the right foot drifted laterally and the distal aspect of the 1st metatarsal bone was prominent.

P.W., born in 1955 (Fig. 1, *III-8*), exhibited only minimal abnormalities. Clinical and x-ray examinations showed ulnar deviation of the distal phalanx of the right 2nd digit. Roentgenograms of the feet and skull were normal. Since both her mother (*V.B.*) and daughter (*I.W.*) were severely affected, this feature was considered a mild expression of the mutant gene. Additionally, at age 17 years, she was noted to have thoracolumbar scoliosis with a 43° curve.

J.W. was examined at age 17 years (Fig. 1, *III-18*). Severe ulnar drift was present. Additionally, there existed a tendency to hyperextension at the PIP joints, radial deviation of 2 terminal phalanges of the left hand and flexion deformity of the right 5th digit. The toes deviated laterally.

B.W., born in 1962 (Fig. 1, *III-24*), had marked ulnar deviation of hands and fingers, with webbing of the thumbs to the palms. Lateral skin tags, the residual of amputated extra digits, were present bilaterally. Polydactyly, inherited through the paternal line, could be documented through 3 previous generations. Simian equivalents were present bilaterally. The feet deviated laterally to a minimal degree.

Y.W., examined at age 7 years (Fig. 1, *III-25*), showed moderate ulnar drift bilaterally, single palmar creases and mild webbing of thumbs to palms. No flexion contractures were present and the feet appeared normal.

I.W., the propositus, weighed 3640 gm at birth following an estimated 36-week gestation (Fig. 1, *IV-4*). The pregnancy, labor and delivery had been uneventful except for double footling breech presentation. The

skeletal malformations noted at birth included marked plagiocephaly, ulnar deviation of hands and fingers 2 to 5, contractures of the thumb against the palm by a soft tissue bridge (Fig. 3A), flexion of the IP joints of the left 3rd digit (Fig. 3B), mild tibial deviation of the toes and limited abduction of the hips. Additionally, there was a 4 cm patch of dark hair over the lower lumbar area, a large mongolian spot over the buttocks and a 2 cm hairy nevus at the left ankle. No bony defects were apparent on x-ray examination. Standard chromosome studies were normal. The father had not been examined but was said by the mother to be without skeletal anomalies.

Family members *I-4*, *II-1*, *III-6* and *IV-1* were not examined. However, they were described by other family members as having some combination of ulnar drift of the hands, flexion contractures and palmar webbing of the thumbs. Three of the 4 were said to be severely affected.

Comment

Features observed in the 8 individuals examined are given in Table 1. Fully expressed, the syndrome has the following features: webbing of the thumb to the palm by a soft tissue bridge, flexion contractures at the IP joints, ulnar deviation of the hands and fingers, simian lines and lateral drift of the toes. These abnormalities produce little functional impairment and do not progress in severity. Ulnar deviation of the hands and fingers is the most common feature; webbing of thumbs to the palms is perhaps the most limiting if not released by surgery. Mentation, facies, visual and auditory acuity, and stature appear normal in all members investigated. Vertical talus, a feature of the digitotalar dysmorph-

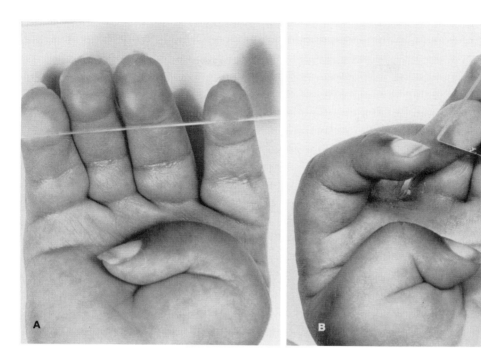

Fig. 3. A and B) Hands of *I.W. (IV-4)* showing contracture of thumbs into palms; B) ulnar deviation and flexion contracture of the left 3rd finger.

ism, was not seen in this kindred. Plagiocephaly, scoliosis, hairy nevi and seizures were each seen in individual patients. Their relationship to the syndrome is not known.

Reference

1. Sallis, J. G. and Beighton, P.: Dominantly inherited digito-talar dysmorphism. *J. Bone Joint Surg. (Br.) 54B*:509, 1972.

Table 1. Findings in Patients with Dominantly Inherited Ulnar Drift Syndrome

Patient	Ulnar Deviation	Webbing of Thumbs	Flexion Deformity of Fingers	Other
M.S.	+	0	+	lateral drift of toes
V.B.	+	0	+	lateral drift of toes
M.W.	+	0	+	seizures, lateral drift of toes
P.W.	0	0	0	scoliosis, ulnar deviation of 1 phalanx
J.W.	+	0	+	— —
B.W.	+	+	+	simian line
Y.W.	+	+	0	simian line
I.W.	+	+	+	lateral drift of toes, midfoot varus, plagiocephaly

A New Familial Metabolic Disorder with Progressive Osseous Changes, Microcephaly, Coarse Facies, Flat Nasal Bridge and Severe Mental Retardation

Bryan D. Hall, M.D. and Francis D. Riggs, M.D.

Normal consanguineous parents produced 6 of 15 offspring (Fig. 1) with a progressive disorder involving a flat nasal bridge, microcephaly, severe mental retardation, short stature, and metaphyseal-epiphyseal abnormalities. The affected members of this family appear to represent a new familial autosomal recessive disorder.

Case Reports

The 6 affected children (Fig. 2) were products of normal gestations with normal birthweight and lengths. None had any difficulties in the nursery and there were no apparent physical differences between the future affected sibs and the unaffected sibs. Three of the affected children (Cases 1, 2, 3) experienced numerous unexplained episodes of vomiting which

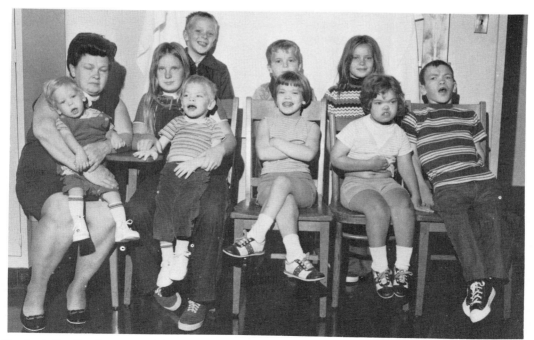

Fig. 1. *A Family:* Front row (left to right) shows *Case 6, Case 5, Case 4, Case 3* and *Case 2.* Mother of the affected children and 4 normal sibs make up the remaining individuals.

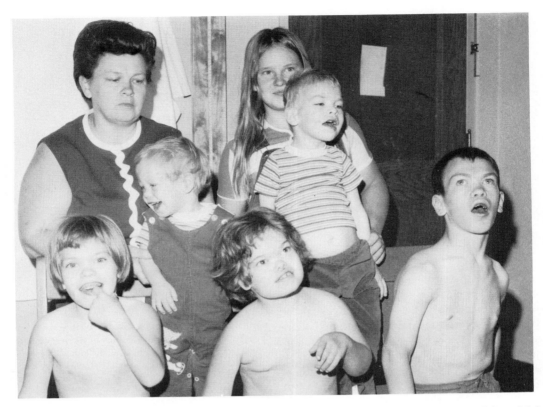

Fig. 2. Close-up of *A Family:* Front row (left to right) shows *Case 4, Case 3, Case 2*, middle row (left to right) shows *Case 6* and *Case 5.* The mother and a normal teenage daughter are in the back row. Note particularly the persistent flat nasal bridges, anteverted nostrils, large lips and progressive worsening of phenotype in the 5 affected sibs.

started at 2-4 weeks of age and persisted until 18 months. Poor linear growth was obvious between 4 and 10 months in the above 3 children, but was not noted in the other 3 affected sibs (*Cases 4, 5, 6*) until 12-18 months of age. Severe delays in psychomotor development were evident by 6 months of age in the affected children. No head circumference measurements were available in any of the children until 16 months of age and no roentgenograms could be obtained prior to 2½ years of age. Total absence of speech was noted in the 6 children, even into adulthood. None of the children had cataracts, corneal clouding, alopecia, skin abnormalities, visceromegaly, joint contractures or lumbar gibbus. The children's parents are first cousins as their mothers are sisters. The family history is otherwise normal.

Case 1

D.L.A. had recurrent pneumonias and seizures his first year of life. His milestone development was delayed. He sat up at 3 years, walked at 3½ to 4 years, and failed to talk by 13 years of age. He was admitted in 1958 to the University of California, San Francisco,

at 13 years of age for evaluation of a neck tumor. Physical examination at that time revealed a height (97 cm) and weight (22 kg) far below the 3rd percentile. He was said to be microcephalic. His facies were unusual in that he had a "saddle nose," anteverted slit-like nares, epicanthal folds and irides heterochromia. The fingers were clubbed, the sternum prominent and there were no secondary sexual characteristics. The trunk-limb ratio was normal. A grapefruit-size right submaxillary tumor was present. Laboratory studies including a PBI, cholesterol, serum calcium and phosphorus, and bone marrow were normal. Roentgenograms of *Case 1* were destroyed and not available for the authors' review; however, they were said to show a delayed bone age (8 years), generalized epiphyseal abnormality described as "epiphyseal lines consisting of densely calcified columnar patterns of cartilage which extended into the metaphyses," and irregular and deformed epiphyses. The femoral necks were broad, short and in a coxa vara position with resultant shallow acetabula. The bony structures of the lumbar spine showed irregular margins.

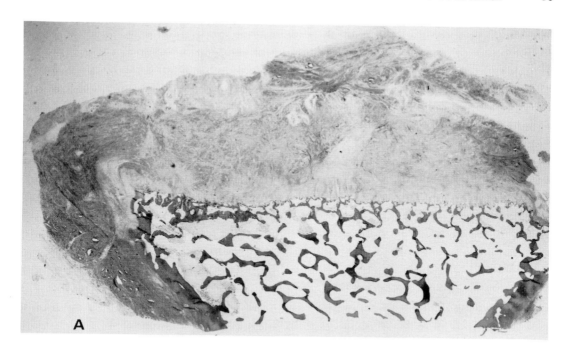

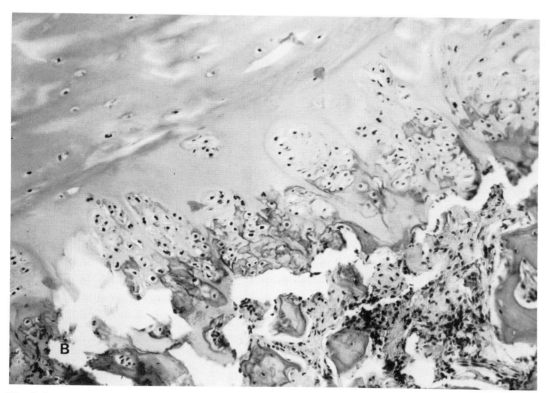

Fig. 3. Bone sections showing thickened epiphysis and variable metaphyseal-epiphyseal alignment of cartilage cells.

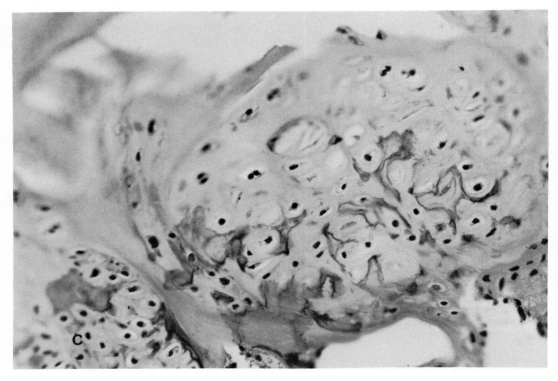

Fig. 3. Continued.

The patient died during the above hospitalization of a nonspecific anaplastic neck tumor which extended into the nasopharynx and pituitary area. Of particular interest relative to the autopsy were the following findings. 1) The brain was normal grossly and microscopically except for the anterior lobe of the pituitary gland which consisted almost exclusively of basophilic cells and chromophobes; 2) the thyroid was small (3.2 gm) showing "hypotrophic hyperplasia"; 3) the small testes (5 gm total) revealed hypomaturation with no evidence of spermatogenesis and a significant decrease in the number of Leydig cells; and 4) hypoplasia of the adrenal cortex, particularly the zona glomerulosa. Bone sections (Fig. 3) showed a normal trabecular pattern. The epiphyseal cartilage appeared thick and the alignment of the cartilage cells at the metaphyseal-epiphyseal junction was variable. The normal columnar arrangement was present in some areas and absent in others. The metaphysis was separated from the epiphyseal cartilage by a thin layer of bone and there was almost complete absence of blood vessel invasion of the epiphyseal cartilage.

Case 2

D.W.A. was initially evaluated at 4 years of age because of psychomotor delay and poor growth. His height (92 cm), weight (12 kg) and head circumference (44.5 cm) were all significantly below the 3rd percentile. He did not sit up until 12 months of age and he could not walk until 5 years of age. Physical examination at 4 years of age revealed a "saddle nose," malformed teeth, hypermobile joints (hypotonia ?), brachydactyly, 4th toe tibial clinodactyly and an IQ of 12. Laboratory studies including serum calcium, phosphorus, alkaline phosphatase, PBI, 17-KS, 17-hydroxycorticoids and an EEG were normal. Roentgenograms showed abnormalities in the epiphyses of the humeral and femoral heads, distal end of the radius, knees and ankles. The epiphyses were described as being irregularly formed with small "bone islands" similar to those seen in hypothyroidism. The femoral necks were broad and short. The spine was normal. Bone age was delayed by 18-24 months.

D.W.A. was reevaluated at 19 years of age (Fig. 4). His height (128 cm), weight (32 kg) and head circumference (51½ cm) were still far below the 3rd percentile. He had moderately severe scoliosis which had started 5 years previously. Except for some scant pubic hair there was no evidence of pubescence. The facies showed a flat nasal bridge and large lips with downturned corners of the mouth. The proximal upper limbs were disproportionally short. There was incomplete elbow extension, and the brachydactylous

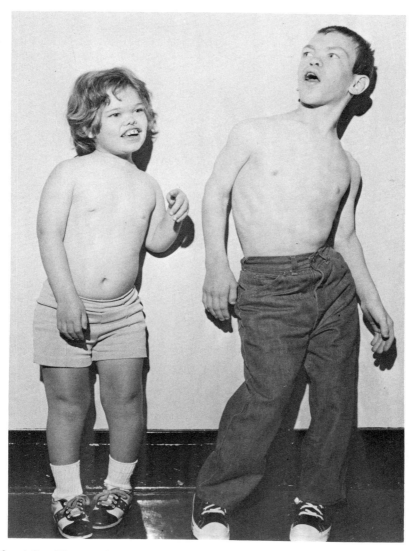

Fig. 4. *Case 3* on left at 17 years of age. Note characteristic facies, slight scoliosis, knock-knees and tibial bowing. *Case 2* at 19 years of age. Note similar facies, moderately severe scoliosis, disproportionately short proximal arms, broad nails and knock-knees.

fingers had short broad nails. There were severe knock-knees, pes planus and valgus foot positioning.

Only roentgenograms of the chest and spine were taken and these showed scoliosis (Fig. 5A) and vertebra (Fig. 5B) which were flat, poorly mineralized and bullet-shaped.

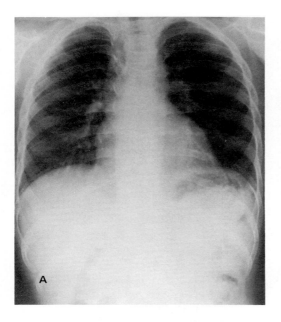

Case 3

L.A. was originally evaluated when she was 2½ years of age. She was not sitting, walking or talking by that time. She had held her head up at 3 months. Her height (8.5 cm), weight (8.6 kg) and head circumference (46 cm) were all below the 3rd percentile. She was described as having a "saddle nose," protruding upper lip, forehead prominence and joint hyperextensibility. The Cattell Infant Intelligence Scale was 21. Laboratory studies including a serum calcium, alkaline phosphatase, PBI and total protein were normal. A serum phosphorus was slightly elevated at 6.4 mg/100 ml. I^{131} uptake studies suggested decreased uptake which showed a good response to uptake after TSH stimulation. The question of hypothyroidism secondary to hypopituitarism arose, but no further studies were pursued. No clinical improvement was noted on thyroid medication during the next year. An EEG showed diffuse dysrythmia despite no clinical seizures until 8 years of age. These grand mal seizures were well controlled until 11 years of age at which time the phenobarbital medication was successfully discontinued.

L.A. was evaluated in 1973 at 17 years of age (Fig. 4) at the University of California, San Francisco. Her height (112 cm), weight (26 kg) and head circumference (48.5 cm) were all far below the 3rd percentile. The inner canthal distance (2.5 cm) was below the 3rd percentile while her interpupillary (5.5 cm) and outer orbital (10 cm) distances were at the 3rd percentile.

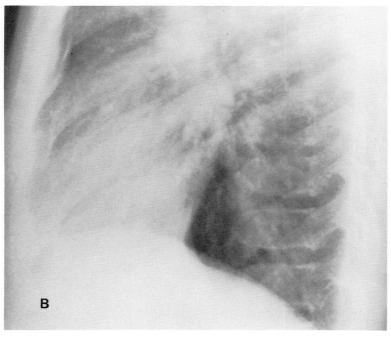

Fig. 5. A) *Case 2's* spine at 19 years of age showing moderately severe scoliosis. B) Note flat bullet-shaped vertebras with sclerotic borders, and poor vertebral mineralization.

She demonstrated an exceedingly flat nasal bridge (saddle nose), anteverted slit-like nares, flat upper philtrum with a prominent lower philtrum, large cupid-bow lips and prominent upper anterior teeth and gums. The arms showed mild proximal shortening while the hands revealed 2nd finger shortening and distal joint radial clinodactyly of the 5th fingers. Tibial bowing, knock-knees, small foot length (16 cm) and equinovarus foot positioning were present. The various joints were slightly hyperextensible and the spine was mildly scoliotic and lordotic. The presence of pubic hair was the only sign of sexual maturation.

Skin fibroblasts showed numerous cytoplasmic inclusions and vacuoles. Roentgenograms showed a normal cranium, sella turcica and facial bones. The vertebras (Fig. 6) showed sclerotic end plates with minimal anterior wedging at multiple levels. The humeral heads were flat and elongated and their normally contoured metaphyses showed vertical striations and small, rounded, oval lucencies (Fig. 7). Similar metaphyseal abnormalities were noted in most other limb areas. The distal femoral epiphyses were poorly formed at the lateral borders and the proximal fibular epiphyses were poorly ossified (Fig. 8). Phalangeal epiphyses (Fig. 9) had irregular sclerotic borders.

Case 4

D.A. had a similar clinical history as her affected sibs. She was hospitalized in 1974 at 12 years of age because of a 2-month history of possible akinetic

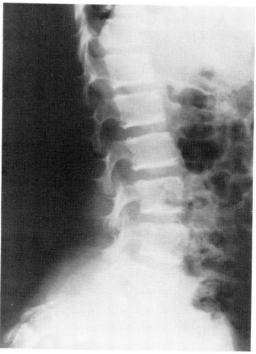

Fig. 6. *Case 3's* spine at 17 years of age showing mild flattening of vertebras with sclerotic borders and lumbar lordosis.

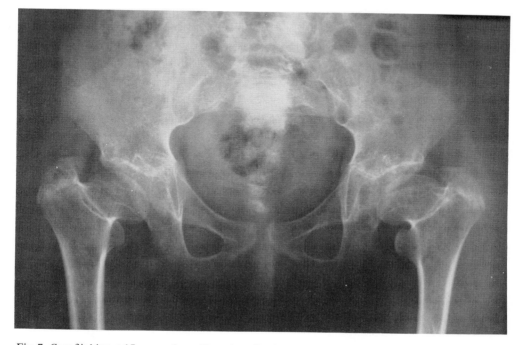

Fig. 7. *Case 3's* hips at 17 years of age. Note short flat femoral necks and vertical metaphyseal striations.

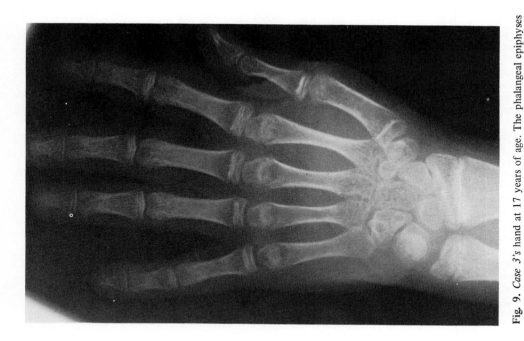

Fig. 9. *Case 3*'s hand at 17 years of age. The phalangeal epiphyses are irregular and have sclerotic borders. The phalangeal metaphyses are similarly involved. The carpal bones may be somewhat small.

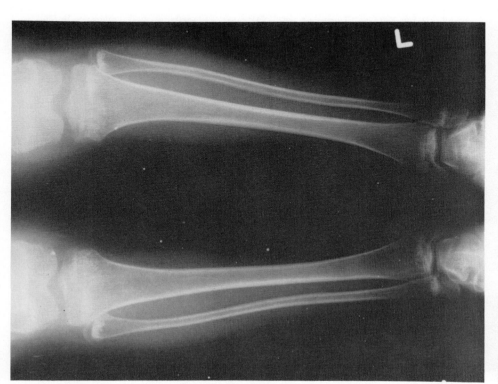

Fig. 8. Note slightly small distal femoral epiphyses with poorly formed lateral and medial borders, poorly mineralized proximal fibular epiphyses, and vertical metaphyseal striations.

seizures. However, a technically poor EEG done at that time was read as normal. Therapy with Dilantin and phenobarbital stopped the above episodes. Her head circumference (51 cm) at this time was at the 3rd percentile while her height (116 cm) and weight (24 kg) were below the 3rd percentile. Physical examination showed Brushfield spots, a flat nasal bridge, a small upturned nose and gingival hyperplasia secondary to gingivitis. In general, her features (Figs. 1 and 2) were less marked than those in the older sibs and there was not any obvious evidence of disproportional limb shortening. Urine studies for metabolic defects including mucopolysaccharides, amino acids and organic acids were negative. No roentgenograms were available for the authors' review.

Case 5

J.A., like his other sibs, was considered normal until about 6 months when his milestone development was noted to be significantly delayed. He did not sit alone or stand with support until 15 months of age and walking did not occur until 4 years. At 41 months of age his mental age was estimated to be 9 months. Growth parameters at 3½ years revealed a height (92.5 cm) at the 3rd percentile, a weight (13.8 kg) at the 10th percentile and a head circumference (46.5 cm) below the 3rd percentile. Laboratory studies at this time revealed borderline elevated serum calcium and alkaline phosphatase and normal thyroid studies, urine and serum amino acids, urine mucopolysaccharides, serum phosphorus and uric acid. A bone age was equal to his chronologic age. An EEG was normal at this time. However, a repeat study one year later showed gross seizure discharge activity.

Evaluation of *J.A.* at 5 years of age revealed a height (96 cm), weight (15 kg) and head circumference (47 cm) which were now below the 3rd percentile. His facial features were similar, but less marked than his older sibs (Figs. 1 and 2). His short stature was proportionate at this time. Laboratory tests including serum calcium and urine metabolic studies were normal. Roentgenograms taken at 3½ years of age showed a probable normal spine (Fig. 10), short femoral neck with a poorly formed femoral epiphysis (Fig. 11), small carpal bones with spotty mineralization and small distal radial epiphyses (Fig. 12). No other areas were x-rayed.

Case 6

E.A. was considered normal until 6 months of age when his milestone development was notably delayed and his weight (7.3 kg) began to drop off. Sitting occurred at 2 years and walking at 2½ years. Crying or screaming episodes at 14 months of age were interpreted by physicians as possible seizures which were treated with phenobarbital and Dilantin. Weight (7.4 kg) and height (73 cm) at 16 months of age were both significantly below the 3rd percentile, while a head circumference of 46.5 cm was on the 3rd percentile

and a similar measurement at 26 months (46 cm) was just below the 3rd percentile. Laboratory studies done between 16 and 26 months of age showed normal thyroid studies, immunoelectrophoresis, serum alkaline phosphatase, serum calcium, phosphorus and uric acid, urine mucopolysaccharides, lipid studies, urine and plasma amino acids, and homovanillic and vanillyl mandelic acid. A serum ammonia level done during a vomiting illness at 16 months of age was elevated at 408 μg%, but was near normal 3 days later.

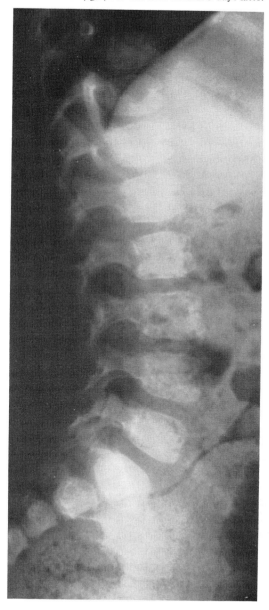

Fig. 10. *Case 5's* spine was considered normal at 3½ years of age.

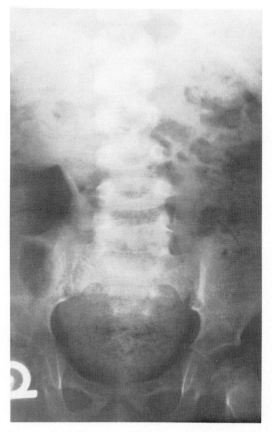

Fig. 11. *Case 5's* hips at 3½ years of age showing the left femoral epiphyses to be poorly formed.

A karyotype showed a normal 46,XY pattern. The Cattell Infant Intelligence Scale was 32 at 2 years of age.

E.A. was evaluated at 2½ years of age (Figs. 1 and 2) at the University of California, San Francisco. His height (81 cm) and weight (9.5 kg) were significantly below the 3rd percentile and his head circumference (47 cm) was just below the 3rd percentile. He had a right epicanthal fold, Brushfield spots, flat nasal bridge, flat philtrum, large lips and prominent gingiva (on Dilantin). There was pes planus and hyperactive reflexes. A skeletal survey was considered normal (Fig. 13).

Discussion

The *A Family* appears to represent a previously undescribed syndrome whose symptoms are postnatal in onset (Table 1). Significant psychomotor delay was obvious by 6 months of age. Poor linear growth and weight gain occurred by 6 to 18 months of age. Microcephaly which was documented as early as 16 months of age became more severe with time. Seizures occurred in at least 4 of the 6 affected children. All of the affected children showed persistently abnormal flat nasal bridges, small upturned nares, large lips and total absence of speech. Three of the teenage children showed no significant sexual development suggesting their overall disorder also affects gonadal function. Metaphyseal and epiphyseal abnormalities were present as early as 3½ years and tended to

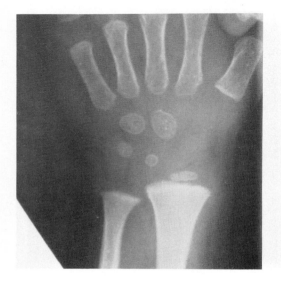

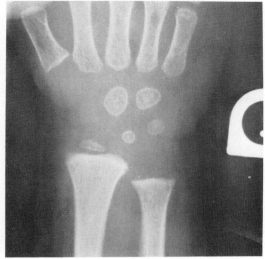

Fig. 12. *Case 5's* hands at 3½ years of age. Note spotty carpal mineralization and some small radial epiphyses.

Table 1. Historic, Clinical and Radiologic Features of the *A Family*

	D.L.A.* Age 13 yrs Case 1	D.W.A. Age 19 yrs Case 2	L.A. Age 17 yrs Case 3	D.A. Age 12 yrs Case 4	J.A. Age 5 yrs Case 5	E.A. Age 2½ yrs Case 6
Historic Features						
Vomiting (first 18 months)	+	+	+	0	0	0
Poor growth (noted by 4 to 10 months)	+	+	+	+	+	+
Psychomotor retardation (noted by 10 months)	+	+	+	+	+	+
Absence of speech	+	+	+	+	+	+
Major Clinical Features						
Microcephaly (noted by 30 months)	+	+	+	+	+	+
Epicanthal folds	+	0	+	+	+	+
Flat nasal bridge (persistent)	+	+	+	+	+	+
Anteverted nares	+	+	+	+	+	+
Large lips	+	+	+	+	+	+
Additional Adolescent Features						
Poor sexual maturation	+	+	+	?	?	?
Scoliosis	0	+	+	0	0	0
Disproportionate short arms	0	+	+	0	0	0
Brachydactyly	0	+	+	0	0	0
Major Radiologic Features						
Delayed bone age	+	+	+	NA	NA	+
Epiphyseal-metaphyseal defects (onset by 3½ years)	+	+	+	NA	+	0
Platyspondyly	0	+	+	NA	0	0
Irregular vertebral margins	+	+	+	NA	0	0
Poorly mineralized vertebra	0	+	+	NA	0	0
Bullet-shaped vertebra	0	+	0	NA	0	0

*Patient died at 13 years, but was first affected sib in *A Family*.
NA - Not applicable because no x-ray films taken.

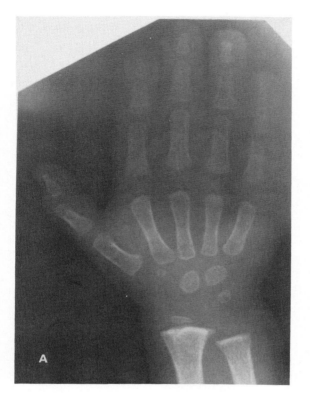

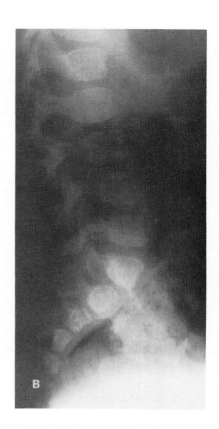

become worse with age. The 2 oldest children (*Cases 2 and 3*) developed scoliosis by 12 to 14 years of age. Disproportionally short arms were noted in *Case 2 and Case 3* at 19 and 17 years, respectively, but not in the younger affected children. This suggests a slowly progressive process relative to the osseous abnormalities.

The sequence of events and the clinical pattern found in this family strongly suggest a metabolic etiology. *Case 3* had numerous cytoplasmic inclusions and vacuoles in her skin fibroblasts which support this assumption. Present preliminary enzyme studies on 2 of the affected children have shown abnormalities of acid-hydrolase in cultured skin fibroblasts with decreased β-glucuronidase and increased N-acetyl-β-glucosaminidase. All serum acid hydrolases were normal. The specific pattern of biochemical abnormalities in this family has not been previously noted in any other metabolic disorder. Further clarification of the biochemical abnormalities is in progress and will be reported elsewhere. Thus, the *A Family* represents a new autosomal recessive metabolic disorder with a recognizable pattern of abnormalities.

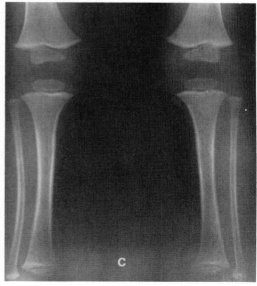

Fig. 13. *Case 6's* skeletal survey at 2½ years of age was considered normal. A) The hands, B) spine, and C) knees are presented for future comparisons.

Lethal Faciocardiomelic Dysplasia–
A New Autosomal Recessive Disorder*

**José-María Cantú, M.D., Alejandro Hernández, M.D., Jorge Ramírez, M.D.,
Manuel Bernal, M.D., Guillermo Rubio, M.D.,
Juan Urrusti, M.D. and Sergio Franco-Vázquez, M.D.**

Concordance for a distinct aggregate of congenital anomalies was observed in 3 male sibs. Parental consanguinity suggests an autosomal recessive pattern of inheritance.

Case Reports

The propositus, *V-46* (Fig. 1), was born on 1/8/74, after a full-term pregnancy complicated by polyhydramnios of 4 l; otherwise the delivery was normal. The birthweight was 2.420 kg and his length 45 cm. On examination (Figs. 2-6) he showed a peculiar facies because of severe microretrognathia, microstomia, epicanthal folds and enlarged auricular lobule, small helix and hypoplastic cymba conchae. Microglossia and glossoptosis were also present. The neck was short

and webbed. The cardiac exploration disclosed intense cardiac sounds in the right hemithorax. Severe hepatosplenomegaly was the only finding in the abdomen. The upper limbs were short mainly because of the mesomelic portion. Both hands were wide and short and deviated to the radial side, and the thumb was hypoplastic and proximally set. The hypoplastic 5th finger showed clinodactyly. The lower limbs were short mainly because of the mesomelic portion. Talipes varus, hypoplastic heels and a wide gap between the 1st and 2nd toes were also found. Cyanosis appeared the second day of life and cardiac failure led the baby to death on the fourth day of life.

Laboratory studies including blood cell count, urinalysis, X-chromatin and karyotype were normal or negative.

Skeletal roentgenograms revealed mandibular hypoplasia, radial and ulnar hypoplasia, brachymeta-

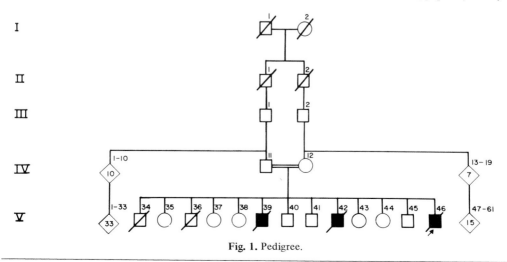

Fig. 1. Pedigree.

*Supported in part by a grant from The Ford Foundation.

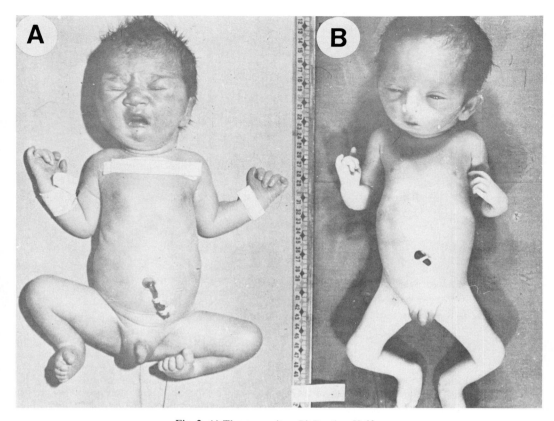

Fig. 2. A) The propositus. B) Brother *V-42*.

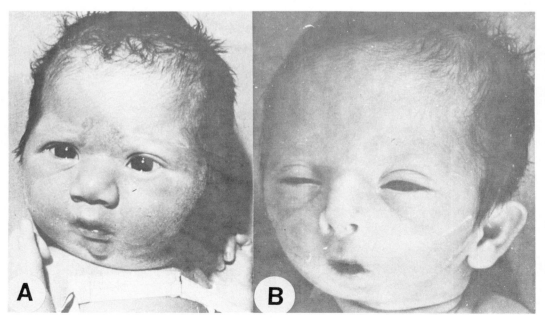

Fig. 3. Facial view. A) The propositus. B) Brother *V-42*.

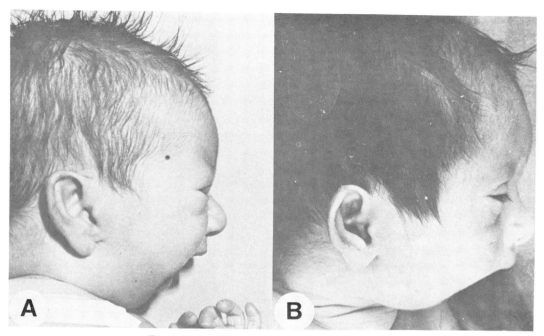

Fig. 4. Profile. A) The propositus. B) Brother *V-42*.

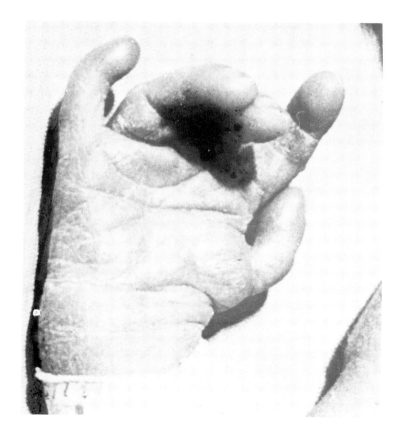

Fig. 5. Close-up of the propositus' right hand.

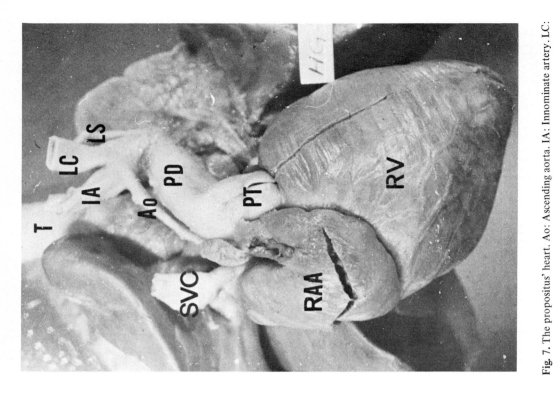

Fig. 7. The propositus' heart. Ao: Ascending aorta. IA: Innominate artery. LC: Left common carotid. LS: Left subclavian. PD: Pulmonary ductus. PT: Pulmonary trunk. RAA: Right atrial appendage. RV: Right ventricle. SVC: Superior vena cava. T: Trachea.

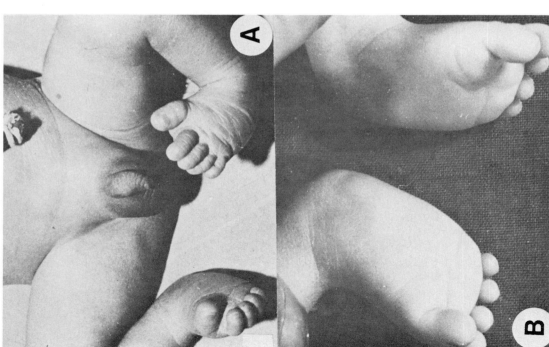

Fig. 6. Lower limbs. A) The propositus. B) Brother *V-42.*

carpalia and brachymetatarsalia, and fibular, tibial and calcaneous hypoplasia, with a bone age corresponding to a 7-month-old fetus.

Postmortem studies confirmed the clinical findings. The heart (Figs. 7 and 8) showed a right atrium markedly enlarged. The right ventricle was dilated, hypertrophic and the free wall measured 0.4 cm in thickness. The left atrium was small and the ventricle hypoplastic. The ascending aorta was very hypoplastic and the valve atretic (0.3 cm in diameter). The pulmonary artery measured 1 cm in diameter and originated from the right ventricle. The interauricular septum was widely open and the mitral valve atretic. There was also a persistence of the left superior vena cava. The remaining organs revealed no gross abnormalities other than chronic congestive processes.

Two male sibs, *V-42 and V-39* (Fig. 1), were retrospectively analyzed and found to have the same clinical manifestations as the propositus (Table 1). Postmortem studies were performed on *V-42* (Figs. 2-4 and 6). The heart showed truncus arteriosus communis, patent ductus arteriosus, patent foramen ovale, high interventricular communication, hypertrophy of the right ventricle and atrium, and hypotrophy of the left heart.

Family Data

The propositus' father and mother, *IV-11 and IV-12* (Fig. 1), were second cousins (inbreeding coefficient 1/64) and were 41 and 35 years old, respectively, at the time of the propositus' birth. Both were normal and have had 10 other children, 7 of whom were considered normal, 1 suffering from aortic coarctation and 2 probably normal but dead during the first year of life from acute GI infections. There was no history of a similar pattern of anomalies in 10 paternal and 7 maternal aunts and uncles, in 33 paternal and 15 maternal cousins, or in ancestors of previous generations.

Discussion

The remarkable similarity among the 3 cases indicates a disorder with a common etiology. As seen in Table 1, the syndrome consists mainly of dwarfism, facial dysplasia, severe cardiac defects and limb malformations. The dwarfism seems to be mesoacromelic because of dysplasia of those limb portions. The

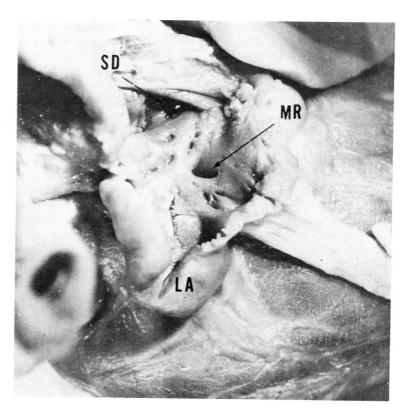

Fig. 8. The propositus' heart. LA: Left atrial appendage. MR: Mitral recess. SD: Septal defect.

Table 1. Clinical Data

Features	Propositus	V-42	V-39
Birthweight (kg)	2.420*	2.140*	2.260*
Length (cm)	45*	41.5*	43*
Head circumference (cm)	33.5	34	34
Polyhydramnios	+	+	+
Dwarfism	+	+	+
Delayed bone age	+	+	+
Epicanthal folds	+	+	+
Abnormal ears	+	+	+
Microretrognathia	+	+	+
Microstomia	+	+	+
Microglossia and glossoptosis	+	+	+
Webbed neck	+	+	+
Severe cardiac defects	+	+	+
Radial and ulnar hypoplasia	+	+	+
Radial deviation of the hands	+	+	+
Brachymetacarpalia (palm simian creases)	+	+	+
Thumb hypoplasia	+	+	+
Fifth finger hypoplasia with clinodactyly	+	+	+
Fibular and tibial hypoplasia	+	+	+
Talipes with hypoplastic heels	+	+	+
Wide gap between 1st and 2nd toes	+	+	+
Age at death (days)	4	4	20

*Below the 3rd percentile.

facial abnormalities could be related to a first arch developmental defect, except for the epicanthal folds. Although the cardiac defects observed in the 2 autopsied cases were different, a common embryopathogenic mechanism is possible, since both anomalies could be explained on the basis of a septation defect of the trunkus and conus.[1,2]

The pedigree analysis suggests an autosomal recessive inheritance because of the presence of the disease in 3 out of 13 children, the lack of phenotypic manifestation in ancestry and the antecedent of parental consanguinity. However, only males were affected, so X-linked recessive inheritance cannot be ruled out.

For differential diagnosis, the pertinent entities from different nosologic reviews were considered by main symptoms.[3-6] The closest resemblance was found in the Pierre Robin syndrome with congenital cardiac defect,[7,8] "false" trisomy 18,[9] Fanconi anemia,[10] the TAR syndrome[11] and the familial aortic atresia.[12,13] It is of interest to mention that the Holt-Oram syndrome,[14] which is produced by an autosomal dominant mutation, also shows malformations of the heart and hands, as if their embryogenetic development had a close relationship.

It can be concluded from the family reported here that a distinct congenital disorder with faciocardiomelic dysplasia and apparent lethality during the newborn period is probably produced by a mutation of a pleiotropic recessive gene located in an autosome.

Summary

Three male sibs from consanguineous parents were found to have a strikingly similar pattern of multiple congenital anomalies. The main features were polyhydramnios; low birthweight; dwarfism; epicanthal folds; abnormal ears; microretrognathia; microstomia; microglossia; glossoptosis; webbed neck; severe cardiac defects; radial and ulnar hypoplasia; radial deviation of the hands; brachymetacarpalia; thumb hypoplasia; clinodactyly and hypoplasia of the 5th finger; simian creases; fibular and tibial hypoplasia; talipes varus with hypoplastic heels; wide gap between 1st and 2nd toes; and delayed bone age. Neonatal death occurred in the 3 babies by severe cardiac failure.

Differential diagnosis permits one to conclude that this is a new type of faciocardiomelic dysplasia with a probable autosomal recessive inheritance.

Acknowledgment

The secretarial assistance of Miss Luz Elena Hernández de Alba is gratefully acknowledged.

References

1. de la Cruz, M. V. and Pio da Rocha, J.: An ontogenic theory for the explanation of congenital malformations involving the truncus and conus. *Am. Heart J. 51*:782, 1956.
2. Maron, B. J. and Hutchins, G. M.: Truncus arteriosus malformation in a human embryo. *Am. J. Anat. 134*:167, 1972.
3. McKusick, V. A.: *Mendelian Inheritance in Man.* Baltimore:The Johns Hopkins Press, 1971.
4. Warkany, J.: *Congenital Malformations. Notes and Comments.* Chicago:Year Book Medical Publishers, 1971.
5. Char, F.: Tables of heritable cardiovascular conditions and associated syndromes. In Bergsma, D. (ed.): Part XV. *The Cardiovascular System*, Birth Defects: Orig. Art. Ser., vol. VIII, no. 5. Baltimore:The Williams and Wilkins Co. for The National Foundation-March of Dimes, 1972, pp. 313-319.
6. Bergsma, D. (ed.): *Birth Defects: Atlas and Compendium.* Baltimore:The Williams and Wilkins Co. for The National Foundation-March of Dimes, 1973.
7. Gorlin, R. J., Červenka, J., Anderson, R. C. et al: Robin's syndrome. A probably X-linked recessive subvariety exhibiting persistence of left superior vena cava and atrial septal defect. *Am. J. Dis. Child. 119*:176, 1970.
8. Bianchine, J. W., Kelemen, M. H., Babitt, H. I. and Lippmann, S.: The Pierre Robin syndrome with congenital cardiac defect. In Bergsma, D. (ed.): Part XV. *The Cardiovascular System*, Birth Defects: Orig. Art. Ser., vol. VIII, no. 5. Baltimore:The Williams and Wilkins Co. for The National Foundation-March of Dimes, 1972, pp. 242-243.
9. de Grouchy, J.: Chromosome 18: A topological approach. *J. Pediatr. 66*:414, 1965.
10. Fanconi, G.: Familial constitutional panmyelocytopathy, Fanconi's anemia (F.A.). I. Clinical Aspects. *Semin. Hematol. 4*:233, 1966.
11. Shaw, S. and Oliver, R. A. M.: Congenital hypoplastic thrombocytopenia with skeletal deformities in siblings. *Blood 14*:374, 1959.
12. Brekke, V. G.: Congenital aortic atresia and hypoplasia of the aortic orifice. *Am. Heart J. 45*:925, 1953.
13. Rao, S. S., Gootman, N. and Platt, N.: Familial aortic atresia in siblings. *Am. J. Dis. Child. 118*:919, 1969.
14. Holt, M. and Oram, S.: Familial heart disease with skeletal malformations. *Br. Heart J. 22*:236, 1960.

Discussion

Dr. Kaufman: I have presented previously at 2 of these conferences, including the last one, families with hypoplastic left heart syndrome. This type of lesion is what we call the obstructive left heart lesions in sibs. In fact, Dr. Shokeir has gone so far as to suggest that it is an autosomal recessive disorder. There were thoracic and duplication renal anomalies which might have been overlooked as normal on many radiographs. I wondered if there were any such findings in family members.

Dr. Cantú: No, we did not find any vertebral anomalies or renal malformations. We have not yet performed renal studies on the family members.

Dr. Antley: We have just reviewed the cases of whistling face syndrome and there are some curious similarities here between them, in that all of the cases which we accepted as whistling face also had microstomia. The hand and feet anomalies in the family that you have presented were very similar to those of the whistling face syndrome. As far as I know, the associated heart anomaly has not been reported. But in a case of aniridia that we had recently seen, we found what we think is whistling face, so there may occasionally be other anomalies associated. Just a thought concerning the similarities between whistling face and the family that you have presented.

Dr. Cantú: In any case, this would be a recessive form. The general component and magnitude of the malformations, I think, could easily differentiate the syndrome.

Dr. Bryan Hall: Did you notice if at the time of birth the children could make facial expressions? There is some similarity between these children and those with the Möbius syndrome.

Dr. Cantú: The facial expressions were normal in the propositus. We have no information in the records on his brothers of abnormalities in that area.

Moderator: The number of inborn errors of morphogenesis is rapidly growing. They have been around for a long time but we are just now starting to recognize them. It is very interesting to see the group from Mexico joining us in this endeavor.

Acrocephalopolysyndactyly, Type Noack, in a Large Kindred

Meinhard Robinow, M.D. and Thomas J. Sorauf, M.D.

We recently studied a family in which several members were affected by a syndrome which we shall refer to as the Noack type of acrocephalopolysyndactyly[1,2] but with equal justification could be classed as acrocephalosyndactyly (ACS) type V (Pfeiffer).[3] We have been impressed by the marked intrafamilial variability of this syndrome.

The propositus was an 8-month-old girl who presented with acroplagiocephaly (Figs. 1 and 2). The shallow orbits, bulging eyes and beaked nose looked somewhat suggestive of Crouzon disease and probably indicated that the sphenoid was also involved in the synostosis. The thumbs showed a minor valgus of the distal phalanx and there was mild webbing of the second interdigital space (Fig. 3). The feet (Fig. 4) showed prominent valgus of the great toes and very broad toenails. Radiographs (Fig. 5) revealed partial duplication of the proximal and distal phalanges. Bilateral metatarsus varus had recently been treated with casting but was not yet fully corrected.

The coronal craniosynostosis was surgically corrected. At 14 months the child's appearance was appreciably improved (Fig. 6) and her development was age-appropriate.

The mother and maternal grandmother were well aware of the fact that the child had inherited a family trait consisting of "flat foreheads" and broad toes, some of which had double toenails. They provided the data for the preliminary pedigree (Fig. 7A). None of the affected individuals had required surgery for acrocephaly and all of them had been mentally normal. Of the 26 direct descendants of the affected woman in the first generation, only 8 were reported to be affected. It is apparent from this pedigree that 2 individuals, considered normal by their family, had carried the gene and passed on the trait. Our rather limited family study picked up one additional affected individual. The corrected pedigree (Fig. 7B) raises the proportion of affected to unaffected to 11:26, a more appropriate ratio for a dominant trait.

The mother of the propositus, who considered herself unaffected, had no discernible acro-

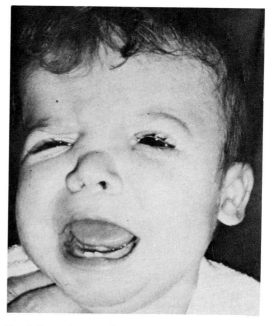

Fig. 1. Propositus, age 9 months. Note the facial asymmetry.

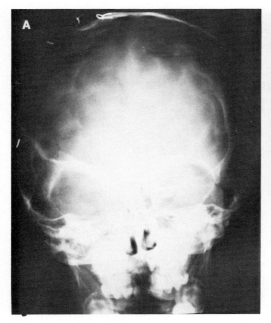
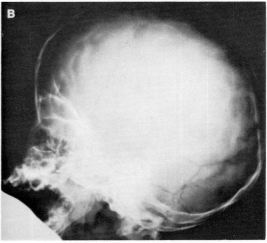

Fig. 2. Propositus, age 9 months. A) PA skull radiograph. Note asymmetry of orbits and of coronal sutures. B) Lateral skull radiograph. Acrocephaly.

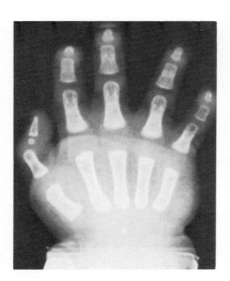

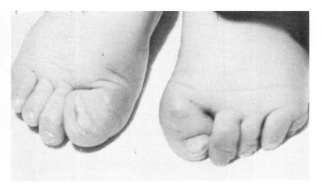

Fig. 4. Propositus. Marked valgus of unduly broad great toes.

Fig. 3. Propositus, age 9 months. Hand radiograph. Note webbing of second interdigital space. The large epiphysis of the distal phalanx of the thumb suggests the presence of a triphalangeal thumb.

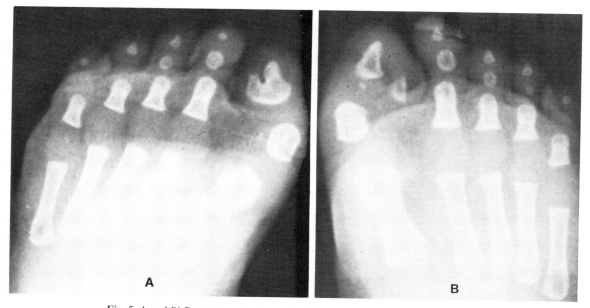

Fig. 5. A and B) Propositus. Radiographs of feet. Partial duplication of great toes.

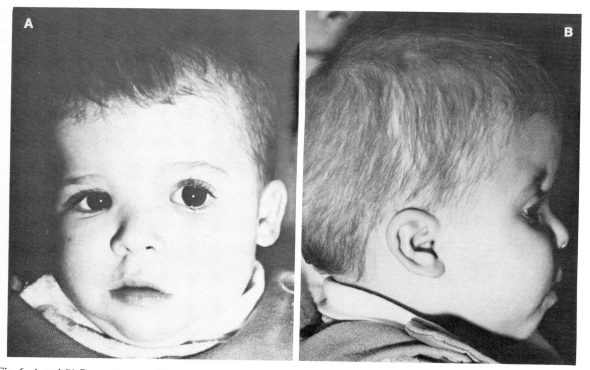

Fig. 6. A and B) Propositus, age 14 months, after surgery for craniostenosis. Appearance improved. Slight facial asymmetry remains.

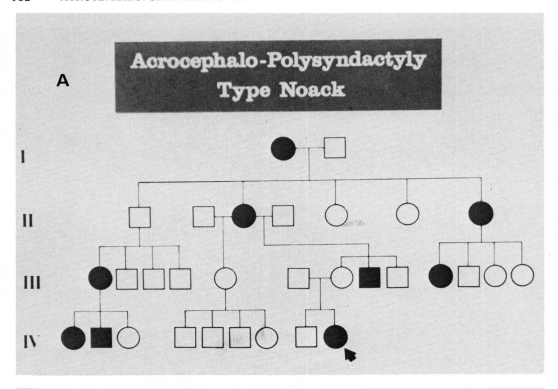

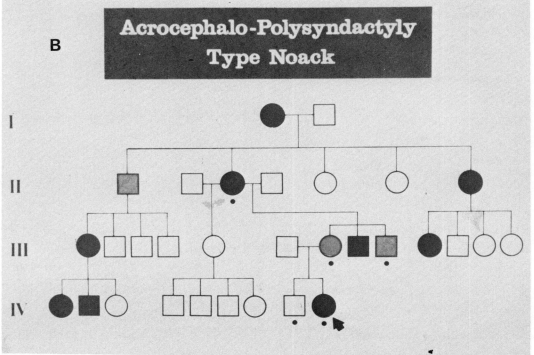

Fig. 7. A) Initial pedigree, as obtained from family. B) Corrected pedigree (see text). Dots indicate individuals actually examined.

cephaly (Fig. 8). Her face seemed unremarkable (Fig. 9). Her great toes (Fig. 10) showed a minor valgus of the distal phalanx but no suggestion of polydactyly. Her hand radiograph (Fig. 11) was normal except for webbing in the second and third interdigital spaces.

The older of her 2 brothers, now in the U. S. Army, had the complete syndrome with double toenails. Her younger brother was said to be unaffected, but his facial appearance (Fig. 12) strongly suggested involvement and his skull radiograph (Fig. 13) demonstrated conspicuous acrocephaly. He did not have polydactyly of the toes, but like his sister, he had interdigital webbing of the hands (Fig. 14).

The maternal grandmother had the full syndrome. Her forehead looked concave in profile (Fig. 15). She had obvious acrocephaly (Fig. 16), an essentially normal hand skeleton (Fig. 17) but webbing in the second interdigital space and preaxial polydactyly of the toes (Fig. 18).

Of the 4 affected individuals we were able to examine, none had polydactyly of the hands, 2 had polydactyly of the toes, 3 had acrocephaly and all 4 had excessive interdigital webbing of the hands, presumably the mildest form of syndactyly.

Summary

ACS was highly variable in this family. At least one affected member could have passed as uninvolved. Others could have been assigned to ACS types III, IV or V. The current classification[3] is probably sound, but great caution is needed to assign individual cases of ACS to any group other than ACS types I or II or the Carpenter syndrome.

The great variability of ACS has obvious implications for genetic counseling.

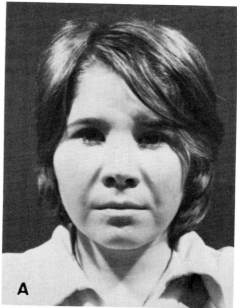

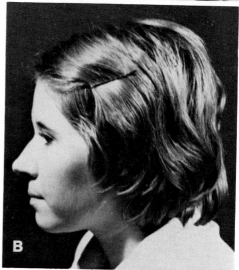

Fig. 9. A and B) Mother of propositus. Normal facial features.

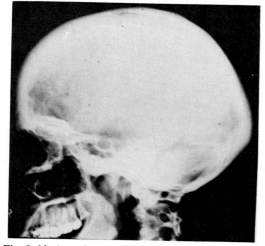

Fig. 8. Mother of propositus. Lateral skull radiograph. No sign of acrocephaly.

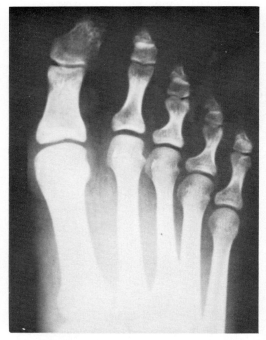

Fig. 10. Mother of propositus. Foot radiograph. Valgus of distal phalanx of great toe.

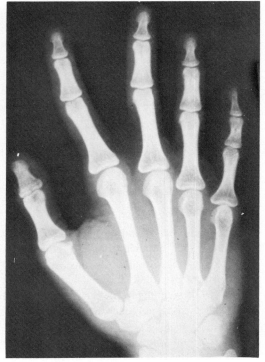

Fig. 11. Mother of propositus. Hand radiograph. Note webbing in second and third interdigital spaces.

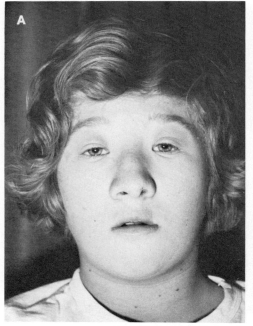

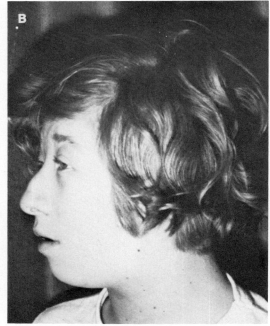

Fig. 12. A and B) Maternal uncle. Characteristic facial appearance.

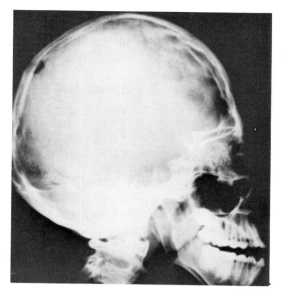

Fig. 13. Maternal uncle. Lateral skull radiograph showing acrocephaly.

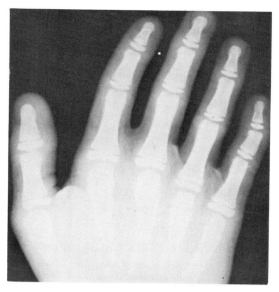

Fig. 14. Maternal uncle. Hand radiograph. Note webbing of second interdigital space.

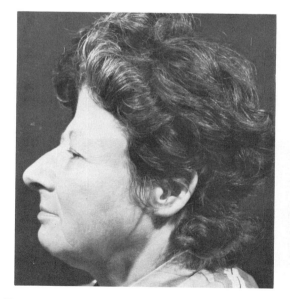

Fig. 15. Maternal grandmother. Note concave contour of forehead.

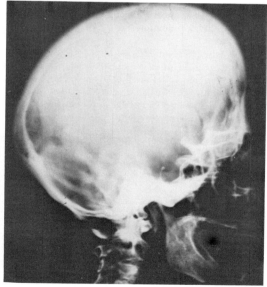

Fig. 16. Maternal grandmother. Lateral skull radiograph. Marked acrocephaly.

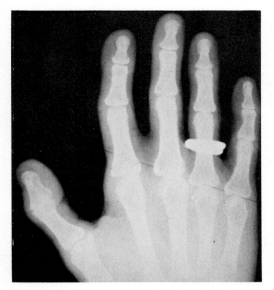

Fig. 17. Maternal grandmother. Hand radiograph. Webbing of second interdigital space.

References

1. Noack, M.: Ein Beitrag zum Krankheitsbild der Akrocephalosyndaktylie. *Arch. Kinderheilk.* *160*:168-171, 1959.
2. Temtamy, S.: Acrocephalopolysyndactyly. In Bergsma, D. (ed.): *Birth Defects: Atlas and Compendium.* Baltimore:Williams & Wilkins Co. for The National Foundation-March of Dimes, 1973, p. 141.
3. Temtamy, S. and McKusick, V. A.: Synopsis of hand malformations with particular emphasis on genetic factors. In Bergsma, D. (ed.): Part III. *Limb Malformations,* Birth Defects: Orig. Art. Ser., vol. V, no. 3. White Plains:The National Foundation-March of Dimes, 1969, pp. 125-184.

Discussion

Dr. Lester Weiss: I think that Dr. Robinow's observation is extremely important. We have had an opportunity to study a large Amish kindred with acrocephaly and, without very careful physical and roentgenographic examinations of the hands and feet, a number of these individuals could have passed for normal, as though they were not carrying this dominantly inherited gene. The abnormalities ranged from minimal, only detected roentgenographically, to syndactyly and polydactyly. I think that the observation Dr. Robinow is making is an important one.

Dr. Jürgen Spranger: Dr. Robinow, I wonder if you could help me differentiate this from the Pfeiffer type of acrocephalosyndactyly. I have great trouble defining the Noack type. I do not think we should credit Mrs. Noack with this inclusion type. If you recall her paper, there were just 2 clinical pictures and not a single radiograph; I could not convince myself that this was any different from what Pfeiffer described with the same type of variabilities. Perhaps you could help me out?

Dr. Robinow: I am in the same situation, namely being unable to distinguish type Noack and type Pfeiffer. But I also suspect that Pfeiffer's cases were heterogeneous, too.

Moderator: Dr. Temtamy, would you comment on this question, specifically the Noack versus the Pfeiffer types.

Dr. Temtamy: I have changed my mind and now consider the Noack and Pfeiffer types as one entity.

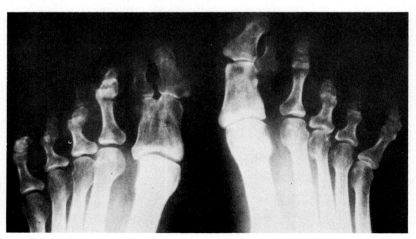

Fig. 18. Maternal grandmother. Radiograph of feet. Duplication of both great toes.

A New Familial Syndrome with Craniofacial Abnormalities, Osseous Defects and Mental Retardation

Art Grix, M.D., Willard Blankenship, M.D., Robert Peterson, M.D.
and Bryan Hall, M.D.

Two Mexican-American brothers with craniofacial abnormalities, large thumbs and halluces, retroverted coccyx, neonatally hypermineralized bones, hypertonicity, psychomotor retardation and poor growth are presented. Their distinct pattern of malformation is easily recognizable and represents a new familial syndrome.

Case Reports

Case 1 was born to a nonconsanguineous 22-year old gravida 3, para 2 mother and a 23-year-old father. The term pregnancy was complicated by first trimester bleeding. Very active fetal motion began between the fourth and fifth months. Labor and delivery were uncomplicated except for a nuchal cord and minimal amniotic fluid. The birthweight was 1985 gm, the length 47 cm and the head circumference 31 cm.

Physical examination at 5 days of age showed (Fig. 1) a large anterior fontanel with widely spaced sutures. Bushy eyebrows and puffy eyelids were noted. The nose was high-set with a bulbous tip and the philtrum was long and simple. A bilateral cleft palate not involving the alveolar ridges was present as were micrognathia, a bifid tongue tip and a short ventral lingual frenulum. The 2nd, 3rd and 5th left ribs were indented anteriorly and hypoplastic radiologically (Fig. 2). Bilateral cryptorchidism and inguinal hernias were noted. He had large thumbs and halluces (Fig. 3 and Fig. 4) without broad nails and the ventral fat

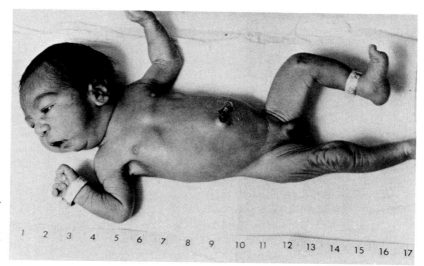

Fig. 1. Full body view of *Case 1* at 5 days of age. Note bushy eyebrows and hypertrichosis of forehead.

107

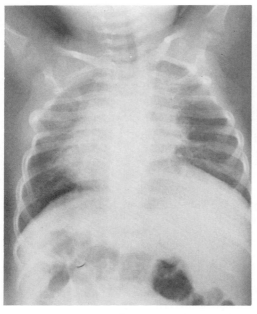

Fig. 2. At 35 months of age. Note rib anomalies as described in text. Note lack of increased bone mineralization that was present earlier in the neonatal period.

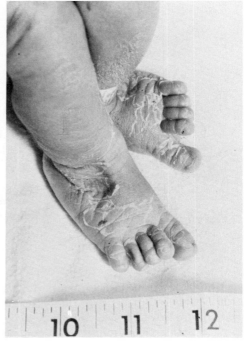

Fig. 4. Large halluces.

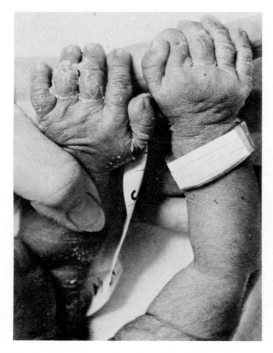

Fig. 3. Note large thumbs, digital fat pads, arm hypertrichosis and desquamating skin.

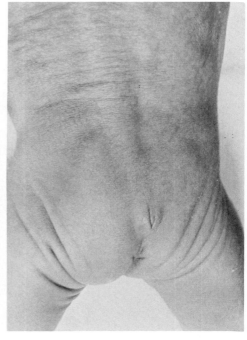

Fig. 5. Pilonidal dimple, decreased gluteal muscle mass and back hypertrichosis.

pads were prominent on the finger tips. The 2nd and 5th fingers overlapped the 3rd and 4th. The skin was dry and peeling with increased body hair and transverse truncal creases. A prominent pilonidal dimple (Fig. 5) was present over the coccyx. He displayed poor feeding, a decreased suck and grasp, and increased irritability and tone.

Laboratory studies included an excretory urogram which showed a nonvisualized right kidney and a large left kidney. A CBC, urinalysis and chemistry panels were normal. Roentgenograms demonstrated coccyx which curved dorsally (retroverted) (Fig. 6) and increased mineralization of the bones (Fig. 7).

At 3½ months of age he had a bilateral hernia repair, repair of his cleft palate, and was treated for a tear duct infection. At 12 months of age he developed a grand mal seizure disorder which was controlled with phenobarbital and Dilantin. He was hospitalized at 23, 34 and 35 months of age for treatment of pneumonia. His height (94 cm) at 35 months of age was at the 10th percentile while his weight (8.5 kg) and head circumference (43½ cm) were below the 3rd percentile. His developmental age at this time was around 4 months. The facies (Fig. 8) demonstrated the same features seen in the newborn period. The rib defect of

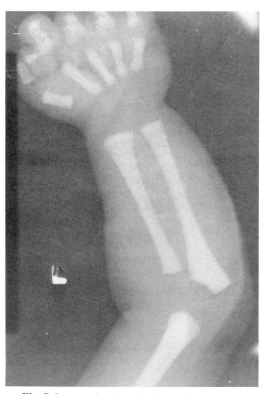

Fig. 7. Increased mineralization at 5 days of age.

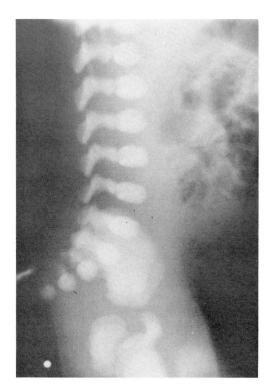

Fig. 6. Increased mineralization and retroverted coccyx.

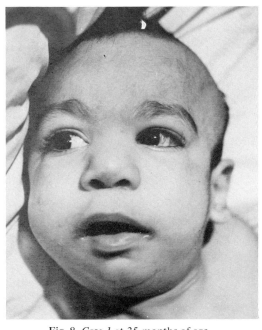

Fig. 8. *Case 1* at 35 months of age.

the left chest was more obvious. He displayed increased gingival hyperplasia, a markedly bifid tongue tip (Fig. 9), was no longer cryptorchid and had significant muscle wasting. The thumbs and halluces were still broad (Fig. 10) and there were excessive creases on the soles (Fig. 11).

Laboratory studies including urine metabolic screens and complete Ig were normal except for a nutritional anemia. Roentgenograms at this time showed normal mineralization (Fig. 2).

The family history was negative except for a short lingual frenulum in one of the 2 normal half-brothers and cleft palate in the paternal grandmother.

Case 2 was born 2 9/12 years after his brother. The pregnancy was term with increased fetal activity which began between the fourth and fifth months. At delivery he required oxygen and mask bagging before normal respirations were established.

When evaluated at 6 weeks of age he was 47 cm in length, weighed 3500 gm and had a head circumference of 34 cm. He had the same facial (Fig. 12) and somatic (Figs. 13-16) characteristics as his brother, but no cleft palate or rib defects. In addition he had a nonpatent nasolacrimal duct and grade 3/6 systolic heart murmur consistent with a ventricular septal defect. His neurologic exam revealed increased irritability and tone but no localizing signs. Although no formal testing was performed, he appeared to have psychomotor delay by 6 months of age.

Laboratory findings at 6 weeks included a normal EEG, serum electrolytes and chemistry panels, as well as normal Ig and thyroid function. His Hb was

9.4 gm %. Metabolic screens for amino acids, mucopolysaccharides, mucolipids and gangliosides were negative as were titers for herpes, cytomegalovirus and toxoplasmosis. Chromosome studies showed a normal 46,XY. Roentgenograms showed a normal bone age with increased generalized skeletal mineralization (Fig. 17) and dorsally curved coccyx (Fig. 18). There were no vertebral or rib defects.

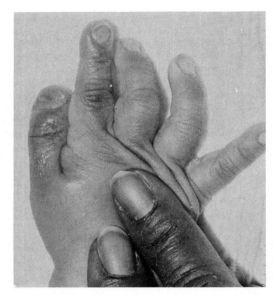

Fig. 10. Note large wide thumb.

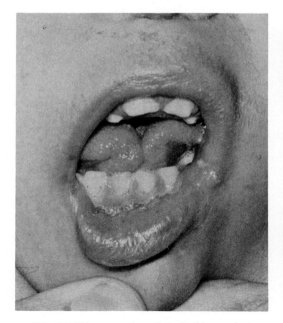

Fig. 9. Bifid tongue tip and gingival hyperplasia.

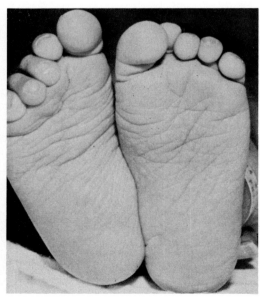

Fig. 11. Large halluces and numerous sole creases.

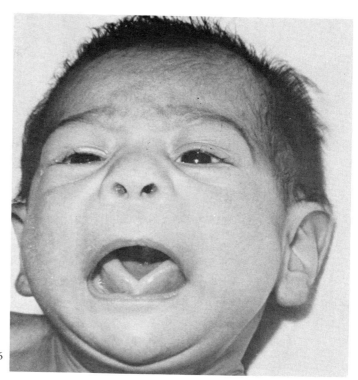

Fig. 12. Facial view of *Case 2* at 6 weeks of age.

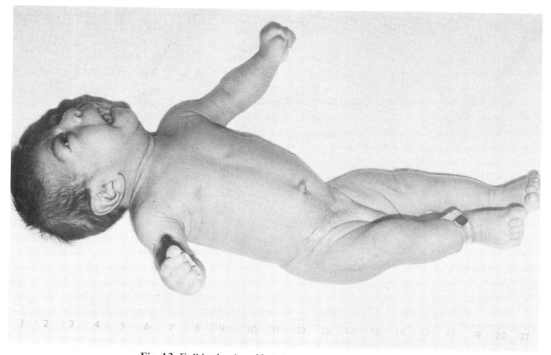

Fig. 13. Full body view. Note transverse truncal creases.

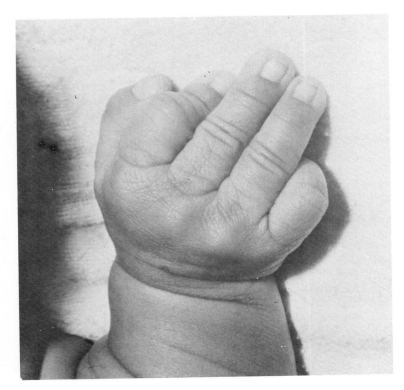

Fig. 14. Note large thumb.

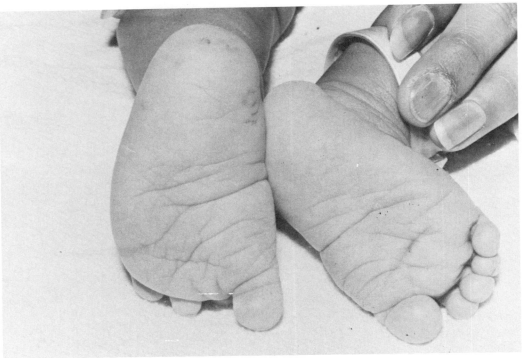

Fig. 15. Large halluces and abnormal sole creases.

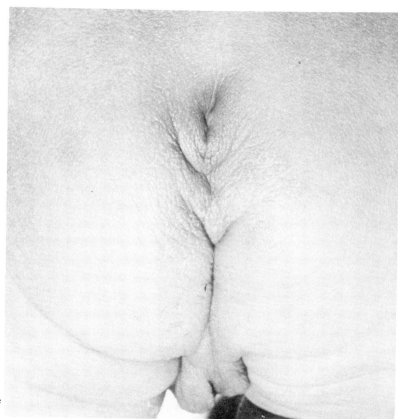

Fig. 16. Pilonidal dimple over coccyx.

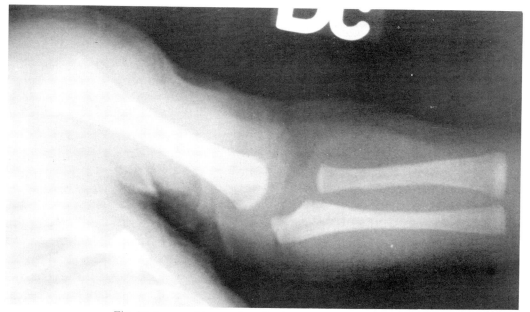

Fig. 17. Increased bone mineralization at 3 months of age.

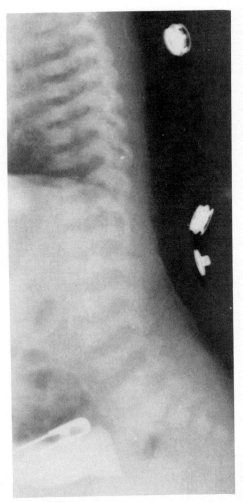

Fig. 18. Retroverted coccyx at 6 weeks of age.

Table 1.

Features	Case 1	Case 2
General		
Increased fetal activity	+	+
Postnatal growth deficiency	+	+
Neurologic		
Psychomotor retardation	+	+
Microcephaly	+	+
Seizures	+	
Hypertonicity	+	+
Facial		
Puffy eyelids	+	+
Nonpatent nasolacrimal duct	?	+
High-set nose	+	+
Bulbous nasal tip	+	+
Long simple philtrum	+	+
Cleft palate	+	
Bifid tip of tongue	+	+
Short ventral frenulum	+	+
Prominent alveolar ridges	+	+
Micrognathia	+	+
Osseous		
Broad thumbs, halluces	+	+
Rib anomalies	+	
Retroverted coccyx	+	+
Increased neonatal bone mineralization	+	+
Skin		
Hypertrichosis	+	+
Pilonidal dimple	+	+
Transverse truncal creases	+	+
Miscellaneous		
Kidney anomalies	+	
Ventral septal defect		+
Inguinal hernias	+	+

Discussion

The major features found in these brothers are listed in Table 1. The pattern of neurologic, osseous and craniofacial characteristics seen in these brothers is unreported to the best of our knowledge and constitutes a new syndrome. Although many of their features can be found in children with storage disorders, neither child demonstrated any associated metabolic abnormalities. Well-established syndromes associated with either broad thumbs,[1] oral bands[2] or increased bone mineralization[3] do not fit our patients' clinical spectrum. The inheritance pattern in our patients appears to be either autosomal recessive or X-linked recessive.

References

1. Rubenstein, J.: The broad thumbs syndrome — progress report 1968. In Bergsma, D. (ed.): Part II. *Malformation Syndromes*, Birth Defects: Orig. Art. Ser., vol. V, no. 2. White Plains:The National Foundation—March of Dimes, 1969, pp. 25-41.
2. Rimoin, D. L. and Edgerton, M. T.: Genetic and clinical heterogeneity in the oral-facial-digital syndromes. *J. Pediatr. 71*:94, 1967.
3. Kozlowski, K. and Yu, J. S.: Pycnodysostosis, a variant form with visceral manifestations. *Arch. Dis. Child. 47*:804, 1972.

Otodental Dysplasia

Ronald J. Jorgenson, D.D.S., Steven J. Marsh, D.D.S.
and Frank H. Farrington, D.D.S., M.S.

Otodental dysplasia is a syndrome of sensorineural deafness and dental anomalies first described by Levin and Jorgenson in 1972.[1] The hearing deficit in the syndrome had a variable age of onset and was progressive. The dental anomalies consisted of altered morphology of the posterior teeth and hypodontia. The crowns of the primary and secondary molars were large and bulbous. The usual developmental grooves on their occlusal surfaces were absent. The roots were short and tapered and some were taurodont in configuration. Premolars were usually absent and when present were decreased in size. The crowns of the primary canines were large and bulbous, but the crowns of the secondary canines were of normal size and shape. The size and shape of the primary and secondary incisors were adjudged to be within normal limits.

The syndrome was documented in 6 consecutive generations of a kindred of northern Italian origin. There were several instances of male-to-male transmission of the syndrome.

A condition similar to otodental dysplasia has been seen recently in 4 generations of family apparently unrelated to the one reported earlier. This second family resides in central South Carolina and is of northern German extraction.

Case Reports

Case 1

D.D., Jr., the proband (Fig. 1), was a white male born on 1/30/70. He was the product of a full-term, uncomplicated pregnancy and weighed 3.1 kg. His mother had had no illnesses during the pregnancy and had used no medications. No abnormalities were noted at birth. He had been hospitalized once only at the age

P 10068

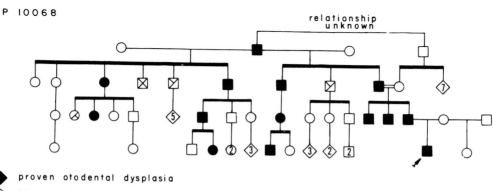

◆ proven otodental dysplasia

⬦ history of deafness

⬦ history of large, bulbous teeth

Fig. 1. Pedigree of family with otodental dysplasia.

of 14 months due to dehydration following the flu. He had had none of the childhood illnesses. At the age of 2 years and again at the age of 3 years, he had suffered from an idiopathic synovitis of the left hip. He had received no medications for significant periods of time for these or other illnesses.

His first tooth to erupt was an upper anterior at the age of 5 months. Three of the primary teeth failed to erupt. He had had no caries, had not complained of toothaches or abscesses and had never developed ulcers of the oral mucosa.

He was examined in April 1974. His facies were symmetric and normognathic (Fig. 2). Skin color was within normal limits, but there were several small, deeply pigmented lesions over the face and scalp. His hair was blonde, straight and normally dense. His helices protruded from his head. No appreciable hearing loss was noted. Fundi were clear and pupils reacted normally to light and accommodation. No soft or hard tissue lesions were noted in the oral cavity. Seventeen primary teeth were present. The lower right molars and the upper right canine were not erupted, but were seen on radiographs (Fig. 3). The crowns of the canines were large and bulbous (Fig. 4). The crowns of the molars were much larger than average, had more than the usual number of well-developed cusps and

lacked developmental grooves and fossae on the cusps (Fig. 5). The remainder of the examination was unremarkable.

No laboratory investigations were carried out. Audiology revealed essentially normal hearing for pure tone and speech discrimination.

Case 2

D.D., Sr. was a white male born on 8/11/30. He was the father of the proband in this pedigree (Fig. 1). Gestational and developmental history could not be recalled with certitude. He had never been hospitalized and recalled having had no serious illnesses. He first noted a decrease in hearing acuity early in the second decade of life. The deficit increased over several years and resulted in the acquisition of a hearing aid by 25 years of age.

The primary teeth were said to have been large and shaped like those of his son. They exfoliated later than average. The secondary teeth were also large and bulbous. Most of the posterior secondary teeth were extracted because of carious lesions which resulted in recurrent toothaches.

He was examined in April 1974. His facies were symmetric and normognathic. There were numerous pigmented nevi over the face and neck. His hair was

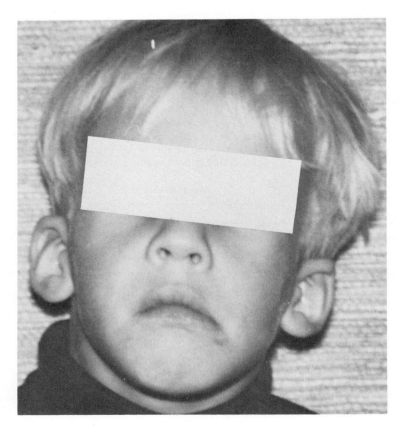

Fig. 2. Facies of *D.D., Jr.*, the proband. Note the large protuberant helices.

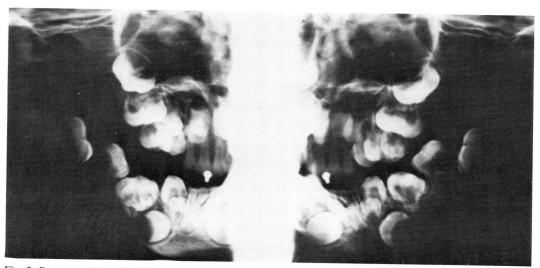

Fig. 3. Panorex radiograph of the proband showing impacted primary teeth, large bulbous crowns of the primary and secondary teeth and "double" pulp chambers in the primary molars.

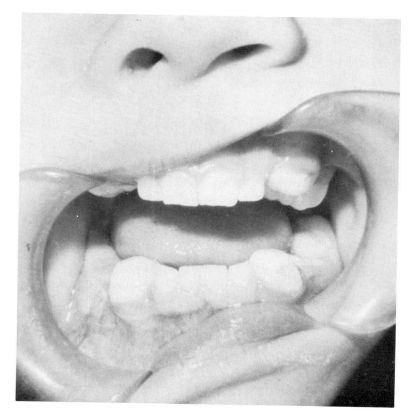

Fig. 4. Anterior view of proband's dentition to show the large crowns of the primary canines.

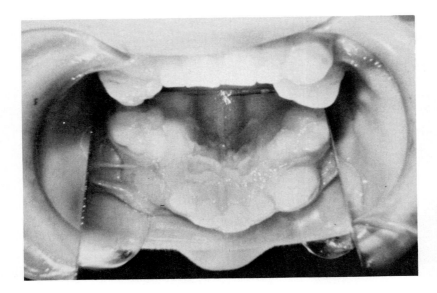

Fig. 5. Occlusal view of the proband's dentitions to show lack of normal occlusal morphology of the primary molars and extra cusps.

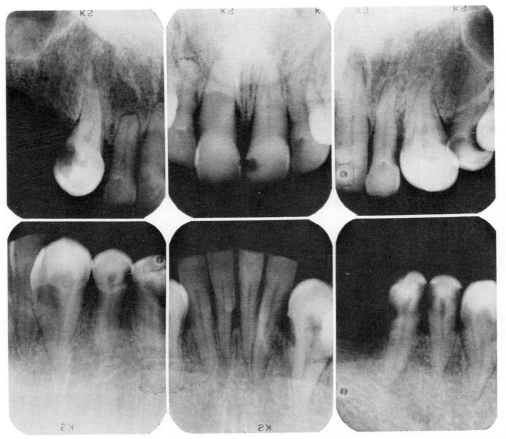

Fig. 6. Intraoral radiographs of the proband's father to show large crowns of the secondary canines and thistle-tube configuration of the pulp chambers of the posterior teeth.

normally pigmented and distributed. His ears were protuberant. No abnormalities were noted in the eyes. No soft or hard intraoral lesions were noted. The gingivae were inflamed and enlarged. There were 18 secondary teeth present. These consisted of the anteriors and several of the premolars. The incisors were well-formed. The canines were larger than average and had bulbous crowns. The premolars were not diminished in size, but their occlusal surfaces were convex with no developmental grooves or fossae. The root structure appeared normal on radiographs (Fig. 6). The pulp chambers had a thistle-tube outline on the radiographs.

There were numerous pigmented lesions over his back and chest. The remainder of the examination was unremarkable.

No laboratory investigations were carried out. Pure tone audiometry indicated a moderate, flat, bilateral sensorineural hearing loss. Speech discrimination revealed moderate loss in the left ear and mild loss in the right ear.

Comments

Deafness and abnormalities of the dentition are frequently reported manifestations of ectodermal dysplasias.[2] Syndromes limited to deafness and dental anomalies have been reported recently.[1,3,4] In each of these reported syndromes, the hearing loss was described as sensorineural.

The dental anomalies in 2 of the reports were similar.[1,3] The posterior teeth were described as large and bulbous. The cusps were irregularly arranged with obliteration of the occlusal grooves and accessory cusps in some cases. In one report, the primary canines were described as malformed and secondary canines as normal.[1] In the other, the primary and the secondary canines were described as malformed.[3] The incisors were reported as normal in size and shape in both cases. The rarity of the anomalies, their association with deafness and an autosomal dominant mode of inheritance in each family suggests that the reports dealt with the same condition, otodental dysplasia.

The dental anomalies described in association with sensorineural deafness by Gorlin and Červenka are fusion of crowns, dens invaginatus, hypodontia and malposed teeth.[4] These findings are different from those of otodental dysplasia.

The constellation of anomalies reported in the present family are identical to those in otodental dysplasia.

The mode of inheritance is also autosomal dominant. It is unlikely that this family is related to the 2 reported previously. The families reside in widely separated geographic areas (New York, Minnesota and South Carolina) and are apparently of different national origins. These findings suggest that there may have been more than one mutation at the locus responsible for otodental dysplasia and that the syndrome is not as infrequent in the population as originally thought.

References

1. Levin, L. S. and Jorgenson, R. J.: Familial otodentodysplasia: A "new" syndrome. *Am. J. Hum. Genet. 24*:61A, 1972.
2. Freire-Maia, N.: Ectodermal dysplasias. *Hum. Hered. 21*:309-312, 1971.
3. Gundlach, K. K. H., Witkog, C. J., Streed, W. J. and Sauk, J. J., Jr.: Globodontia — a new inherited anomaly of tooth form. (Abstract no. 10) *Proceedings of the American Academy of Oral Pathology*, 1974.
4. Gorlin, R. and Červenka, J.: New oral syndromes. (Abstract no. 11) *Proceedings of the American Academy of Oral Pathology*, 1974.

Autosomal Dominant Branchiootorenal Dysplasia*

Michael Melnick, D.D.S., David Bixler, Ph.D., D.D.S., Kenneth Silk, M.D.,
Huen Yune, M.D. and Walter E. Nance, M.D., Ph.D.

Several families have previously been reported in which anomalies of the embryonic branchial arch system and hearing impairment have been transmitted as an autosomal dominant trait with variable gene expression.[1-4] The common features of these families included malformed external ears, preauricular pits, branchial cleft cysts and deafness which may be sensorineural, conductive or mixed.

In an interesting case reported by Fara et al,[5] a father and 3 offspring had branchial anomalies and associated hearing impairment. They also reported that 1 of the 4 affected family members presented with agenesis of the right kidney. Since the latter occurred in only one of those affected, it was considered as an isolated finding. However, in light of the family presented here, it may have more significance.

The present report concerns a family of 9 (Table 1) in which the father and 3 of the 6 living children had a mixed hearing loss with associated branchial abnormalities (Figs. 1-3) in a pattern that was consistent with autosomal dominant inheritance. IVP studies revealed that all 4 affected individuals had an unusual bilateral renal dysplasia with distinctive anomalies of the collecting system.

Table 1. Summary of Phenotypic Findings

	Clinical Findings	Subjects*						
		II-4	II-5	III-3	III-4	III-5	III-6	III-7
General	Asthenic habitus	+	-	-	±	+	+	-
	Long narrow facies	+	±	-	+	+	+	±
Head	Constricted palate	+	-	-	+	+	+	-
	Deep overbite	+	-	-	+	+	+	-
	Cup-shaped anteverted pinnas	+	-	-	+	+	+	-
	Bilateral prehilical pits	+	-	-	+	+	+	-
	Aplasia of lacrimal ducts	+	-	-	+	-	-	-
Hearing	Mixed hearing loss	+	-	-	+	+	+	-
	Mondini type cochlear defect	+	-	-	+	+	+	-
	Stapes fixation	+	-	-	+	+	+	-
Neck	Bilateral branchial fistula	+	-	-	+	+	+	-
Urologic	Renal dysplasia (bilateral)	+	-	-	+	+	+	-
Vision	Myopia	+	+	+	+	+	+	÷

*See Figure 8.

*This is publication number 74-29 from the Department of Medical Genetics and was supported in part by Indiana University Human Genetics Center PHS P01 GH 21054 and a USPHS Individual Fellowship DE 01274.

121

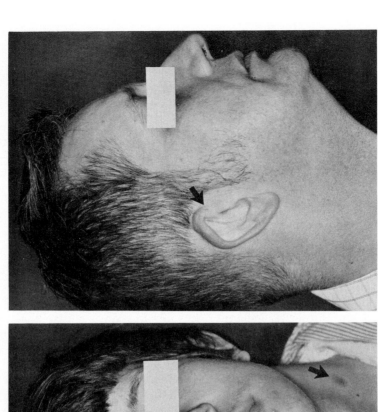

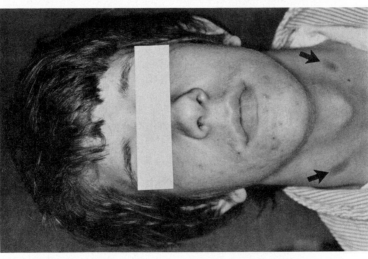

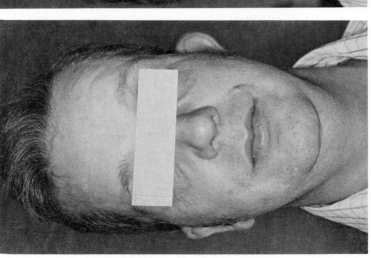

Fig. 1. *II-4.* Note the cup-shaped anteverted left pinna and the surgically corrected right ear.　**Fig. 2.** *III-4.* Note the bilateral infected branchial fistulas.　**Fig. 3.** *II-4.* Note the prehelical pit.

Case Reports

Case 1

II-4 was a 44-year-old white male who was first noted to have a hearing loss at about age 5 and had plastic surgery performed on both external ears. At the time of examination, he wore a hearing aid, and still had difficulty in communicating. He was of above average intelligence and was a college graduate employed in a managerial job.

Examination of the head and neck revealed a long narrow facies, small ears with cup-shaped anteverted pinnas, bilateral prehelical ear pits and bilateral branchial cleft fistulas below the level of the hyoid and just anterior to the sternocleidomastoid muscle. Examination of the eyes revealed bilateral aplasia of the inferior lacrimal ducts; the patient complained that his eyes fill up with tears at unpredictable and inappropriate times. Intraoral examination revealed only a moderately constricted palate and a very deep overbite (90%).

This father had a mixed hearing loss (Table 2). There was no atresia of the external meatus. Tympanometry produced curves that were within normal limits but no acoustic reflex was elicited from either side, strongly suggesting stapes fixation. AP and lateral tomography of both ears revealed hypoplasia of the apex of the cochlea (Mondini deformity). There was no evidence of atresia of the oval window.

An IVP (Fig. 4) on this man revealed an unusual configuration to the superior pole of both kidneys, in that they were more sharply tapered than the inferior poles. This tapering was associated with a craniad projection of the renal pelvis along the medial border of the kidney and a generalized blunting of the calyces. The blunted calyces could not be explained on the basis of papillary necrosis or chronic pyelonephritis. It should be noted that this man had no renal symptoms, and kidney function tests showed no abnormalities.

Case 2

III-4 was the 15-year-old son of *II-4*. His external ear anomalies, similar to those of his father, were noted at birth but hearing loss was not suspected until some time later. He wore a hearing aid intermittently with some benefit. He had some speech difficulties but was of average intelligence and was, at the time of this examination, attending high school.

Examination of the head and neck revealed a long narrow facies with cup-shaped anteverted pinnas, bilateral prehelical pits and bilateral branchial cleft fistulas in exactly the same location as in the father. A unilateral aplasia of the right lacrimal duct was noted, but this caused no trouble for the patient. He too had a moderately constricted palate and a very deep overbite (90%).

Audiologic studies revealed a mixed hearing loss (Table 2) similar to that of the father. There was no atresia of the external meatus. AP and lateral tomography of both ears revealed hypoplasia of the cochlea that was similar, but somewhat less severe, than the defect noted in the father. Tympanometry was consistent with bilateral fixation of the stapes footplate, the acoustic reflex having been absent in both ears.

Table 2. Audiologic Studies

| | Puretone Average, dB (500-2000 HZ) | | | | Speech Reception Threshold, dB | | Speech Discrimination | |
| | Bone | | Air | | Air | | | |
	R	L	R	L	R	L	R	L
II-4 (Father)	35	43	68	47	60	38	100	98
III-6 (Daughter)	17	17	58	45	58	40	100	100
III-5 (Daughter)	53	33	95	60	82	50	76	96
III-4 (Son)	35	50	77	57	60	48	82	82
II-5 (Mother)	2	*	3	2	0	-4	98	98
III-3 (Daughter)	2	*	2	2	0	0	100	100
III-7 (Daughter)	-2	-2	2	12	0	2	100	98

*Could not test

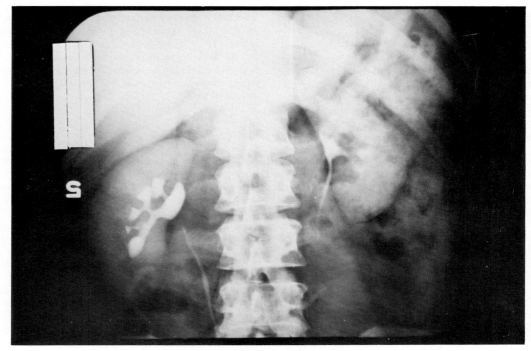

Fig. 4. *II-4.* Renal IVP.

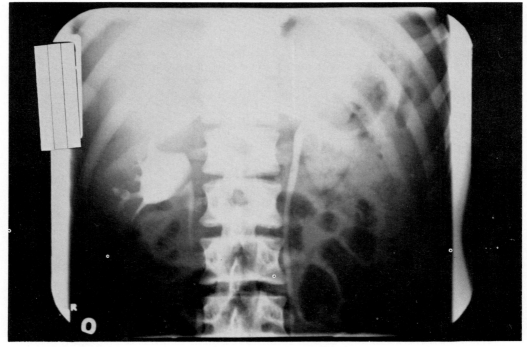

Fig. 5. *III-4.* Renal IVP.

IVP (Fig. 5) revealed unilateral hypoplasia of the left kidney. The right kidney showed an incompletely fused renal lobe forming a larger than usual kidney with a separate second superior pole 3 cm below the higher superior pole. Also on the right, the lateral group of the inferior pole calyces seemed to be situated a little more superficially and one of these calyces was slightly blunted suggesting a calyceal diverticulum. The right renal pelvis was large and mostly extrarenal. The patient had no renal symptoms, and renal function tests showed no abnormalities.

Case 3

III-5, the 13-year-old daughter of *II-4*, was known to have had a hearing loss since early in life and a hearing aid which she used infrequently. She recently had an exploratory tympanotomy because the clinical finding indicated that there was a significant conductive component to her hearing impairment. At surgery, congenital fixation of the stapes footplate was found but its mobilization has not resulted in dramatic improvement in the audiogram. *III-5* also had a history of psychomotor seizures and was on medication (phenobarbital tid).

Examination of the head and neck revealed a long narrow facies with cup-shaped anteverted pinnas of the ears, bilateral prehelical pits and bilateral branchial cleft fistulous scars in the identical location as in her father and brother. No lacrimal duct anomalies were noted. A moderately constricted palate and very deep overbite (90%) were present.

Of all the affected family members, she had the most severe mixed hearing loss (Table 2). AP, oblique and lateral tomography revealed that the ossicles were more horizontally oriented than usual. The cochlea was hypoplastic as evidenced by a small cochlear diameter. A small bulbous radiolucency at the apical turn indicated a Mondini deformity. The audiologic studies were consistent with a mixed hearing loss, supported by little apparent improvement in hearing since mobilization of the stapes.

IVP studies (Fig. 6), including renal tomography, revealed an extremely hypoplastic but normally functional right kidney and ureter. The ureteropelvic junction on the right side was abnormally peaked cranially. The superior pole of the left kidney showed a segmental hypoplasia with a sharply tapering configuration toward the superior pole and reduced renal parenchymal volume. Many of the minor calyces in the left kidney showed blunted calyceal fornices but with no signs of chronic pyelonephritis or papillary necrosis.

Case 4

III-6 was the 12-year-old daughter of *II-4* and was noted to have multiple anomalies of the head and neck

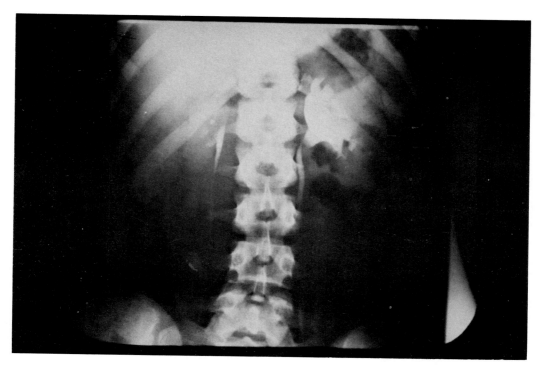

Fig. 6. *III-5.* Renal IVP.

at birth. A hearing loss was suspected before she went to school and she has used a hearing aid intermittently since the third grade.

The head and neck findings of *III-6* were identical to those of *III-5*. She has a mixed hearing loss similar in degree to her father's (Table 2). AP and lateral tomography of both ears showed the ossicles to be slightly rotated and situated slightly more anterior to the cochlea than usual, although the malleus and incus appear to be well-formed. The cochleas were hypoplastic and only 1½ turns of cochlea could be identified on both sides. The internal auditory canals were short. In general, the ear defects noted in *III-6* were less pronounced than in the other affected family members but a Mondini deformity of the cochlea was noted again. An absent acoustic reflex suggested the presence of a bilateral fixation of the stapes footplate.

IVP studies (Fig. 7) revealed that the right kidney was smaller than the left and that the number of calyces was reduced in both. All minor calyces were blunted but the kidney outlines were quite smooth. The cortical thickness was somewhat greater than normally observed. Finally, there was an unusual deformity in both renal pelves with a craniad outpouching along the medial border of the kidney. As in the other family members, the renal function was normal.

The remaining available members of the family, *II-5* (age 41, mother), *III-3* (age 18, daughter) and *III-7* (age 9, daughter), were also admitted to the Clinical Research Center for detailed examination. Diagnostic studies revealed them all to be normal females in good general health, specifically without kidney or ear malformations and with essentially negative past medical histories. There is one son, *III-1* age 22, who was living in another state and was unavailable for examination. The parents report that he does not facially resemble the affected family members nor was he known to have any of the clinical stigmata of the syndrome. This did not rule out the possibility of renal dysplasia, although it seemed unlikely.

Family History

As Figure 8 illustrates, the father (*II-4*) was the first known affected member of either the paternal or maternal relatives. There were no relatives known to have any of the many stigmata characterizing the syndrome. Since male-to-male transmission was present, the pedigree supported autosomal dominant transmission of the disorder.

Discussion

The physical, radiographic and audiologic findings in affected family members were re-

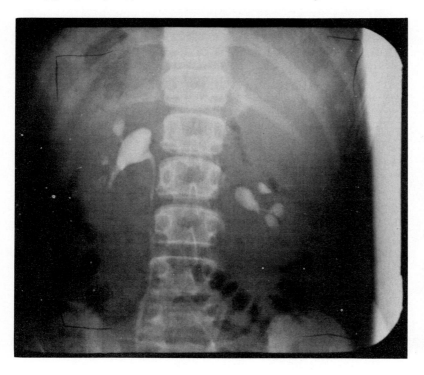

Fig. 7. *III-6.* Renal IVP.

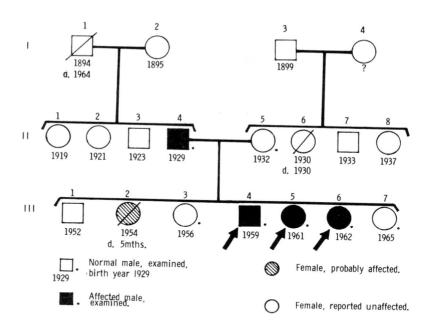

Fig. 8. Pedigree of reported family with b r a n c h i o o t o r e n a l dysplasia.

markably constant; all had 1) mixed hearing loss with a Mondini type cochlear malformation on tomography and evidence for stapes fixation on impedance audiometry, 2) cup-shaped anteverted pinnas with bilateral prehelical pits, 3) bilateral branchial fistulas opening inferior to the hyoid and anterior to the sternocleidomastoid, 4) moderately constricted palate with deep overbite and 5) bilateral renal dysplasia. In this family we have what can be called autosomal dominant branchiootorenal dysplasia, designating a defect in the growth and differentiation of the branchial arches, otocyst and renal primordia.

It has been suggested by McKusick[6] that preauricular pits and branchial cleft anomalies represent separate autosomal dominant mutations, because most families present with either one or the other. However, there are a growing number of families in the literature that exhibit both traits in an autosomal dominant pattern. Hunter[7] states that this represents a third autosomal dominant mutation. Several additional families[1-4,8] have been reported in which branchial cleft anomalies, preauricular pits and malformed auricles have been associated with deafness, in what may represent a fourth autosomal dominant mutation. Finally, Hilson[9] described 4 families in which an autosomal dominant mutation caused malfunctions of the external ear and kidney but no other branchial anomalies or hearing loss.

It is apparent that the genetics do not help distinguish the 6 disorders because they are all autosomal dominant. If one were recessive or X-linked we could then say that they are different mutations, but this is not the case. However, whether multiple alleles or mutations of separate loci are involved remains uncertain. Future understanding of this group of syndromes will benefit by: 1) a comprehensive and more uniform work-up including IVPs of all patients who present with one or more of the stigmata in this grouping in order to rule out the remaining ones (this will probably serve to reduce the number of types) and 2) linkage studies on patients (and their families) who fall into any of the 6 classifications in an attempt to confirm or refute allelism.

In any case, as a clinical geneticist, it is important to remember that significant kidney malformations may be found in patients with inherited branchial abnormalities even in the absence of overt renal symptoms.

References

1. Fourman, F. and Fourman, J.: Hereditary deafness in family with ear pits (fistula auris congenita). *Br. Med. J. 2*:1354, 1955.
2. McLaurin, J. W. et al: Hereditary branchial anomalies and associated hearing impairment. *Laryngoscope 76*:1277, 1966.
3. Wildervanck, L. S.: Hereditary malformations of the ear in three generations. *Acta Otolaryngol. (Stockh.) 54*:553, 1962.
4. Bourguet, J., Mazeas, R. and LeHuerou, Y.: De L'Atteinte de deux premieres fentes et des deux premiers arcs branchiaux. *Rev. Otoneuroophthalmol. 38*:161, 1966.
5. Fara, M., Chlupackova, V. and Hrivnakova, J.: Dismorphia oto-facio-cervicalis familiaris. *Acta Chir. Plast. 9*:255, 1967.
6. McKusick, V. A.: *Mendelian Inheritance in Man*, 3rd Ed. Baltimore:Johns Hopkins Press, 1972, p. 38.
7. Hunter, A. G. W.: Inheritance of branchial sinuses and preauricular fistulae. *Teratology 9*:225, 1974.
8. Rowley, P. E.: Familial hearing loss associated with branchial fistulas. *Pediatrics 44*:978, 1969.
9. Hilson, D.: Malformation of ears as a sign of malformation of genito-urinary tract. *Br. Med. J. 2*:785, 1957.

A Familial Syndrome of Aniridia and Absence of the Patella

Arthur E. Mirkinson, M.D. and Natalie K. Mirkinson, M.S.

Congenital aniridia is thought to have an incidence of 1:50-90,000 in the population and to follow an autosomal dominant inheritance with no sex predilection. It has been associated with many somatic abnormalities, the most well known of which is Wilms tumor, in approximately one of 70 aniridics. Aniridia has been associated with only one bone abnormality, mesodermal and ectodermal dysgenesis, where it acts occasionally as a dominant trait and is not present at birth, appearing in the 2nd decade. Aniridia has also been reported in one case of Laurence-Moon-Biedel-Bardet-like syndrome with obesity and polydactly.[1] There are no reported familial occurrences of bone dysplasia associated with abnormalities of the iris. The nail and patellas are linked in a syndrome, and at least one case of mental retardation has been associated with chromosomal abnormalities and absence of the patella.[2]

The present case report is that of the combined occurrence of congenital aniridia and absence of the patellas, in 3 generations (Fig. 1). It started spontaneously with the grandmother (III-2) of the proband and was clearly delineated through 3 generations (III-2, IV-3, V-2). No individual expression of either of the defects has been noted in other members of this kindred.

The survey was quite fortunate in having access to the great grandmother of the proband (II-11) who was clearly able to describe members of generations I and II. We were assured that no

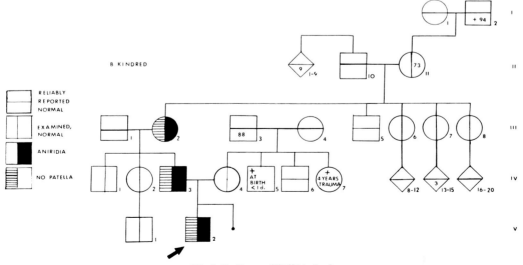

Fig. 1. Pedigree of "B" kindred.

129

incidence of either of these defects was present in those family members.

Case Reports

The proband is a 5-year-old boy (*V-2*), the product at the time of conception of a 38-year-old mother and a 28-year-old father. The couple had one other conception which ended at 5 months' gestation in a spontaneous abortion.

The child was noted to be a thin, hypotonic infant at birth. The birthweight was 6 pounds and 3 ounces. The length 50 cm. The head was 35 cm and the chest 32.5 cm in diameter. When it was noted shortly after birth that the infant had aniridia, closer examination then revealed that the newborn had absence of patellas, bilateral inguinal hernias and bilateral cryptorchidism.

At the age of three months the child had a bilateral herniorrhaphy performed for correction of the hernias and undescended testicles. The testes were examined and found to be normal in appearance.

Physical examination has been found to reveal no gross abnormalities and to be within essentially normal limits with the exception of a short systolic functional murmur and the described ophthalmic and bone disorders. His developmental milestones have been normal.

Because of the close relationship between aniridia and Wilms tumor, the child has been under close scrutiny for that problem, but no evidence of tumor has been found.

The patient's ophthalmologic problems came under early and continuing medical supervision. He has been examined on numerous occasions, once under general anesthesia, at which time the retina was noted to be normal. His visual acuity is 20/60 bilaterally. He has a significant bilateral lid ptosis. No glaucoma or increased pressure has ever been noted.

Because of the problems associated with his behavior pattern, the patient was referred to the Association for the Help of Retarded Children for evaluation and in turn was sent to the Genetics Laboratory at the North Shore Hospital for investigation. It was revealed that the patient had an IQ of approximately 103 and a social quotient of 79. It was felt that this child was a hyperkinetic child with normal intelligence, but with a severe behavioral disorder. Chromosomal analysis revealed a normal male karyotype, 46,XY. Amino acid screening revealed no abnormality.

The patient's father is 32 years old. He also had been found to have congenital aniridia. Subsequently amblyopia was found to be present in the right eye. There were no cataract or glaucomatous changes present. The only positive physical finding on examination has been the x-ray demonstration of markedly hypoplastic patellas, the right more than left. On the right, it is 3 cm in its greatest dimension and the upper pole is bipartite.

The paternal grandmother (*III-2*) has a history of congenital aniridia which appears in this kindred for the first time. At the present time she is considered legally blind due to progressive retinal degeneration and glaucoma. Her weight was well over 300 pounds. Her attending physician felt that this was due to an undetermined endocrine disorder due to the presence of a marked enlargement of the pituitary sella. X-ray films of her knees have revealed bilateral absence of the patellas.

The paternal great-grandmother of the proband is alive at the age of 77. She has been examined and found to have normal patellas and irides. She was able to give a clear and precise history of both of her parents, her husband's family and of the sibs and offspring of the rest of her children and grandchildren. In no case has there been any evidence of eye or bone dysfunction or abnormality noted.

The mother of the proband was one of 4 children. One of her sibs died one day after birth of unknown causes. Another died at 4 years of age of trauma. The maternal grandparents were normal. A maternal granduncle of the proband was reported to have had nocturnal epilepsy.

Summary

This is the first report of a syndrome of aniridia and aplasia of the patella. The origin of the defect arises spontaneously in the grandmother of the proband and must be assumed to be a de novo mutation. There is no associated chromosomal abnormality or overt biochemical or other somatic defect. This is an extremely rare mutation exhibiting a dominant autosomal form of inheritance. The gene for aniridia is a dominant gene whose penetrance here is 100%. The combination of aniridia and bone malformations in general is very rare. This linked defect probably represents one of the most rare of human genetic abnormalities. The penetrance of the combined abnormality seems to follow that of the more well-known aniridia gene.

References

1. Bornstein, M. B.: Bilateral aniridia with polydactyly. The relationship of ocular anomalies (colobomata) with an atypical Bardet-Biedel syndrome. *J. Genet. Hum. 1*:211, 1952.
2. Nakagome, R., Warkany, J. and Rubenstein, J. H.: Mental retardation, absence of patella and chromosomal mosaics. *J. Pediatr. 72*:695, 1968.

Discussion

Moderator: I could not see the state of the iris very well in the slides. Was it totally absent?

N. Mirkinson: There is a very thin rim.

Moderator: All of the way around?

N. Mirkinson: Yes, all the way around.

Moderator: But only a thin rim?

N. Mirkinson: The grandmother uses medication for glaucoma and there is an irregular formation of what appears to be minimal iris tissue.

Moderator: Has anyone seen this syndrome? This combination of abnormalities?

Dr. DuMars: I had an unrelated question, Dr. McKusick. Following several of these children with aniridia or hemihypertrophy and looking for Wilms tumor, I guess that I am looking for reassurance that this is something that we should be doing, as far as radiographs are concerned. What is the medical follow-up, looking for Wilms tumor? Has any Wilms tumor been found in a prospective study of those individuals with aniridia or with hemihypertrophy?

Dr. Kaufman: I am not responding to that question. But do I understand the association correctly? Is not the autosomal dominant form of aniridia unassociated with Wilms tumor? Is it not only the sporadic cases that are associated with Wilms tumor? Is this really necessary to do this in this family?

Moderator: I have the impression that aniridia is heterogeneous. Every time you see aniridia does not mean that you have this simple, autosomal dominant variety. We have heard that it could be perhaps aniridia patella aplasias syndrome. I have the same impression that Dr. Kaufman has, I guess, that it is mainly sporadic cases of aniridia that have the Wilms tumor and which have the hemihypertrophy and so on. But does anyone have any solid information on what the risk is and how much follow-up is necessary in these cases?

Dr. Weiss: I cannot answer the question on follow-up. But the question on has it been found prospectively; the answer is yes. The people in Philadelphia have followed some cases who were examined because of aniridia and who subsequently were found because of the investigation to have Wilms tumor. I know of at least two such cases.

Combined Limb Deficiencies and Cranial Nerve Dysfunction: Report of Six Cases

Martin Steigner, D.D.S., Ray E. Stewart, D.M.D., M.S. and Yoshio Setoguchi, M.D.

Combined limb deficiencies and cranial nerve dysfunction have been reported in a number of syndromes. Limb malformations associated with a spectrum of orofacial anomalies consisting of micrognathia, hypoglossia, microstomia, hypodontia, oral bands and syngnathia have been reported. Hall[1] proposed a classification based on the occurrence of hypoglossia for oromandibular and limb hypogenesis syndromes.

Cohen et al[2] also emphasized the heterogeneity which exists within each one of these diseases suggesting that many of these conditions presently regarded as separate syndromes may in fact represent the same formal genesis syndrome. The extensive variability may be due to some as yet unknown intrauterine insult occurring at slightly different times. Orofacial anomalies associated with absence deformities of the limbs suggest a developmental correlation between the limbs and the first visceral arch.[3] With interference in normal formation occurring during the second month of gestation, these anomalies would be expected to occur together.[1]

Of the syndromes listed in Table 1, only Moebius syndrome, or congenital facial diplegia, consistently has been reported as having multiple paresis of muscles innervated by cranial nerves. Classically, Moebius syndrome consists of nonprogressive facial paralysis which is usually bilateral, but often asymmetric, involving structures innervated by the sixth and seventh cranial nerves. Approximately 75% of patients with this syndrome have sixth nerve paralysis affecting the lateral rectus muscles which tends to be bilateral and complete.[4-10] Most patients reveal no family history of the disorder and there is no unanimity of opinion regarding the genetics involved.[4] Henderson, however, alludes to a few cases of affected sibs.[6]

This report documents 6 previously unreported cases, all male, ranging in age from one to 20 years, who demonstrate variable orofacial anomalies and limb deficiencies but have in common cranial nerve dysfunction resulting in facial paralysis. Table 2 lists the presence of the disorders in each of the six cases.

Case Reports

Case 1

M.B. (Fig. 1), a 4-year-old white male, was the product of the first pregnancy of a 36-year-old woman and her 38-year-old husband. The pregnancy was uneventful except for trauma from the steering column

Table 1. Syndromes of Oromandibular and Limb Hypogenesis[1] (Type)

Moebius syndrome
Aglossia-adactylia syndrome
Hanhart syndrome
Ankyloglossum superius syndrome
Amniotic band syndrome
Charlie M. syndrome

Table 2. Case Reports: Table of Multiple Features

	Facial paralysis VII nerve	Abducens paralysis VI nerve	Hypo-glossia	Micro-gnathia	Hypo-dontia	Oral bands webs or hypertrophic frena	Sygnathia	Congenital amputations or disarticulation	Streeter bands (Amniotic bands)	Mental retardation	Pectoral hypoplasia	Epiphora	Speech Problems
Case 1 (M.B.)	+ (asymmet.)	+	±	+	-	-	-	+	-	-	-	-	-
Case 2 (D.K.)	+	+	+	+	+	+	-	+	-	-	-	-	+
Case 3 (S.M.)	+ (asymmet.)	+	±	+	-	-	-	+	-	-	-	+	+
Case 4 (S.S.)	+	+	±		-	-	-	+	-	-	-	+	+
Case 5 (N.T.)	+ (asymmet.)	+	+		-	-	-	+	-	-	+	+	-
Case 6 (G.W.)	+	+	+	+	-	-	-	+	-	-	+	-	-

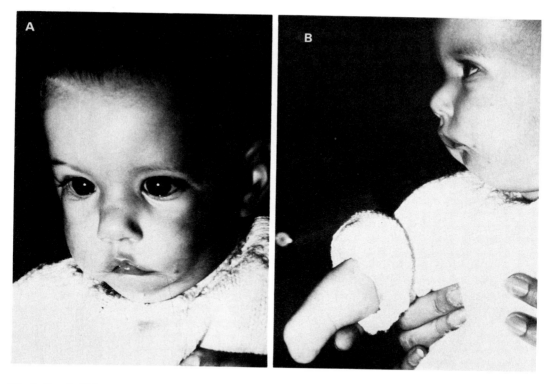

Fig. 1. *Case 1, M.B.*, at about one year of age. A) His left facial palsy is not apparent. B) Severe micrognathia and half of the congenital bilateral wrist disarticulation can be seen.

contacting the abdomen as a result of an auto accident. However, no vaginal bleeding or overt injury was noted. There was a history of an upper respiratory infection. A single dental extraction was accomplished with local anesthesia only at 4 months' gestation. There was also a history of ingestion of Clomid during the first 10 days of pregnancy. *M.B.* was delivered by C section and was noted to have bilateral disarticulation (acheira) and facial palsy at birth.

Examination revealed facial palsy was present primarily affecting the left side of his face. He had bilateral sixth cranial nerve palsy and could not move his eyes laterally. He could not close his left eye totally. He had a small mandible and consequent dental malocclusion in his primary dentition. His upper lip could not be controlled as there was no voluntary muscle activity in his obicularis oris. The left corner of his mouth drooped and allowed saliva to escape. The family history revealed twin maternal cousins with cleft lip.

The limb deficiency was congenital bilateral wrist disarticulation for which he had been treated with prosthetic devices. The patient also had bilateral genu valgum. He had normal motor development and appeared well-coordinated and his speech was assessed as normal.

Case 2

D.K. (Fig. 2), a 10-year-old white male, was the product of a full-term pregnancy. In the first trimester an auto accident of unknown severity occurred. Vitamins were the only medicines taken during the pregnancy. The family history was negative for other congenital malformations or birth defects.

D.K. had bilateral facial paralysis and extreme micrognathia resulting in a severe dental malocclusion. His upper lip was paralyzed or flaccid and his lower lip had to compensate for his "open-mouth" breathing and swallowing characteristics. His tongue was atrophic and was fixed to the floor of the mouth and alveolar ridge in the anterior portion. During infancy it was noted that *D.K.* had an alveolar ridge cleft in the midline as well as a partial cleft at the anterior tip of the tongue. Radiographs revealed congenitally missing lower incisors. His speech was defective, but he had compensated well and was not difficult to understand. There was a convex facial profile due largely to his small mandible. He was unable to abduct either eye or to close his left eye totally.

The limb deficiencies were classified as congenital right upper limb wrist disarticulation, congenital left upper limb partial acheira and congential bilateral lower limb apodia.

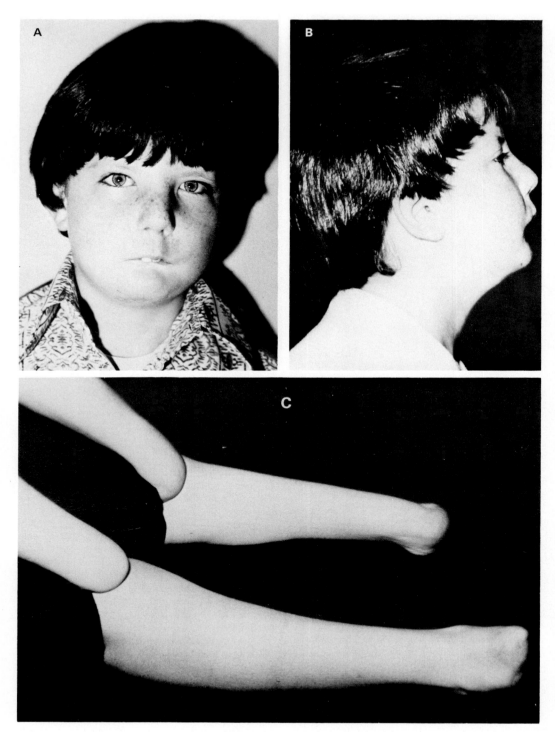

Fig. 2. *Case 2, D.K.* A) Lower lip compensation for a severe dental malocclusion is apparent. A fixed atrophic tongue complicated his bilateral facial paralysis. B) Lateral view displaying extremely hypoplastic mandible. C) Limb disarticulation of all 4 limbs.

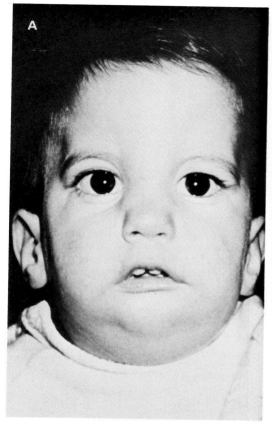

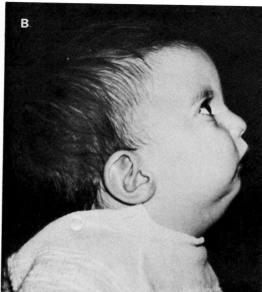

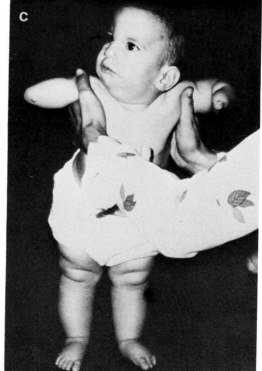

He did well in school. He was ambulatory and handled his limb prostheses adequately.

Case 3

S.M. (Fig. 3), a one-year-old white male, was hypoxic at birth and became cyanotic. The respiratory distress resolved spontaneously. Multiple congenital anomalies were noted including limb deficiencies and facial palsy.

He had paralysis of the right side of his face, severe micrognathia and an abnormally shaped head with significant frontal bossing. No premature fontanel closing was observed. His ears were low-set. The left ear was noticeably smaller than the right, but his hearing was clinically normal. He was unable to move either eye laterally. His mother noted that he had excessive tearing, especially when excited or eating. His facial profile was extremely convex owing largely to the small mandible.

Oral examination revealed a high-arched palate with no apparent cleft, and 7 primary incisors. A thick mucous saliva seemed to cause problems with swallowing as well as hindering respiration. His tongue was apparently normal. His right upper lip and right corner

Fig. 3. *Case 3, S.M.* A) Unilateral facial palsy with a wide nasal bridge leading to a frontal bossing at the central forehead area. B) Micrognathia and low-positioned ears are apparent. C) Upper limb disarticulation in this one-year-old.

of the mouth were flaccid and there was drooling. He had no speech at that time. There was moderate trismus but skull films did not indicate any pathology of hard tissue. His motor development was delayed possibly due to the upper limb abnormalities. However, he sat up well and was a responsive alert child.

The limb anomalies consisted of congenital bilateral terminal transverse hemimelia of the upper limbs. He suffered from right wrist disarticulation and left elbow disarticulation. His karyotype revealed multiple chromosome breaks suggesting a possible diagnosis of Fanconi syndrome; however, this was not borne out clinically.

Case 4

S.S. (Fig. 4), a 10-year-old white male, was the product of a normal pregnancy, except that labor was induced 3 weeks postterm. The only medicines taken during the gestation were nonprescription antitussives and decongestants (Allerest, Tranquil Aid, Pertussin, Anafin Decongestant, Dristan, Cēpacol, Sucrets, Preofarin, Isophrin, Parazets, Cheracol, Supernapac, Coricidin). His maternal grandmother had arthrogryposis; otherwise, the family history was negative.

The patient was small for his age but he was reportedly a healthy active child. He presented with a mask-like, expressionless facies due to bilateral facial paralysis. He was unable to move his eyes laterally and

was unable to close them. There was a characteristic open-mouth facies due to his inability to move the upper lip over his protrusive maxillary incisors. His mandible was small and he had a convex facial profile. His palate was highly arched and he had a moderately severe dental malocclusion. Speech was abnormal as it was difficult to produce labials since he was unable to bring his lips together.

The limb anomalies were limited to the upper limbs and included congenital right wrist disarticulation and missing digits on the left hand (partial adactylia).

A seizure of 3 minutes' duration in July 1971 was the only other positive finding in his history. He was performing adequately in school.

Case 5

N.T. (Fig. 5), an 11½-year-old white male, was born with unilateral facial paresis, a limb deficiency and pectoral agenesis. He was the third of 3 children. He had a left facial paralysis and was unable to abduct either eye. An expressionless appearance was noted when he was quite young. He had a slight internal strabismus and had been wearing corrective lenses since he was 4 years old. Excessive tearing had been noted. It had been suggested, but not confirmed, that he had had a blocked nasolacrimal passage. He had a slightly small tongue and the left corner of his mouth drooped due to the facial paralysis.

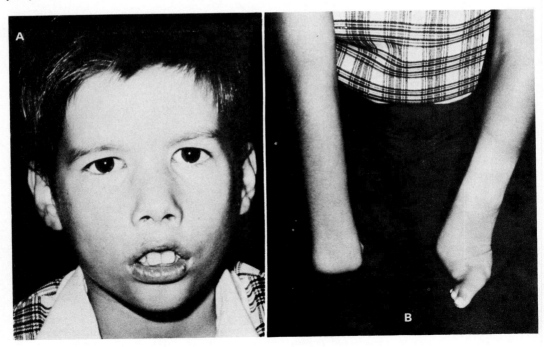

Fig. 4. *Case 4, S.S.* A) Expressionless, open-mouth facies with protrusive maxillary dentition and flaccid upper lip. B) Upper limb malformations.

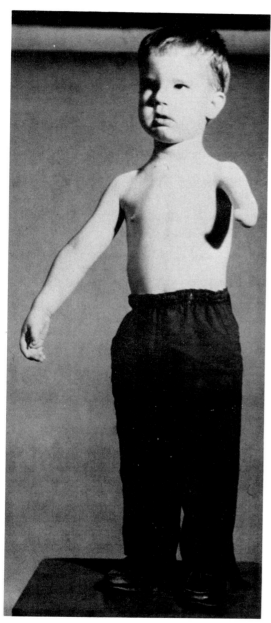

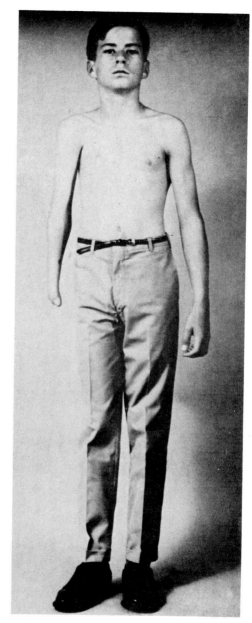

Fig. 5. *Case 5, N.T.* Full-body view at about 5 years of age. Anomalies include left facial paralysis and left upper limb congenital amputation.

Fig. 6. *Case 6, G.W.* Full-body view at about 15 years of age. The pectoral muscle aplasia and wrist disarticulation are evident.

His limb deficiency was limited to his upper left limb where he suffered from a congenital left transverse amputation above the elbow. He also had agenesis of his left pectoral muscle mass. He tolerated his prosthesis well.

Physical development had been slow and he had had problems with short attention span and with being easily distracted. Consequently, he had been labeled as hyperkinetic. He was adjusting well in public school.

Case 6

G.W. (Fig. 6), a 20 9/12-year-old white male, was the product of an uncomplicated second pregnancy. At birth he was noted to have an absent right hand, a defect of the lower jaw and a defect of the rib cage. The limb anomaly was classified as congenital right wrist disarticulation (acheira). He also suffered from absence of movement of his right pectoral muscle mass due to absent pectoralis and intercostal muscles. His face was immobile due to bilateral facial paresis. There was no family history of similar or other anomalies.

In addition to the hand, facial and pectoral anomalies, there was sixth cranial nerve paralysis and he was not able to move his eyes laterally. He had a recessive lower jaw and a maxillary protrusion possibly related to a lack of upper lip pressure secondary to seventh cranial nerve paralysis. The patient complained of being unable to open his mouth widely and had a grossly abnormal swallowing pattern.

Oral examination revealed an atrophic tongue that deviated to the right and had a deep groove at the midline on protrusion. Dysphagia had been a problem and there was a history of rampant dental caries.

Discussion

Individually, certain of these cases seemed to fit well into one or another of the syndromes listed in Table 1. Others demonstrated multiple features each of which was previously considered to be pathognomonic of one of these syndromes (Table 2).

These patients and many of those reported in the literature [1,2,5,8,11] lend support to the hypothesis that the various syndromes featuring the simultaneous occurrence of orofacial anomalies and congenital limb malformations, once considered to be nosologically distinct, may in fact represent variable expressions of a single dysmorphic syndrome.

The anomalies observed in these patients and those reported as specific syndromes featuring limb malformations associated with orofacial defects occur in a pattern which suggests an intrauterine insult (environmental, genetic, or both) at between 3½ to 8 weeks, giving rise to an array of structural defects, the specificity of which depends on the precise time at which the insult occurs.

Summary

Six cases have been presented with combined limb deficiencies and cranial nerve dysfunctions. The major features are congenital disarticulation and congenital amputation associated with various orofacial deficits. Anatomic variations in limb and facial anomalies in these cases, as well as in other cases previously reported, seem to indicate that they are part of a single dysmorphic syndrome rather than a group of distinct clinical syndromes as reported in the past.

References

1. Hall, B. D.: Aglossia-adactylia. In Bergsma, D. (ed.): Part XI. *Orofacial Structures,* Birth Defects: Orig. Art. Ser., vol. VII, no. 7. Baltimore:Williams & Wilkins Co., for The National Foundation-March of Dimes, 1971, pp. 233-236.

2. Cohen, M. M., Pantke, H. and Siris, E.: Nosologic and genetic considerations in the aglossy-adactyly syndrome. In Bergsma, D. (ed.): Part XI. *Orofacial Structures*, Birth Defects: Orig. Art. Ser., vol. VII, no. 7. Baltimore:Williams & Wilkins Co., for The National Foundation-March of Dimes, 1971, pp. 237-240.

3. Temtamy, S.: Association of absence deformities of the extremities with oral-facial malformation. In: *Congenital Genetic Factors in Hand Malformatiion, I.* Dissertation submitted for Ph.D. to The Johns Hopkins University, 1966, pp. 77-80.

4. Gorlin, R. J. and Pindborg, J. J.: *Syndromes of the Head and Neck.* New York:McGraw-Hill, 1964.

5. Hannissian, A. S., Fuste, F., Hayes, W. T. and Duncan, J. M.: Möbius syndrome in twins. *Am. J. Dis. Child. 120*:472-475, 1970.

6. Henderson, J. L.: The congenital facial diplegia syndrome: Clinical features, pathology, and etiology. *Brain 62*:381-403, 1939.

7. Pitner, S. E., Edwards, J. E. and McCormick, W. F.: Observations on the pathology of Moebius syndrome. *J. Neurol. Neurosurg. Psychiatry 28*:362-374, 1965.

8. Uribe, J. D. and Epps, C. H.: The Moebius syndrome: A report of three cases. *Inter-Clinic Infor. Bull. 13*:17-23, 1974.

9. Van Allen, M. W. and Blodi, F. C.: Neurologic aspects of the Mobius syndrome. *Neurology (Minneap.) 10*:249-259, 1960.

10. Warkany, J.: *Congenital Malformations Year Book.* Chicago:Medical Publishers, 1971.

11. Jorgenson, R. J.: Moebius syndrome, ectrodactyly, aypoplesia of tongue and pectoral muscles. In Bergsma, D. (ed.): Part XI. *Orofacial Structures,* Birth Defects: Orig. Art. Ser., vol. VII, no. 7. Baltimore:Williams & Wilkins Co., for The National Foundation-March of Dimes, 1971, pp. 233-236.

Discussion

Moderator: Dr. Bryan Hall, you have been interested in this pattern of associated anomalies. Would you like to comment?

Dr. Hall: I am glad that somebody took the effort to look at the classification that I proposed when I was very idealistic. The one point that I wanted to make is that as far as the Charlie M. and Hanhart syndromes are concerned, I am not sure that they are related to the oral mandibular hypoplasia-limb anomalies classification. As far as being related to the Moebius and the aglossia-adactylia syndromes, I personally have seen overlaps between the aglossia-adactylia syndrome and the Moebius syndrome. Whether they are all caused by the same etiology, I do not know. But certainly it is important to identify the presence or absence of facial palsies because those patients without facial palsies who have those abnormalities are rarely mentally retarded, while those with facial palsies are often retarded.

Dr. Steigner: We did not find mental retardation in any of our 6 cases. I agree with your aglossia-adactylia/Moebius idea.

Moderator: A doctor from Crete, I am sorry but I cannot remember his name at the moment, has one patient from a set of identical twins with the aglossia-hypodactylia syndrome. This discordance would go along with the idea that it could have been some kind of a singular insult which culminated in this pattern. I would appreciate any thoughts of yours on what might be the single kind of defect?

Dr. Steigner: I am sorry but I have no idea of what it might be. Our cases are all sporadic. There was no consanguinity.

Familial Presacral Teratomas

Keith W. Ashcraft, M.D., Thomas M. Holder, M.D. and David J. Harris, M.D.

A tumor complex consisting of at least a presacral teratoma and a sacral deformity has been found in 23 patients occurring in a familial pattern. Many of the patients have also had anorectal stenosis, postanal abscesses, urinary tract anomalies and skin dimpling as part of the tumor complex. In addition, 7 patients in these families had either sacral defects by roentgenogram, a history of recurrent perianal abscesses or both sacral defect and skin dimples but did not have palpable tumors. The age of discovery of this tumor has ranged from 1 month to 89 years. Thirteen of 23 patients with the tumor have been female and 10 male.

In most instances, the predominant symptom has been constipation associated with anorectal stenosis. Five patients have presented with postanal abscesses. Nine of the tumor patients have been without symptoms, discovered only as a result of examination of other family members.

Physical examination revealed a palpable tumor in 23 patients varying from a 1.5 cm discoid mass in the hollow of the coccyx to an extremely large tumor extending well up out of the pelvis into the lower abdomen. The upper extent of most tumors, however, has been entirely palpable on rectal examination. Associated anorectal stenosis prevented rectal exam, and thus, palpation of the tumor in some of the very young patients resulted in a delay in diagnosis of the tumor in several instances. The tumor abscesses have all been located immediately posterior to the anus with the exception of one presenting on the left buttock. Three patients without history of abscesses have had an interesting dimple in the immediate postanal area. One patient who

has had a tumor and her sister (who does not have the tumor) had a laterally placed dimple on the buttock. These skin dimples have proved to be a cutaneous attachment of the tumor in those instances where resection has been carried out.

Roentgenologic findings included anterior displacement of the rectum because of the tumor mass in the sacral hollow. In all tumor patients and in some without palpable lesions, a sacral deformity of greater or lesser degree has been noted. This usually consisted of unilateral absence of the lower sacral segments. Seven of the patients have been noted to have associated urinary tract anomalies. One had a neurogenic bladder and 6 patients were noted to have vesicoureteral reflux. Calcification in the tumor has been noted in only the one patient whose specimen was radiographed after removal, although careful preoperative radiograph failed to reveal any evidence of the fine calcification which was later proved to be present. In no instance have recognizable bony structures or teeth been seen in these tumors.

Of the 19 patients who have undergone operation for this tumor, 18 had resections. One patient underwent incision and drainage of a postanal abscess 10 years prior to a diverting colostomy done for complete rectal obstruction. She died within several months of disseminated adenocarcinoma originating in this presacral teratoma — the only instance of malignancy in the series. Several of the patients underwent operation many years ago at various hospitals and operative details are unavailable. In the 14 patients upon whom we have operated, firm attachment of the tumor to the perichondrium of the coccyx has been noted in all. The tumor has been intimately attached to the rectum in all patients whether or not they had anorectal stenosis. In 8 patients it has been necessary to resect the full thickness of the rectal wall because the tumor could not be completely removed otherwise. In 6 patients it was possible to sharply dissect through the rectal muscle layers leaving the mucosa and submucosa of the rectum intact. The tumor was intimately attached to the skin in those patients with abscess or with skin dimples. In at least 4 patients, dural attachment was noted. In one, the communication with the subarachnoid space was recognized and closed. In another, operated upon many years ago from an anterior approach, failure to recognize the spinal fluid communication resulted in the postoperative death of the patient from meningitis. All tumors were removed from the posterior approach except for those 3 whose size necessitated a combined anterior-posterior approach.

Pathologic examination of all the recent tumors has demonstrated elements of 3 germ layers providing a diagnosis of teratoma. In 2 of the early instances where the lesion was predominantly cystic, the pathologic diagnosis has been dermoid cyst. The lesions have been predominantly cystic, although some solid elements were noted in those carefully examined. There has been only one instance of malignancy in the 19 patients undergoing resection. Two patients operated upon many years ago have had benign recurrence. One of those currently awaits reoperation.

In addition to the 23 patients with palpable tumors, there were 7 patients who demonstrated part of this tumor complex. Four of these had sacral defects only. Two patients, now deceased, had a history of recurring perirectal abscesses. The remaining patient with partial symptom complex consisting of a sacral defect and a lateral dimple on the buttock was a 10-year-old sib of 2 patients who have had the tumor and the daughter of a man who has had the tumor. Repeated careful rectal examinations in this group of patients with the partial tumor complex have failed to reveal any evidence of a mass lesion in the area.

The 30 patients came from 6 kindreds (Figs. 1-3). In one instance, the child was illegitimate

and was treated some 10 or 12 years ago prior to our being aware that this was a familial lesion. We have been unable to locate the patient or family. In another family, the youngest child had a tumor. His older male and female sibs do not have it. His mother was free of sacral defect or palpable tumor. The father has declined examination. In still another family, mother and daughter have had the tumor (the mother died of malignant tumor). Father and son have been examined and found to be free of tumor. No further family members were available. In one kindred, the grandfather died of emphysema and was noted at the time to have a tumor in or near his rectum. The father and 2 daughters had the typical presacral tumor and one daughter had a lateral sacral dimple and sacral defect but no palpable tumor. In a 5th kindred (Fig. 2), 2 brothers have been noted with the tumor. One of the brothers had no children; the other had 9. Of the 9 children, 3 are known to have the tumor — 2 have been resected and 1 awaits resection. Offspring of the 2 sons with the tumor have not been in for examination. The youngest female sib had a tumor but her child did not. There has been one granddaughter with the tumor. Her father had a known sacral defect with no palpable tumor on repeated examinations. The most extensively examined family was headed by an 89-year-old man (*J.L.M.*) found to have a tumor

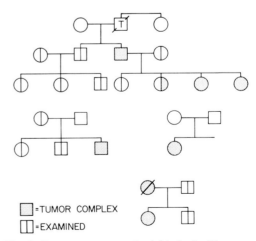

▢ =TUMOR COMPLEX
▯ =EXAMINED

Fig. 1. Tumor occurrence in 4 kindreds. The square containing the T represents the parent who died with an undiagnosed type of rectal tumor. The half-shaded circle represents a sib with sacral defect and skin dimple but without palpable tumor.

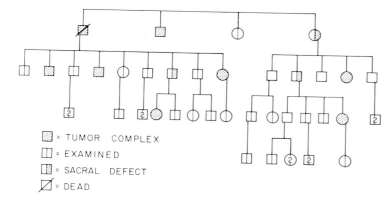

= TUMOR COMPLEX

= EXAMINED

= SACRAL DEFECT

= DEAD

Fig. 2. Tumor occurrence in the *R Family*. Half-shaded figures represent patients with unequivocal sacral deformity but without palpable tumors.

(Fig. 3). He had been constipated all his life and had anorectal stenosis. He had a brother, now deceased, who had a history of perirectal abscesses. *J.L.M.* had 7 children — 2 of whom had the tumor and one with a history of rectal abscesses. The offspring of both sons have had instances of partial or total tumor complex as noted.

In the sibships at risk and examined, 23 of 50 persons had the tumor. In all instances where examination was possible, the parent either had the tumor complex or had a sacral defect without a palpable tumor. The tumor complex fulfills the following criteria for dominant inheritance: 1) vertical transmission; 2) transmission from male to female and male; 3) transmission from female to male and female; 4) equal sex ratio and 5) occurrence of tumor complex in 23 of the 50 at risk sibs.

These tumors appeared to differ considerably from usual sacrococcygeal teratoma. First, they were not visible on inspection with the exception of those which present as abscesses and one which presented as a lower abdominal mass. Secondly, they occurred with equal incidence in males and females. Thirdly, the incidence of malignancy was only 5%.

In addition to our original report,[1] review of the literature has revealed several papers reporting what may be comparable lesions. Sacral defects have been described in 6 female members of one family — 3 of whom had anal stenosis and 4 of whom had soft presacral tumors.[2] Two of these tumors were demonstrated to be anterior sacral meningoceles on spinal contrast studies. Others have not been studied or resected. None of our patients were demonstrated to have sacral meningoceles, although in 2 there was communication with the subarachnoid space. There have, in addition, been 9 patients reported in one family with sacral defects — 4 of whom were females with sacral tumors.[3] One was a meningocele and one was a dermoid. Two patients remained undiagnosed. Eklof reported a 5-year-old boy with teratoma in the presacral region, anal

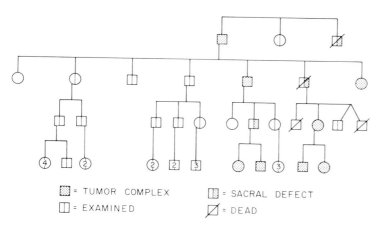

= TUMOR COMPLEX

= EXAMINED

= SACRAL DEFECT

= DEAD

Fig. 3. Tumor occurrence in the *M Family*. The 2 deceased half-shaded figures represent patients with recurrent rectal abscesses presumed to represent a partial tumor complex. The half-shaded figure still living has a sacral defect but no palpable tumor.

stenosis and a sacral defect.[4] No other family history was available in this instance. A mother and daughter combination have been described by the Mayo Clinic with presacral dermoid tumors but with no mention of anal stenosis or sacral defect.[5]

Genetic linkage studies are being carried out in this group of patients and in the kindred. Examination of other family members continues.

Summary

A tumor complex consisting of presacral teratoma and sacral deformity was described along with its occurrence in 6 kindreds. In addition to the tumor and the sacral defect, some patients have had recurrent abscesses, rectal stenosis and skin dimples as manifestation of the tumor. Urinary tract anomalies have also been found to be associated in some patients. The tumor differed considerably from the usual sacrococcygeal teratoma. Only one of the 19 resected tumors had proved to be malignant, although 2 have recurred in a benign manner. This appears to be inherited as a dominant characteristic.

References

1. Ashcraft, K. W. and Holder, T. M.: Congenital anal stenosis with presacral teratoma. *Ann. Surg.* *162*:1091-1095, 1965.
2. Cohn, J. and Bay-Nielsen, E.: Hereditary defect of the sacrum and coccyx with anterior sacral meningocele. *Acta Paediat. Scand. (Suppl.) 58*:268-274, 1969.
3. Kenefick, J. S.: Hereditary sacral agenesis associated with presacral tumours. *Br. J. Surg. 60*:271-274, 1973.
4. Eklof, O.: Roentgenologic findings in sacrococcygeal teratoma. *Acta Radiol. (Diagn.) (Stockh.) 3*:41-48, 1965.
5. Theuerkauf, F. J., Hill, J. R. and Remine, W. H.: Presacral developmental cysts in mother and daughter. *Dis. Colon Rectum 13*:127-132, 1970.

Variable Limb Malformations in the Brachmann-Cornelia de Lange Syndrome

Hermine M. Pashayan, M.D., F. Clarke Fraser, M.D., Ph.D.
and Samuel Pruzansky, D.D.S.

The Brachmann-Cornelia de Lange (BCDL) syndrome[1-3] is one of the many snydromes of multiple congenital anomalies. To date numerous aspects of the syndrome have been shown to be variable, ie mental retardation,[4,5] stature[5] and the age at which the characteristic facial features become most apparent.[6,7] The abnormalities of the upper limbs have long been known to vary from phocomelia, with complete absence of a hand and 1 or 2 long bones, to a low-placed thumb in an otherwise slightly micromelic hand.

The purpose of this report is to document the variable abnormalities of the upper limbs in patients who are obvious cases of the BCDL syndrome and to define syndrome specific hand anomalies that can be of diagnostic value in the not so obvious or atypical case of the syndrome.

Case Reports

The features common to all the cases presented in this report are listed in Table 1. The limb abnormalities are listed separately for each case.

Case 1. A.M.C. (MCH 328151)(Fig. 1)
  Micromelia (hands and feet)
  Clinodactyly of the 5th digits
  Hypoplastic middle and distal phalanges of 5th digits
  Single crease on 5th digits
  Short 1st metacarpals
  Low insertions of the thumbs
  Short proximal end of the radii

Case 2. L.T. (MCH 264771)(Fig. 2)
  Micromelia (hands and feet)
  Clinodactyly of 5th digits
  Hypoplastic middle and distal phalanges of 5th digits
  Single crease on left 5th digit
  Short 1st metacarpals
  Low insertion of the thumbs
  Flattening of the distal ossification centers of the radius
  Overconstriction of the long bones of upper limbs
  Fusion of ribs (1st and 2nd left)
  Flat iliac crests

Case 3. E.S. (MCH 238151)(Fig. 3)
  Micromelia (hands and feet)
  Clinodactyly of the 5th digits
  Single crease on 5th digits

Table 1. Features Common to the 10 Patients

Brachymicrocephaly
Shortness of stature
Bushy eyebrows with synophrys
Long eyelashes
Flat nasal bridge
Upturned tip of nose exposing the nares to front view
Increased distance from nose to vermilion of upper lip
Narrow high-arched palate or cleft palate
Large squared incisors
Micrognathia
Low-set ears
Low hairline (anterior)
Hirsutism (shoulders, lower back and limbs)
Some degree of mental retardation
Small feet
Variable degree of upper limb malformations

147

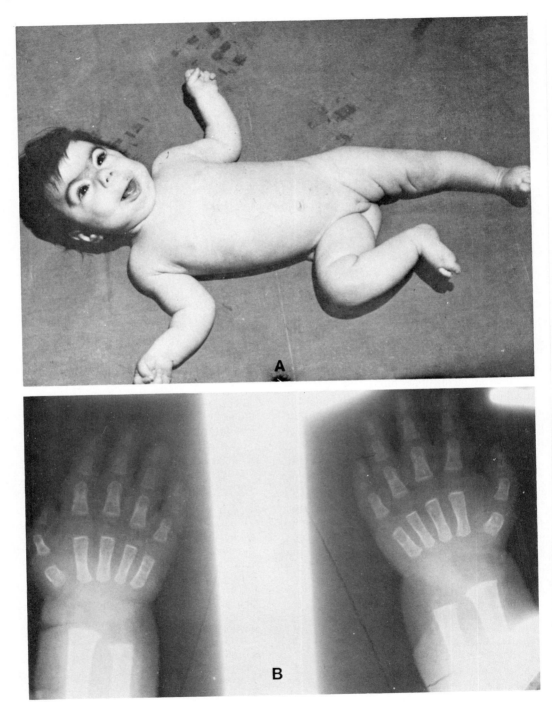

Fig. 1. A) *Case 1* showing the typical facial features of the BCDL syndrome and the 4 limbs; B) x-ray films of hands showing clinodactyly of the 5th digits with hypoplasia of the middle and terminal phalanges of the 5th digits. Also note the short and broad 1st metacarpals.

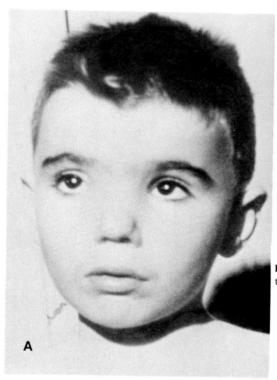

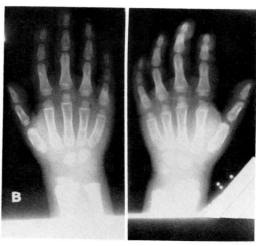

Fig. 2. A) *Case 2,* facial features; B) roentgenogram of the hands showing similar features as *Case 1.*

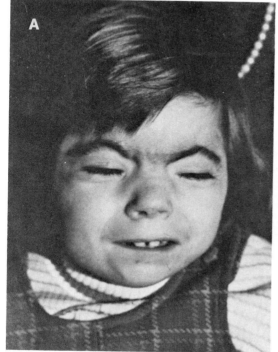

Fig. 3. A) *Case 3*, typical facial features; B) left hand.

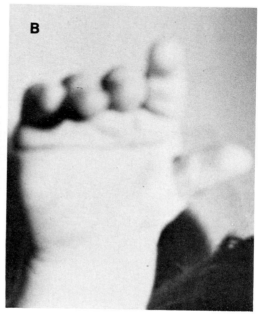

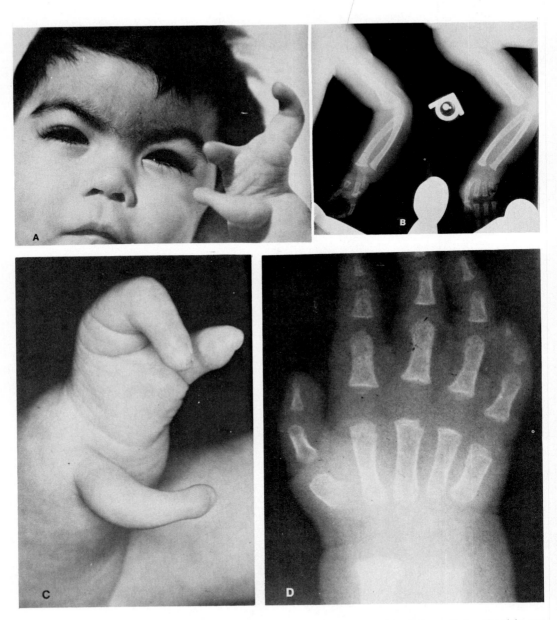

Fig. 4. A) *Case 4*, typical facial features and right hand; B) roentgenogram of both upper limbs: the right arm showing missing phalanges and metacarpals, and short radius and ulna; the left arm showing narrow radius with deformity of the proximal end. C) Close-up of right hand; D) roentgenogram of left hand showing clinodactyly of the 5th digit and hypoplasia of the middle and distal phalanges. Very short and wide 1st metacarpal.

Hypoplastic middle and distal phalanges of 5th
digits
Short 1st metacarpals

Case 4. A.M.F. (MCH 380835)(Fig. 4)
Micromelia of feet and left hand
Left hand: Clinodactyly of 5th digit
Hypoplastic middle and distal phalanges of 5th
digit
Single crease on 5th digit
Short 1st metacarpal
Right hand: Lobster claw deformity with 3 digits
Very short 1st metacarpal with 2 phalanges
Two other metacarpals with 3 hypoplastic
phalanges each
Short proximal end of radius

Case 5. A.C. (MCH 408594)(Fig. 5)
Micromelia of feet only
Bones of hands limited to a single digit on either
side (3 phalanges on the left and 2 phalanges
on the right)
Single bone replacing the ulna or radius
Limitation of extension of the elbow
Short ribs
Cleft of the thoracic vertebras
Delayed bone age at birth

Case 6. J.B. (MCH 444508)(Fig. 6)
Micromelia of left hand and feet
Left hand: Clinodactyly of 5th digit
Hypoplastic middle and distal phalanges of 5th
digit
Single crease on 5th digit
Short 1st metacarpal
Proximal radial metaphyseal abnormality with
subluxation (left)
Right hand: Claw hand deformity with 3 digits
Hypoplastic ulna and radius

Case 7. L.B. (CCFA 3059)(Fig. 7)
Micromelia (hands and feet)
Clinodactyly of 5th digits
Hypoplastic middle and distal phalanges of 5th
digits
Clinodactyly of the 2nd digits
Short 1st metacarpals
Deformity of the proximal radial metaphysis

Case 8. L.W. (Chicago 001)(Fig. 8)
Micromelia of feet
Hypoplastic radii and ulnas

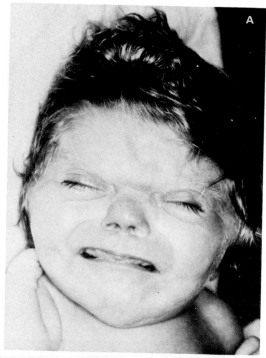

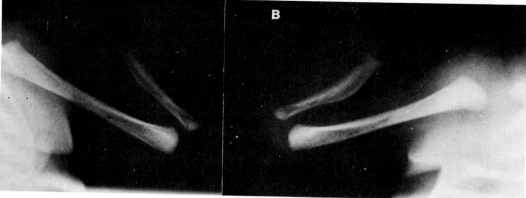

Fig. 5. A) *Case 5*, typical facial features. Note the severe malformations of the upper limbs. B) Roentgenograms of the upper limbs showing a single small bone replacing the radius and ulna. The single digits noted clinically do not appear on roentgenography.

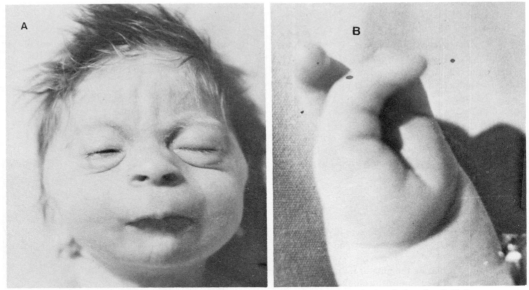

Fig. 6. A) *Case 6*, typical facial features; B) close-up view of right hand showing 3 digits.

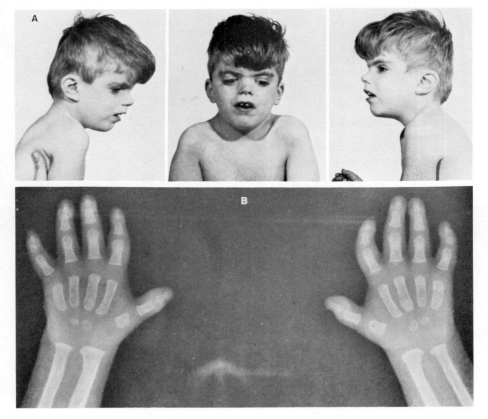

Fig. 7. A) *Case 7*, typical facial features; B) roentgenograms of the hands showing clinodactyly of the 2nd and 5th digits with hypoplasia of the 5th middle and terminal phalanges. The 1st metacarpals are short and wide.

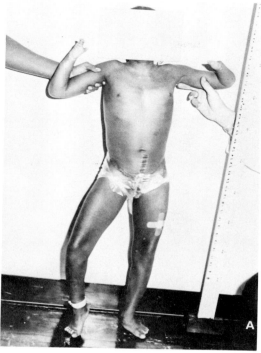

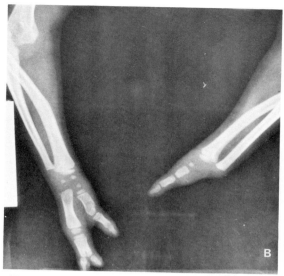

Fig. 8. A) *Case 8,* note malformed hands; B) roentgenogram of upper limbs showing numerous missing metacarpals and phalanges, and short right radius and ulna.

Deformity of the proximal radial metaphysis
Limitation of extension of the elbows
One digit with hypoplastic phalanges on left
Three hypoplastic digits on right with bony syndactyly of the proximal phalanges of 2 digits

Case 9. F.S. (Chicago 1516)(Fig. 9)
Micromelia of feet
Oligodactyly with 2 hypoplastic digits on the left and 3 hypoplastic digits on the right
Limitation of extension of the elbows
Narrow and short ulnas and radii

Case 10. M.B. (Chicago 554)(Fig. 10)
Micromelia (hands and feet)
Clinodactyly of 5th digits
Hypoplastic middle and distal phalanges of 5th digits
Short 1st metacarpals
Low insertion of the thumbs
Single crease on the left 5th digit
Deformity of the proximal radial metaphysis with subluxation

Comments

Ten patients were included in this study. The group consisted of 5 girls and 5 boys. Five were in an institution, 4 were at home and 1 died at an early age. Six of the patients are from the Montreal Children's Hospital (McGill University) files and 4 are from the files of the Center for Craniofacial Anomalies (University of Illinois). Eight of the children are white, 1 is black (*Case 8*) and 1 is oriental (*Case 4*).

The purpose of the study was to outline the variable abnormalities of the upper limbs, therefore only patients showing the characteristic facial features of the BCDL syndrome were used. Table 1 lists the features common to the 10 patients and photographs demonstrating the facial features document the diagnosis.

Results of the clinical, photographic and roentgenographic evaluation of 20 upper limbs revealed the following findings: 8/12 upper limbs studied showed extensive malformations including a missing long bone and absent fingers, metacarpals and carpals. Of the remaining 12 upper limbs, the most frequent findings were as follows: *clinically* — micromelia, clinodactyly of the 5th digits (12/12), single crease on the 5th digits (8/12), proximal insertion of the thumb (12/12); *roentgenographically* — hypoplastic middle and distal phalanges of the 5th digits (12/12), short and unusually broad 1st metacarpal (12/12), deformity of the proximal radial metaphysis ± sub-

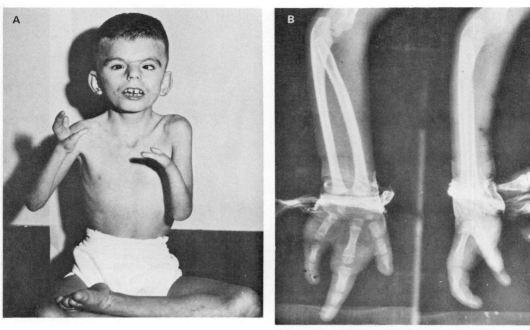

Fig. 9. A) *Case 9*, characteristic facial features and severe abnormalities of the upper limbs; B) roentgenogram of the upper limbs showing the numerous missing metacarpals and phalanges.

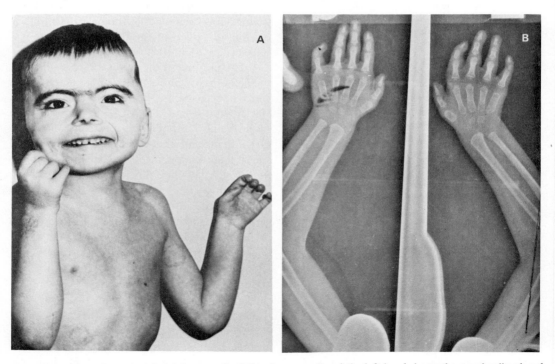

Fig. 10. A) *Case 10*, typical facial features. Both hands are small and the left hand shows the proximally placed thumb. B) Roentgenogram of the upper limbs showing clinodactyly of the 5th digits with hypoplasia of the 5th middle and distal phalanges. The 1st metacarpals are short and wide.

Table 2. Summary of the Clinical and Radiologic Findings

Case No.	Sex of patient	Nose – small with anteverted tip	Mouth – thin upper lip with downgoing angles	Long philtrum	Ears – low-set and malformed	Brachycephaly	Microcephaly	Synophrys	Long eyelashes	Hirsutism – forehead	CP/wide-spaced teeth	Micromelia	Clinodactyly of 5th digit	Proximally placed thumb	One crease on 5th digit	One digit missing	More than 1 digit missing	Rudimentary hand	One forearm bone missing	Simian crease	Short 1st metacarpal	Hypoplastic 5th middle and distal phalanges	Proximal radial metaphyseal abnormality	Micromelia of feet	Downturned toes
						Face						Minor				Major				Radio-logic				Lower Limb Malfor-mations	
1	F	+	+	+	+	+	+	+	+	+	+/-	+	+	+	+	-	-	-	-	+	+	+	+	+	+
2	M	+	+	+	+	+	+	+	+	+	-/+	+	+	+	+L	-	-	-	-	+R	+	+	+	+	+
3	F	+	+	+	+	+	+	+	+	+	-/+	+	+	+	+	-	-	-	-	+	+	+	+	+	-
4	F	+	+	+	+	+	+	+	+	+	-/-	+L	+L	+L	+L	-	+R	+R	-	+L	+L	+L	+	+	+
5	F	+	+	+	+	+	+	+	+	+	-/-	-	-	-	-	+	+	+	-	-	-	+	+	+	+
6	M	+	+	+	+	+	+	+	+	+	-/-	+L	+L	+L	+L	-	+R	+R	-	+L	+L	+L	+	+	-
7	M	+	+	+	+	+	+	+	+	+	-/+	+	+	+	-	-	-	-	-	+	+	+	+	+	+
8	F	+	+	+	+	+	+	+	+	+	-/+	-	-	-	-	-	+	+	-	-	-	+	+	+	+
9	M	+	+	+	+	+	+	+	+	+	-/+	-	-	-	-	-	+	+	-	-	-	+	+	+	-
10	M	+	+	+	+	+	+	+	+	+	-/+	+	+	+	+L	-	-	-	-	+	+	+	+	+	+

Key:

M = male
F = female
L = left
R = right

\+ = present
\- = absent

luxation (12/12). The humeral and radial deformities were variable and included: short, broad humeri, elongated humeral neck, subluxation and dislocation of the radii with rounding and hypoplasia of the proximal radial metaphyses. Table 2 summarizes the above findings.

It is interesting to note that in 1967 Kurlander[8] described these same roentgenographic findings as being "syndrome specific." The authors would like to suggest that these be looked for and documented for all cases of the typical BCDL syndrome and for the so-called atypical cases where the presence of these features could help substantiate the diagnosis.

References

1. Brachmann, W.: Ein Fall von symmetrischer Monodaktylie durch Ulnadefekt, mit symmetrischer Flughautbildung in den Ellenbergen, sowie anderen Abnormitäten (Zwerghaftigkeit, Halsrippen, Behaarung). *Jb. Kinderheilk.* 84:225, 1916.

2. de Lange, C.: Sur un type nouveau de dégénération (typus amstelodomensis). *Arch. Méd. Enf.* 36:713, 1933.

3. de Lange, C.: Nouvelle observation du "typus amstelodomensis" et examen anatomo pathologique de ce type. *Arch. Méd. Enf.* 41:193, 1938.

4. Pashayan, H., Whelan, D., Guttman, S. and Fraser, F. C.: Variability of the de Lange syndrome: Report of 3 cases and genetic analysis of 54 families. *J. Pediatr.* 75:853, 1969.

5. Barr, A. N., Grabow, J. D., Mathews, C. G. et al: Neurologic and psychometric findings in the Brachmann-de Lange syndrome. *Neuropädiatrie* *3*:46, 1971.

6. Pashayan, H., Levy, E. P. and Fraser, F. C.: Can the de Lange syndrome always be diagnosed at birth. *Pediatrics* *46*:940, 1970.

7. Passarge, E., Mecke, S. and Altragge, H. C.: Cornelia de Lange syndrome: Evaluation of the phenotype. *Pediatrics* *48*:833, 1971.

8. Kurlander, G. J. and deMeyer, W.: Roentgenology of the Brachmann-de Lange syndrome. *Radiology* *88*:101, 1967.

Epilepsy Anticonvulsants and Malformations

John F. Annegers, Ph.D., Lila R. Elveback, Ph.D., W. Allen Hauser, M.D.
and Leonard T. Kurland, M.D.

A number of recent reports suggest that there is an increased rate of malformations in the offspring of women with epilepsy taking anticonvulsant medications (chiefly diphenyl-hydantoin and phenobarbital). However, the relative contributions of epilepsy per se, genetic factors and the medications are not known.

The many reports of the last few years on maternal epilepsy and congenital anomalies are not strictly comparable. These studies differ in the types of populations studied and the methods of ascertainment of congenital malformations. The results suggest an increased rate of malformations among the children of women taking anticonvulsants although the overall risk is still low. Limited data on untreated maternal epilepsy do not show an increased rate, but the number of pregnant women with epilepsy not taking anticonvulsants is small. In addition these pregnancies may differ in regard to the type and severity of the convulsive disorder. The increased incidence of malformations among the children of women on anticonvulsants appears to result chiefly in elevated rates of cleft lip and palate and congenital heart disease.

Patients with a diagnosis of epilepsy and pregnancy from 1939 through 1972 were identified through the Rochester-Olmsted records linkage facility at the Mayo Clinic. The histories that were identified were reviewed for the epilepsy status and anticonvulsant usage during each pregnancy which resulted in a delivery at a Rochester hospital. The case histories of these 284 births were reviewed for malformations noted at birth or later in life. The pregnancies were classified into 4 groups (Table 1): 1) those with epilepsy and anticonvulsant usage, 2) those with epilepsy but who were untreated, 3) those pregnancies occurring before the onset of epilepsy and 4) those after the remission of epilepsy.

There were 10 malformations in the 141 deliveries to women who took anticonvulsants during the first trimester (Table 2). Five of these had ventricular septal defects (2 had additional cardiac anomalies), 2 had cleft palate (one with cleft lip) and one had an atrial septal defect and a cleft palate. One case of Down syndrome and one of microphthalmia were noted. There was only one malformation, agenesis of a testicle, among the 56 births to women with untreated epilepsy. There were no malformations among the 87 births occurring before the onset or after the remission of maternal epilepsy.

The numbers of malformations in those on (10/141) and off (1/56) anticonvulsants were not significantly different. However, the findings of 6 cases of congenital heart disease and 3 of cleft lip or palate were significantly higher than that expected on the basis of incidence rates of these anomalies among births in Rochester (Table 3).

Three of the anomalies were familial. One of the mothers of an infant with congenital heart disease had undergone surgical repair of an atrial septal defect. The father of a child

Table 1. Number of Malformations in the Children of Mothers with Epilepsy Born in Rochester, Minnesota 1939-1972*

Mother's Status	No. of Mothers	No. of Births	Stillbirths	Infant Deaths	No. with Malformations
Pregnancy following the remission of epilepsy	13	26	0	0	0
Pregnancy before the onset of epilepsy	30	61	3	2	0
Epilepsy without anti-convulsants during first trimester	36	56	0	0	1
Epilepsy and taking anti-convulsant medication during first trimester	78	141	0	8	10
Total	138†	284	3	10	11

*Adapted from *Arch. Neurol. 31*:370, 1974.
†Some mothers had pregnancies which occurred under more than one classification.

Table 2. Types of Anticonvulsant Medication Taken by Mothers During First Trimester of Pregnancy and Congenital Malformations in Offspring

Therapy	No. of Live-born Infants	No. of Live-born Infants			
		CHD*	CP	CHD + CP	Other
Diphenylhydantoin alone	24			1†	2‡
Diphenylhydantoin with					
Phenobarbital	58	2 (1 yr, 2 yrs)§			
Mephobarbital	11				
Phenobarbital, mephobarbital	1				
Phenobarbital, paramethadione	1				
Mephenytoin	1				
Primidone	1				
Bromide	1				
Phenobarbital alone	28	2 (5 mos, 4 yrs)	1		
Phenobarbital with					
Mephenytoin	4				
Primidone	1	1 (1 mo)			
Aminoglutethimide	1				
Methoximide	1				
Mephobarbital alone	5		1		
Mephobarbital, trimethadione	1				
Phensuximide alone	2				
Total	141	5	2	1	2

*CHD indicates congenital heart disease; CP, cleft palate.
†This infant also had bilateral equinus deformities.
‡One infant had Down syndrome, and one had corneal opacity and microphthalmia.
§Age at diagnosis in parenthesis, given when not at birth or neonatal period.

Table 2 reprinted from *Arch. Neurol. 31*:371. Copyright 1974, American Medical Association.

Table 3. Cleft Lip and Palate and Congenital Heart Disease in the Children of Women Taking Anticonvulsants

	Expected Number	Observed Number
Cleft lip and/or palate	0.3*	3‡
Congenital heart disease	0.8†	6‡

*Based on a rate of 1.9 per 1,000 births among all births at Mayo Clinic hospitals, 1935-1971.
†Based on a rate of 5.7 per 1,000 births among Olmsted County, Minnesota, 1950 1969.
(Mayo Clinic Proc. 46: 794-799, 1971)
‡p <.01.

with cleft lip and palate had cleft palate and in the case of cleft palate alone, the father's aunt and her children were reported to have clefts.

This study was extended to the children of males with epilepsy. Eight malformations were found in 200 cases. There were no cases of cleft lip or palate and only one of congenital heart disease. There was no specific pattern of malformations and the occurrence did not relate to the status of the father's epilepsy or anticonvulsant usage at conception (Table 4).

Conclusions

Our study of maternal epilepsy is consistent with others in reporting an increased incidence of certain malformations in the offspring of women taking anticonvulsants. We did not find an increased frequency of anomalies in the untreated pregnancies of women with epilepsy or in the children of males with epilepsy.

Discussion

Dr. Poznanski: In your series, did you evaluate the presence of distal digital hypoplasia and nail absence? As you know, we have reported 3 affected children who have had short distal phalanges and the Australian group reported 7 cases.

Dr. Annegers: No, we did not.

Moderator: Dr. Poznanski, was Dilantin used in all 3 of your cases?

Dr. Annegers: In our series, we could not detect any difference between Dilantin and phenobarbital or the combination of the two, as far as the occurrence of malformations, although, of course, the number was small in each treated group.

Table 4. Paternal Epilepsy and Malformations Among Children Born in Rochester, Minnesota 1939-1972

Pregnancy Classification	No. of Fathers	No. of Births	Still-births	Infant Deaths	Malformations No.	Type	Age at Dx
Epileptic on Medication	43	76	1	1	3	Spina bifida myelomeningocele and hip dysplasia	Birth
						Syndactylism (2nd and 3rd toes)	Birth
						Hyperplasia of both feet	Birth
Epileptic without medication	16	31	0	1	1	Pulmonary stenosis	15 yrs
Before the onset of epilepsy	26	54	1	0	2	Hypospadias	Birth
						Hypospadias	3 mos
After the remission of epilepsy	18	39	1	0	2	Ureteral atresia and renal dysplasia	5 days
						Hypospadias	Birth
Total	91*	200	3	2	8		

*Some of the fathers had children under more than one classification.

Dr. Poznanski: Our cases had both Dilantin and phenobarbital, so we could not tell which was at fault. However, we have seen the same digital findings in some children who did not have this. We have had some in association with anal atresia and other anomalies, where the same digital manifestations were present and no maternal history of anticonvulsant drugs was present.

Dr. Aase: To further complicate the picture, we have a family study which combines Dr. Poznanski's recent comments with those of others, reporting familial aggregation of distal digital abnormalities, which seems to be aggravated by the presence of anticonvulsants in the mother.

Dr. Lieber: I may have missed this, but did all of your epileptic parents have idiopathic epilepsy to begin with?

Dr. Annegers: No, probably 90% were idiopathic and 10% were symptomatic. One malformation occurred in a case where the mother had symptomatic posttraumatic epilepsy. The others were all cases of idiopathic epilepsy.

Diagnostic Criteria for the Whistling
Face Syndrome

Ray M. Antley, M.D., Naoki Uga, M.D., Norbert J. Burzynski, D.D.S.,
Richard S. Baum, M.D. and David Bixler, Ph.D., D.D.S.

Thirty-four probands with whistling face syndrome (WFS) have been reported with over 60 anatomic anomalies of the face, head, hands, feet and other organ systems noted. The large number of malformations associated with this disease tends to obscure the presence of those few more significant malformations which appear to serve as potent indicators of the disease without introducing disease heterogeneity. It is our purpose to analyze the reported cases, adding 3 new probands with this syndrome with the expectation of detecting patterns of anomalies. The goal of this analysis is the exploration and detection of patterning of various anomalies with a view to simplifying the diagnostic criteria for the WFS. Such a technique could be useful for other syndromes as well.

Case Reports

Case 35

J.W. was a white female born to unrelated parents (mother 34 years old, father 37 years old) after 41 weeks' gestation with a birthweight of 3520 gm. There was no history of maternal exposure to irradiation, drugs or viral infections. The pregnancy was complicated by mild toxemia which responded to treatment. The patient was referred to the neonatology unit at Methodist Hospital of Indiana because of cyanosis with feeding. The infant had difficulty nippling due to her small mouth and mandible. She became cyanotic with feeding for reasons which were not specifically identified, and her weight gain was slow, requiring 3 weeks to regain her birthweight. On the third day of life she began to have myoclonic seizures which were

subsequently controlled with phenobarbital. She was last seen at 17 weeks of age with continuing poor weight gain, increasing evidence of developmental retardation, developing asymmetry of the skull and increasing scoliosis.

The child was the youngest of 4 sibs. Her parents, as well as her 3 older brothers, are well, exhibiting none of the stigmata evident in the proposita. The proband had the whistling face appearance (Fig. 1); micrognathia; long philtrum; H-shaped defect in the soft tissue of the lower lip; flattened facies; full cheeks; small nose; broad nasal bridge; hypoplasia of the alae nasi without coloboma; supraorbital swelling; deep-set eyes; blepharophimosis; antimongoloid-slanted eyes; and primary telecanthus without epicanthus. Two findings previously unreported in this syndrome are bilateral microtia and extremely hypoplastic irides. The joint and skeletal anomalies consisted of metacarpophalangeal and interphalangeal contractures of the hands; elbow and knee contractures; and ulnar deviation of the fingers. Syndactyly of toes 2 and 3 was present bilaterally. There was no talipes equinovarus deformity.

Radiologic studies showed a left scoliosis with the 9th and 10th thoracic vertebras being variants of hemivertebras. Skull radiographs showed a steeply inclined anterior fossa, as previously noted in this syndrome (Fig. 2). IVP and cardiac films were normal. X-ray films of the upper limbs showed ulnar deviation of fingers 3, 4 and 5 with radial deviation of 2 and finger contractures without bony abnormalities (Fig. 3).

Case 36

K.B. was a white female born 7/6/64 to unrelated parents (mother 30 years old, father 31 years old). Neither parent nor her 2 older sibs showed any stigmata of the syndrome. The pregnancy, labor and delivery were uneventful except labor was induced.

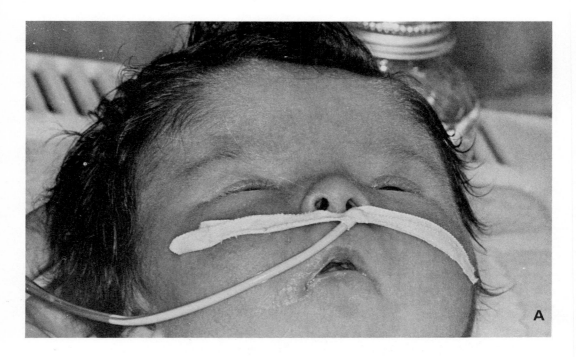

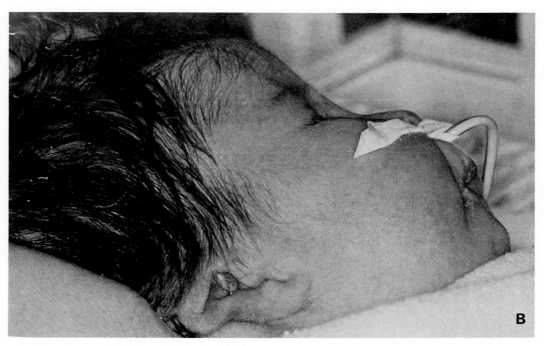

Fig. 1. Patient *J.W.* (*Case 35*) at 1 week of age. A) Note facial features of small mouth, hypoplastic nose with broad nasal bridge, giant rounded cheeks, supraorbital swelling, blepharophimosis and small H-defect in lower lip. B) Note whistling face appearance, deep-set eyes, flattened facies and microtia.

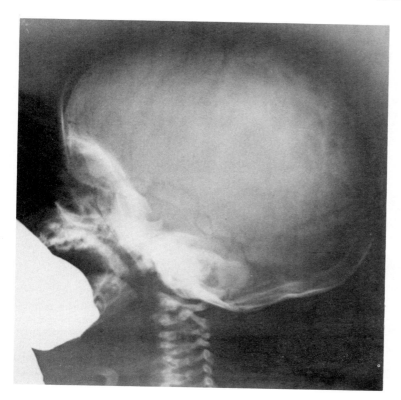

Fig. 2. *Case 35.* Roentgeno-gram of skull, lateral view, at 17 weeks of age. Note the steep anterior cranial fossa.

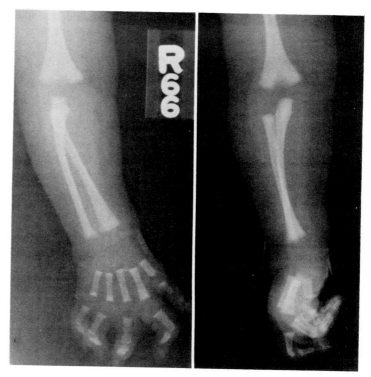

Fig. 3. *Case 35.* Ulnar devi-ation of fingers 3, 4 and 5 with unusual radial devi-ation of finger 2. Finger contractures are evident and there is no bony change seen.

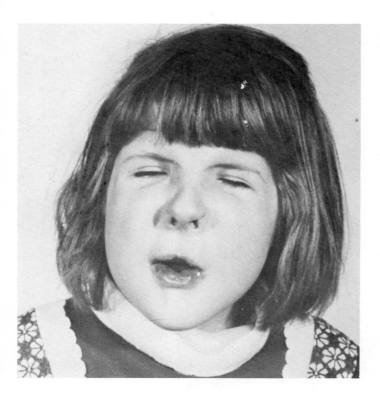

Fig. 4. Patient *K.B.* (*Case 36*) at 8 years of age. Note the whistling face appearance, the small mouth, notched nostrils, deep-set eyes and broad nasal bridge.

The child was first examined at the Child Evaluation Center, University of Louisville, at 8½ years. She had a height of 43 2/3 inches (<3rd%) and weight 19.5 kg (<3rd%). The clinical features included the whistling face appearance (Fig. 4); microstomia; long philtrum; H-shaped defect of the chin; small nose; no epicanthus; broad nasal bridge; supraorbital swelling; deepset eyes; flattened facies; and deep furrowing of the skin over the forehead. Inner canthal distance was 33 mm (75th%). Intraoral examination revealed normal dentition and fissuring of the tongue. She had an anterior open bite and a Class II malocclusion. The following joint and skeletal abnormalities were found: finger and thumb contractures; ulnar deviation of fingers; contractures of hands, wrist and ankles; marked kyphoscoliosis of the thoracic spine without abnormality of the vertebral bodies; flattened left side of the chest; and bilateral talipes equinovarus deformity. There were fusiform enlargements of the metacarpophalangeal and interphalangeal joints of the fingers bilaterally. The gastrocnemius muscles are hypoplastic bilaterally. The feet appear disproportionately small. Behavioral evaluation indicates a bright cooperative child with an IQ of 107.

Case 37

J.P., a 12-year-old white male, was first brought to the University of Louisville Health Sciences Center because of multiple congenital anomalies. He was the fourth of 5 sibs. One elder sib had died of multiple GI anomalies at 5 days of age. An older male sib, age 16, was retarded and the cause was undetermined. According to the description provided by the family, this sib had none of the signs of WFS. His parents and other 3 sibs were well and exhibited none of the stigmata evident in the propositus. Parental consanguinity was denied. The mother and father were 23 and 28 years old, respectively, at the birth of the proband. The pregnancy, labor and delivery which resulted in the birth of the proband in 1961 were said to be uncomplicated. Birthweight was 3290 gm. During the newborn examination, unusual facies, hand deformities and clubbed feet were noted. At the time of the examination (4/25/74), the proband weighed 30 kg (3rd%) and measured 50½ inches tall (<3rd%). The propositus had the whistling face appearance; a small mouth; H-shaped defect of the chin; long philtrum; small nose; coloboma of the nostrils; deep-set eyes; epicanthic folds; and a short neck with a suggestion of webbing (Fig. 5). The skull was brachycephalic in shape. OFC was 51 cm (10th%). There was a narrowing of the palate and irregularity of position of the dentition. The following joint and skeletal abnormalities were found: finger and thumb contractures; ulnar deviation of the fingers; contractures of the palms with limitation of pronation; scoliosis to the right;

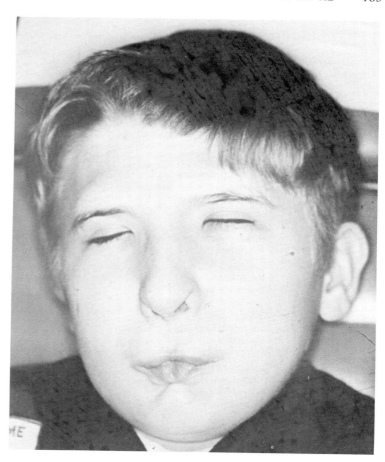

Fig. 5. Patient *J.P.* (*Case 37*) at 12 years of age. Note the whistling face appearance, small mouth, H-shaped soft tissue defect in the chin, long philtrum, notched nostrils and epicanthus.

shortened left leg; and talipes equinovarus deformity. Mild hearing loss was found unilaterally. Behavioral evaluation indicated a pleasant friendly boy with nasal speech and an IQ of 85.

Analysis of Malformation Frequencies

We reported these cases largely to investigate the frequency of anomalies in WFS with the intention of reducing and simplifying the diagnostic criteria. (An excellent qualitative review of the syndrome has previously been published.[1]) For this analysis, we used 26 individually described cases including our 3. A list of all reported malformations was compiled for tabulation. All case reports were reviewed and the malformations found for each proband were recorded, both on the basis of the authors reporting and the basis of photographs. When no mention of the anomaly was made and the photographs were not clearly informative, an entry of missing data was made. Borderline or indefinite findings were included as negative findings in the final tabulation, but were used for correlation studies. Tabulations are expressed as the number of positive factors per 26 cases, and no correction has been made for missing data (Table 1). A matrix was then constructed of individuals by malformation and a set of standard analyses including frequency counts, cross tabulations and Pearson correlations were performed on the data.

Approximately one half of the 60 malformations had been reported less than 9 times (in 26 cases) in WFS; consequently, we did not consider them to be major indicators of the condition. When the 24 most prevalent malfor-

Table 1.

Anomaly	Our Cases			Frequency of Anomaly in 26 Probands
	35	36	37	
Microstomia	+	+	+	26
Long philtrum	+	+	+	24
Ulnar deviation of the hand or fingers	+	+	+	22
Small nose	+	+	+	21
Finger contractures	+	+	+	21
Talipes Equinovarus	0	+	+	19
Growth retardation	+	+	+	19
Kyphosis or scoliosis	+	+	+	18
H-shaped defect in chin	+	+	+	18
Deep-set eyes	+	+	+	16
Joint contractures (excluding 5,6,8 & hips)	+	+	+	16
Micrognathia	+	0	0	15
Epicanthus	0	0	+	14
Broad nasal bridge	+	+	0	14
High-arched palate	+	0	0	14
Whistling face	+	+	+	14
Supraorbital swelling	+	+	0	13
Full cheeks	+	0	0	13
Skull changes	+	0	0	13
Coloboma of nostrils	0	+	+	13
Antimongoloid-slanted eyes	+	0	0	12
Flattened facies	+	+	0	12
Hypertelorism	+	0	0	11
Short neck	0	0	+	11

mations are arranged in descending order of their frequency (Table 1), a number of consistent anomalies are evident. Microstomia occurs in all cases. Long philtrum, ulnar deviation of the hands and fingers, small nose and hand contractures constitute an impressive list of almost standard anomalies. Furthermore, these anomalies are not independent of one another; patterns of related anomalies can be appreciated. There appear to be 3 interrelated facial complexes. Microstomia was associated with the whistling face appearance, an H-shaped defect in the chin and micrognathia. There was an association between long philtrum, coloboma of the nostrils and nasal hypoplasia. In addition there was a group of findings including broad nasal bridge, epicanthus and hypertelorism which are compatible. Growth retardation was a prominent general feature. The classic whistling face appearance was specifically mentioned or obvious from pictures in 14 of the probands. The observations of deep-set eyes, full cheeks, antimongoloid slant to the palpebral fissures and flattened facies admittedly are subjective in nature but contribute significantly to the syndrome gestalt. Further analysis indicated that there are significant correlations between supraorbital soft tissue swelling and flattened facies ($r = .61$, $p < .03$). There was a complete correspondence between the reporting of full cheeks and both supraorbital soft tissue swelling and flattened facies. The correlation between supraorbital swelling and deep-set eyes did not prove to be significant, contrary to the earlier suggestion of Weinstein and Gorlin.[1]

Of considerable interest to us was the reporting of hypertelorism. This finding was recorded in 10 of the 26 cases, and yet in no unequivocal case has true bony hypertelorism been established by radiographic examination. The obvious anatomic relationship between hypertelorism, epicanthus, blepharophimosis and a broad nasal bridge points to the problems intrinsic to a study based upon analysis of literature cases (multiple examiners). For example, data analysis showed that hypertelorism was positively correlated with a broad nasal bridge (r = .62, p < .01) and epicanthus (r = .11, p < .33) but was negatively correlated with blepharophimosis (r = -.35, p < .1). These results suggested different descriptive reporting of the same phenomena. It appears that observers reported either hypertelorism (and broad nasal bridge) or blepharophimosis. When hypertelorism was noted, epicanthus was randomly observed (r = 0, p = .50). However, if these 4 observations are considered to belong to the category of primary telecanthus as suggested by numerous authors, then 24 out of the selected 26 probands were positive. This sign, primary telecanthus, turned out to be one of the most consistent findings in the syndrome.

Consistent joint anomalies were present in the hands. Ulnar deviation of the hands and thumbs with finger contractures were found in practically every case. Of note was that kyphosis or scoliosis are as common as talipes equinovarus. The latter had been reported in every case published prior to Weinstein and Gorlin's case in 1969. A number of other joints were affected but are consistently associated with hand, ankle and vertebral column contractures. Further analysis of the important variables as to their association and clustering have lead us to reduce the signs in WFS to 4 clinically descriptive categories: 1) microstomia, 2) hypoplastic nose and alae, 3) primary telecanthus and 4) multiple joint contractures.

Comments on the Case Reports

The facial features of these 3 cases exhibit the characteristic features of the WFS: small mouth, hypoplastic nose and deep-set eyes. Two anomalies previously unreported are aniridia and microtia, found in *Case 35*. The significance of these latter malformations, embryologically and etiologically, is unknown, but they do illustrate a new variation in the basic computation of signs in WFS. They may

represent a chance occurrence or be illustrative of a heterogeneity in this syndrome which is still to be identified. The skeletal changes exhibited by these cases illustrate in typical fashion the growth retardation; joint contractures of the fingers and thumbs; ulnar deviation of the fingers without bony abnormalities; and scoliosis found in other previously reported cases.

While previous cases have mostly been of normal intelligence, our 3 cases illustrate again that mental retardation is not an uncommon feature of the syndrome. Although usually thought of as being cosmetically disfiguring and as rendering the affecteds somewhat handicapped in motor activities, this syndrome has not been emphasized as life-threatening. There are, however, 3 infants reported in the literature who suffered respiratory deaths in association with severe developmental retardation.[2-4] We suggest that our patient *J.W.* (*Case 35*) may represent a particularly lethal form of this syndrome characterized by the typical anatomic features, accentuated feeding difficulty, severe developmental retardation and ultimately death due to respiratory complication at an early age. At this time, however, there appears to be no valid reason for creating a separate category of WFS designated as "severe."

Genetics

The majority of the cases reported have been sporadic, as have all 3 of the cases reported here.

Eight of the 37 probands described or mentioned in the literature have been familial cases.[5-10] In each case, there was parent-to-child transmission and there are no reports of multiple affected sibs without an affected parent. Consanguinity has been reported in one case.[11] Since a greater than normal disparity in the father's and mother's age has been reported in some diseases thought to be etiologically linked to new dominant mutations, we wished to evaluate WFS for parental age differences. For sporadic probands, there were age data on 14 mothers and 12 fathers. The average ages were 27.8 and 31.0, respectively. The difference between maternal and paternal age is less than the 4- to 6-year difference noted in achondroplasia.[12] With the limited data available, we were unable to substantiate a paternal age effect. The parental ages observed were not strongly supportive of new mutations as the cause of sporadic cases of WFS. Further support for this idea comes from the observations on the familial cases. In each instance the parent was much less severely affected than the offspring, suggesting amelioration of signs with time. Thus, older affecteds may remain undiagnosed thereby increasing the number of sporadic cases.

References

1. Weinstein, S. and Gorlin, R. J.: Cranio-carpotarsal dysplasia of the whistling face syndrome. *Am. J. Dis. Child. 117*:437, 1969.

2. Rintala, A. E.: Freeman-Sheldon's syndrome; carnio-carpo-tarsal dystrophy. *Acta Paediatr. Scand. 57*:553, 1968.

3. Marden, P. M. and Walker, W. A.: A new generalized connective tissue syndrome. *Am. J. Dis. Child. 112*:225, 1966.

4. Buchta, R. and Mace, J.: Craniocarpotarsal dysplasia, a syndrome which may be more prevalent than hitherto appreciated. *Clin. Pediatr. (Phila.) 9*:5, 1970.

5. Pitanguy, J. and Bisaggio, S.: A chiro-cheilopodalic syndrome. *Br. J. Plast. Surg. 22*:79, 1969.

6. Fraser, F. C., Pashayan, H. and Kadish, M. E.: Cranio-carpotarsal dysplasia. *JAMA 211*:1374, 1970.

7. Walker, B. A.: Whistling face-windmill vane hand syndrome (craniocarpotarsal dystrophy, Freeman-Sheldon syndrome). In Bergsma, D. (ed.): Part II. *Malformation Syndromes*, Birth Defects: Orig. Art. Ser., vol. V, no. 2. White Plains:The National Foundation-March of Dimes, 1969, pp. 228-230.

8. Gross-Kieselstein, E., Abrahamov, A. and Ben-Hur, N.: Familial occurrence of the Freeman-Sheldon syndrome. *Pediatrics 47*:1064, 1971.

9. Pfieffer, R. A., Amnermann, M., Baisch, C. and Bollhoff, G.: Das Syndrom Von Freeman und Sheldon. *Z. Kinderheilkd. 112*:43, 1972.

10. Temtamy, S. A.: *Genetics Factors in Hand Malformations.* Thesis, The Johns Hopkins University, Baltimore, 1966.

11. Hashemi, G.: The whistling-face syndrome. *Indian J. Pediatr. 40*:23, 1973.

12. Stern, C.: *Principles of Human Genetics*, 3rd Ed. San Francisco:W. H. Freeman, 1973, p. 569.

Chromosomal Syndromes

Mechanisms of Chromosome Banding*

David E. Comings, M.D.

The discovery of chromosome banding has made it clear that there are still a number of things that we do not know about chromosome structure. These techniques have stimulated a number of investigations into the mechanisms of banding and the results of some of these will be described.

There are 3 major types of chromatin. Biochemical and cytologic studies indicate that the chromosome is basically composed of 3 different types of chromatin: 1) centromeric constitutive heterochromatin, 2) intercalary constitutive heterochromatin and 3) euchromatin (Table 1).[1-4] The different banding techniques basically involve distinguishing between these different types. Centromeric constitutive heterochromatin is usually localized around the centromere but may also occasionally occur at the telomere or in blocks in the chromosome arms. It is late replicating, genetically inactive, condensed during interphase and detected by C-banding. If an organism possesses satellite DNA, it is usually localized to centromeric-type heterochromatin. In some cases, however, this type of heterochromatin contains nonrepetitious DNA.[5,6] Intercalary constitutive heterochromatin occurs predominately in the chromosome arms and is

Table 1. Three Major Types of Chromatin*

	Centromeric Constitutive Heterochromatin	Intercalary Constitutive Heterochromatin	Euchromatin
Location	Usually pericentromeric	Chromosome arms	Chromosome arms
Detection	C-banding	G-banding Q-banding	G- and Q-interbands
DNA replication	Late	Late	Early
Interphase state	Condensed	Condensed	Usually diffuse
Genetic activity	Inactive	Inactive	Usually active
Satellite DNA	Usually present	Usually absent	Absent
AT-rich, nonrepetitious DNA	±	+	-
Resistant to extraction by 0.07 N NaOH in fixed chromosomes	+++	±	-

*Facultative heterochromatin (inactive X) not included.

*Supported by NIH grant GM-15886 and the Norman V. Wechsler Research Fund.

detected in these regions by Q- or G-banding. It is also late replicating[7-9] and condensed onto the inner surface of the nuclear membrane during interphase.[4] It is slightly AT-rich, not significantly enriched in repetitious sequences and is less methylated than euchromatin.[10-13] Euchromatin is early replicating, potentially genetically inactive, dispersed and forms the interbands of G- and Q-banding. Since no single characteristic distinguishes these 3 types of chromatin, it should not be surprising that there is no single mechanism responsible for chromosome banding. Rather, one or more of the characteristics of each type of chromatin also play a role in determining how they can be specifically elicited by the different banding techniques. The following general statements can be made about mechanisms of banding.

Histones are not involved. It has been suggested by some that histones play a role in chromosome banding. This, however, seems unlikely since treatment of chromosomes for up to 4 hours with 0.2 N HCl does not affect either Q-banding[14] or G- or C-banding.[15] This statement cannot be considered proved, however, until it is shown that the acid treatment really does extract histones from fixed, dried chromatin preparations. To demonstrate this, purified mouse interphase nuclei were fixed with methanol-acetic acid, dried onto slides and extracted with 0.2 N HCl for 4 hours. The nuclei were scraped off, solubilized in sodium dodecyl sulfate (SDS) and electrophoresed. This indicated that the histones had indeed been completely removed.[15]

Repetitious DNA is not involved. The initial C-banding technique arose as a consequence of the in situ hybridization studies by Pardue and Gall.[16] In their procedure to anneal radioactive satellite DNA onto mouse chromosomes, the fixed chromosomes were first treated with sodium hydroxide. They found that after staining the chromosomes with Giemsa there was intense staining of the centromeric heterochromatin. This led to the development of the C-banding technique by Arrighi and Hsu.[17] The relationship between repetitious DNA and centromeric heterochromatin implied that the repetitious DNA played some direct role in the

mechanism of C-banding. However, the following observations indicate that this is not the case. 1) Under various conditions, C-banding can be produced not only when the centrometric DNA is double-stranded and the DNA in the arms is single-stranded, but also when both are single-stranded or both double-stranded, and even when the centromeric DNA is single-stranded and the DNA in the arms is double-stranded.[18] 2) In the Chinese hamster about 10-15% of the genome stains as C-band heterochromatin but there is less than 1% satellite DNA.[6] More directly, it has been shown by in situ hybridization that some of the C-band heterochromatin in the Chinese hamster does not contain highly repetitious sequences (Hsu, personal communication). Presumably the presence of repetitious satellite DNA is indirectly involved in that it is associated with certain types of nonhistone proteins that are not present in the euchromatin. The repetitiousness per se seems not to be involved in C-banding. Once the satellite DNA is excluded there is no significant difference in the degree of repetitiousness of early and late replicating DNA,[19] making it unlikely that repetitious sequences play a role in G-banding either.

The mechanism of C-banding. In C-banding, as performed by the Arrighi-Hsu technique, the primary factor is the extensive extraction of DNA in the chromosome arms while the DNA of the centromeric heterochromatin is protected from extraction presumably by nonhistone proteins.[18] Efforts are presently underway to identify these protective proteins. While a similar protection of intercalary heterochromatin in the chromosome arms may be partially responsible for G-bands, it does not play the major role that it does in C-banding since G-bands can be produced without extracting significant amounts of chromosomal DNA.[18,20]

Base composition plays only a minor role. There are several lines of evidence which indicate that the DNA of G-bands is slightly more AT-rich than the DNA of interbands. This evidence is based on: A) ultracentrifugation studies which show that late replicating DNA is relatively AT-rich and early replicating DNA is relatively GC-rich,[10,12,13] B) studies with anti-nucleoside antibodies which suggest that the G-band material is AT-rich[21] and C) studies with acridine-orange banding which are also consistent with this interpretation.[2,18,22] Further evidence suggesting a role of base composition in Q-banding comes from the studies of Weisblum and deHaseth[23] and Pachmann and Rigler.[24] They demonstrated that AT-rich DNA enhances quinacrine fluorescence (QF) while DNA containing guanine quenches QF. This, in combination with the studies by Ellison and Barr[25] showing intense QF of a region of *Samoaia* chromosomes containing highly AT-rich satellite DNA, would seem to indicate that base composition was very important in Q-banding. However, we have observed that when the mouse DNA is fractionated into a GC-rich midband, AT-rich and satellite fractions by cesium chloride or cesium sulfate ultracentrifugation, all 4 fractions quench QF to the same degree.[26] This indicates that within the range of base composition found in any given organism the differential fluorescence is not sufficient to account for the chromosome banding. Thus, we would suggest that with the exception of some highly AT-rich satellite DNA, base composition per se plays a minor role in Q-banding.

Q-banding and nonhistone proteins. A further indication of the role of DNA protein interactions in Q-banding is shown by the fact that there are regions of heterochromatin in the mouse, human and muntjac which contain DNA that is either AT-rich or has the same base composition as main band DNA and yet fluoresce very poorly with QF.[14,27-29] When DNA and histones are combined in vitro, the presence of histones has no significant effect on inhibiting QF. Histones appear to bind in the large groove of DNA.[30-32] When the DNA is complexed with polylysine, polyarginine or spermine which bind in the small groove of DNA,[33-35] there is a significant inhibition of the binding of quinacrine to DNA. When mouse nuclei were subfractionated into 5 different chromatin fractions, a fraction rich in constitutive heterochromatin and in nonhistone proteins and a second fraction, rich in euchromatin

and in nonhistone proteins, showed an absolute decrease in the number of binding sites for quinacrine.[26] When DNA was isolated from these fractions, it bound to quinacrine just as well as DNA from the remaining fractions. Studies by Gottesfeld et al[36] have also shown that the different chromatin fractions quench fluorescence to different degrees, while the DNA from these fractions quench it to the same degree. Our interpretation of these findings is that the regions of the chromosome which stain poorly with quinacrine are due to the presence of nonhistone proteins binding in the small groove and inhibiting the intercalation of quinacrine.[26] This is consistent with the findings of Limon[37] that the ability to produce good banding is dependent in part upon the size of the group at the 9 position of quinacrine. Banding was absent when this group contained less than 3 CH_2 groups. Presumably the large group at position 9 lies in the small groove and when nonhistone proteins lie in the same groove it inhibits quinacrine binding.

The role of differential condensation. When trypsin treated chromosomes are stained with Feulgen, there is very little differential staining, while after staining with Giemsa, marked banding is apparent.[14] This indicates that variations in the amount of DNA along the metaphase chromosome are not the primary factor in chromosome banding. However, in some cases whole mount electron microscopy,[38,39] Feulgen staining[40-43] or phase contrast microscopy[44] have shown that there is some degree of differential condensation corresponding to the banded regions in mitotic chromosomes. This is borne out by the observation that in both the human[45] and Chinese hamster[46] there is an excellent correlation between the chromomeres of meiotic pachytene chromosomes and C- and G-bands of mitotic chromosomes. This indicates that the centromeric and intercalary constitutive heterochromatin, which are condensed during interphase, tend to remain differentially condensed during mitosis and meiosis.

G-banding. Giemsa is a complex dye composed of the oxidation products of methylene blue, which include azure A, B, C and thionin. These all belong to a group of dyes called the thiazins and have different numbers of methyl groups. We have found that all of them, except thionin, produce good C- and G-banding and that eosin is not necessary to produce banding. The thiazin dyes are highly metachromatic, which means that their absorption spectra change upon binding to chromotropes or upon increasing the concentration of the dye. This is due to a shift from monomer to dimer or polymer configuration of the dye. When these dyes are exposed to films of gelatin or gelatin plus DNA they undergo marked metachromatic shift. For example, with methylene blue the absorption peak at low concentrations is 660 nm while when bound to gelatin films it is 580 nm. When azure A and thionin are bound to gelatin films, the peak absorption is 560 nm. This indicates that the magenta complex described by Sumner et al[47] is due to marked metachromatic shifts of the thiazin dyes and is only minimally dependent upon the presence of eosin. A thorough knowledge of the mechanisms of G- and R-banding will only come from in vitro studies of kinetics of dye binding to isolated heterochromatin and euchromatin samples treated by the various techniques and then electrophoresed to determine the effect of the salts on specific proteins. These studies are in progress.

References

1. Comings, D. E.: The structure and function of chromatin. In Harris, H. and Hirschhorn, K. (eds.): *Advances in Human Genetics.* New York: Plenum Press, 1972, p. 237.
2. Comings, D. E.: Biochemical mechanisms of chromosome banding and color banding with acridine-orange. In: *Chromosome Identification — Techniques and Applications in Biology and Medicine.* Nobel Symposium. New York: Academic Press, 1973, vol. 23, p. 293.
3. Comings, D. E.: The structure of human chromosomes. In Busch, H. (ed.): *The Cell Nucleus.* New York:Academic Press, 1973, vol. 1, p. 537.
4. Comings, D. E. and Okada, T. A.: DNA replication and the nuclear membrane. *J. Mol. Biol.* 75:609, 1973.
5. Mattoccia, E. and Comings, D. E.: Buoyant density and satellite composition of DNA of mouse heterochromatin. *Nature (New Biol.)* 229:175, 1971.
6. Comings, D. E. and Mattoccia, E.: DNA of mammalian and avian heterochromatin. *Exp. Cell Res.* 71:113, 1972.
7. Ganner, E. and Evans, H. J.: The relationship between patterns of DNA replication and of quinacrine fluorescence in the human chromosome complement. *Chromosoma* 35:326, 1971.
8. Zakharov, A. F. and Egolina, N. A.: Differential spiralization along mammalian mitotic chromosomes. I. BUdR-revealed differentiation in Chinese hamster chromosomes. *Chromosoma* 38:341, 1972.
9. Pathak, S., Hsu, T. C. and Utakoji, T.: Relationships between patterns of chromosome banding and DNA synthetic sequences: A study of the chromosomes of the Seba's fruit bat, *Carollia perspicillata. Cytogenet. Cell Genet.* 12:157, 1973.
10. Comings, D. E.: Replicative heterogeneity of mammalian DNA. *Exp. Cell Res.* 71:106, 1972.
11. Comings, D. E.: Methylation of euchromatic and heterochromatic DNA. *Exp. Cell Res.* 74:383, 1972.
12. Tobia, A. M., Schildkraut, C. L. and Maio, J. J.: Deoxyribonucleic acid replication in synchronized cultured mammalian cells. I. Time of synthesis of molecules of different average guanine + cytosine content. *J. Mol. Biol.* 54:499, 1970.
13. Bostock, C. J. and Prescott, D. M.: Buoyant density of DNA synthesized at different stages of the S phase of mouse L cells. *Exp. Cell Res.* 64:267, 1971.
14. Comings, D. E.: Heterochromatin of the Indian muntjac: Replication, condensation, DNA ultracentrifugation, fluorescent and heterochromatin staining. *Exp. Cell Res.* 67:441, 1971.
15. Comings, D. E. and Avelino, E.: Mechanisms of chromosome banding. II. Histones are not involved. *Exp. Cell Res.* 86:202, 1974.
16. Pardue, M. L. and Gall, J. G.: Chromosomal localization of mouse satellite DNA. *Science* 168:1356, 1970.
17. Arrighi, F. E. and Hsu, T. C.: Localization of heterochromatin in human chromosomes. *Cytogenetics* 10:81, 1971.
18. Comings, D. E., Avelino, E., Okada, T. A. and Wyandt, H. E.: The mechanism of C- and G-banding of chromosomes. *Exp. Cell Res.* 77:469, 1973.
19. Comings, D. E. and Mattoccia, E.: Replication of repetitious DNA and the S period. *Proc. Natl. Acad, Sci. USA* 67:448, 1970.
20. Pathak, S. and Arrighi, F. E.: Loss of DNA following C-banding procedures. *Cytogenet. Cell Genet.* 12:414, 1973.
21. Schreck, R. R., Warburton, D., Miller, O. J. et al: Chromosome structure as revealed by a combined chemical and immunological procedure. *Proc. Natl. Acad. Sci. USA* 70:804, 1973.

22. Bobrow, M. and Madan, K.: The effects of various banding procedures on human chromosomes, studied with acridine orange. *Cytogenet. Cell Genet.* 12:145, 1973.

23. Weisblum, B. and deHaseth, P. L.: Quinacrine, a chromosome stain specific for deoxyadenylate-deoxythymidylate-rich regions in DNA. *Proc. Natl. Acad. Sci. USA* 69:629, 1972.

24. Pachmann, U. and Rigler, R.: Quantum yield of acridines interacting with DNA of defined base sequence. *Exp. Cell Res.* 72:602, 1972.

25. Ellison, J. R. and Barr, H. J.: Quinacrine fluorescence of specific chromosome regions. Late replication and high AT content in *Samoaia leonensis*. *Chromosoma* 36:375, 1972.

26. Comings, D. E., Kovacs, B. W., Avelino, E. and Harris, D. C.: Mechanisms of chromosome banding, III. Quinacrine banding. *Chromosoma*. (Accepted for publication.)

27. Jones, K. W. and Corneo, G.: Location of satellite and homogeneous DNA sequences on human chromosomes. *Nature (New Biol.)* 233:268, 1971.

28. Caspersson, T., Zech, L., Johansson, C. and Modest, E. J.: Identification of human chromosomes by DNA-binding fluorescent agents. *Chromosoma* 30:215, 1970.

29. Rowley, J. D. and Bodmer, W. F.: Relationship of centromeric heterochromatin to fluorescent banding patterns of metaphase chromosomes in the mouse. *Nature (Lond.)* 231:503, 1971.

30. Simpson, R. T.: Interaction of a reporter molecule with chromatin. Evidence suggesting that the proteins of chromatin do not occupy the minor groove of deoxyribonucleic acid. *Biochemistry* 9:4814, 1970.

31. Farber, J., Baserga, R. and Gabbay, E. J.: The effect of a reporter molecule on chromatin template activity. *Biochem. Biophys. Res. Commun.* 43:675, 1971.

32. Olins, D. E. and Olins, A. L.: Model nucleohistones: The interaction of F1 and F2a1 histones and native T7 DNA. *J. Mol. Biol.* 57:437, 1971.

33. Feughelman, M., Langridge, R., Seeds, W. E. et al: Molecular structure of deoxyribonucleic acid and nucleoprotein. *Nature* 175:834, 1955.

34. Suwalsky, M., Traub, W. and Subirana, J. A.: An x-ray study of the interaction of DNA with spermine. *J. Mol. Biol.* 42:363, 1969.

35. Wilkins, M. H. F.: Physical studies on the molecular structure of deoxyribonucleic acid and nucleoprotein. *Cold Spring Harbor Symp. Quant. Biol.* 21:75, 1956.

36. Gottesfeld, J. M., Bonner, J., Radda, G. K. and Walker, I. O.: Biophysical studies on the mechanism of quinacrine staining of chromosomes. *Biochemistry*. (In press.)

37. Limon, J.: Fluorescence of chromatin-bound acridine derivatives. *Exp. Cell Res.* (In press.)

38. Bahr, G. F., Mikel, U. and Engler, W. F.: Correlates of chromosomal banding at the level of ultrastructure. In: *Chromosome Identification — Techniques and Applications in Biology and Medicine*. Nobel Symposium. New York: Academic Press, 1973, vol. 23, p. 280.

39. Golomb, H. M. and Bahr, G. F.: Correlation of the fluorescent banding pattern and ultrastructure of a human chromosome. *Exp. Cell Res.* 84:121, 1974.

40. Rodman, T. C. and Tahiliani, S.: The Feulgen banded karyotype of the mouse: Analysis of the mechanisms of banding. *Chromosoma* 42:37, 1973.

41. Rodman, T. C.: Human chromosome banding by Feulgen stain aids in localizing classes of chromatin. *Science* 184:171, 1974.

42. Heneen, W. K. and Caspersson, T.: Identification of the chromosomes of rye by distribution patterns of DNA. *Hereditas* 74:259, 1973.

43. Yunis, J. J. and Sanchez, O.: G-banding and chromosome structure. *Chromosoma* 44:15, 1973.

44. McKay, R. D. G.: The mechanism of G and C banding in mammalian metaphase chromosomes. *Chromosoma* 44:1, 1973.

45. Ferguson-Smith, M. A. and Page, B. M.: Pachytene analysis in human reciprocal (10:11) translocation. *J. Med. Genet.* 10:282, 1973.

46. Okada, T. A. and Comings, D. E.: Mechanisms of chromosome banding, III. Similarity between G-bands of mitotic chromosomes and chromomeres of meiotic chromosomes. *Chromosoma* 48:65, 1974.

47. Sumner, A. T., Evans, H. J. and Buckland, R. A.: Mechanisms involved in the banding of chromosomes with quinacrine and Giemsa. *Exp. Cell Res.* 81:214, 1973.

Inherited Partial Trisomy 2: 46,XX,1p+;t(1;2) (p36;q31)

Richard J. Warren, Ph.D., Elma G. Panizales, M.D. and Ronald J. Cantwell, M.D.

The proband in our report is a female child who presents with serious psychomotor retardation. The mother's pregnancy with this child was full-term and uneventful. The birth was spontaneous with a good Apgar score. The birthweight and head circumference were in the 3rd percentile and length was in the 25th percentile. The child has suffered no trauma or serious illnesses since birth.

The child (Fig. 1) was first seen at 14 months of age because of delayed motor development and peculiar facies. She was ex-tremely floppy, unable to hold her head steady and unable to sit up even with support. At that time she did not respond to visual stimulation. At 22 months she continued to have generalized hypotonia and was still unable to sit up by herself. Her head size fell below the 3rd percentile, but her height remained at the 25th and her weight was at the 50th percentile. Her head was shortened in the AP diameter, the ears were low-set and placed backwards and downwards (Fig. 2). Her forehead was prominent but not unusually high. The chin receded but was

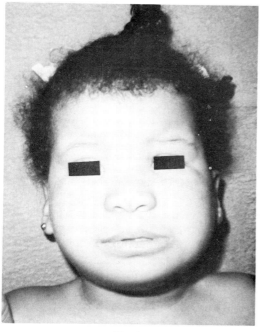

Fig. 1.

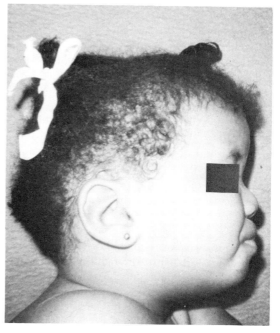

Fig. 2.

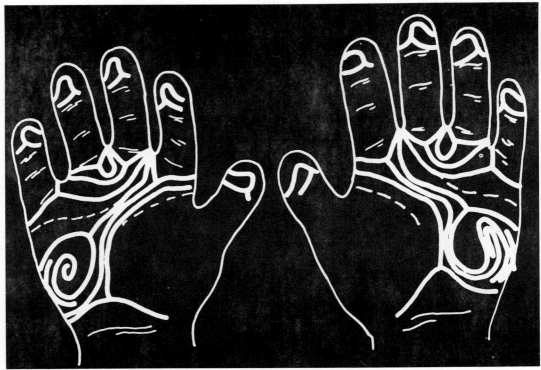

Fig. 3.

not hypoplastic and the posterior hairline was low.

The eyes had an antimongoloid slant, with bilateral epicanthal folds. She had hypertelorism. The pupils were equal in size and equally reactive to light. She had full extraocular movements but an A-pattern esotropia was seen. She had an inconsistent response to visual stimuli in that she resisted having her eyes covered but would not gaze at an object presented to her, nor would she follow one consistently. Her fundi were normal. The nasal bridge was flat and broad. The nasolabial philtrum was flattened. There was no labial nor palatal defect. She had only 4 erupted teeth at 22 months of age.

The neck was short but not webbed. Chest and abdomen were normal. There was a café-au-lait spot just below the right costal margin. Patches of depigmentation on the diaper area, secondary to diaper rash, were observed.

The hands were chubby and short with bilateral clinodactyly of the 5th fingers. There were clubfeet. Dermatoglyphics were abnormal (Fig. 3). Radial loops were seen on the 1st, 2nd

and 4th digits of the right hand and on the 2nd and 5th of the left hand. The atd angles were bilaterally elevated with t″ triradii. A large S pattern was present in the right hypothenar area and a large whorl pattern was seen on the left.

The skeletal survey mainly confirmed the clinical findings of equinovarus of the right foot and the shortened midphalanx of both 5th fingers. This was compatible with the clinodactyly. An IVP showed extra calyceal structures on the right upper pole, suggesting the presence of a cyst or diverticulum.

Psychometrics showed that she was functioning in the severely retarded level. She smiled spontaneously, put her hands together, but did not reach for any object presented to her. Speech was at a level of 3 months. Hearing tests were normal.

Reflexes were hypotonic and she had bilateral Babinski reflexes. Neck righting reflex was present, but she did not have a parachute response.

Chromosome studies revealed an abnormal number 1 chromosome (Fig. 4) that had extra

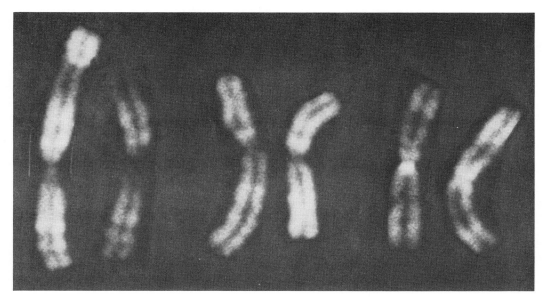

Fig. 4.

material translocated to its short arm. The mother's karyotype was normal. The father's karyotype, however, revealed a balanced translocation between number 1 and number 2 chromosomes (Fig. 5) and we think the description to represent the break points should be 46,XX,t(1;2)(p36;q31).

The family history, briefly, is that the mother is 32 and the father is 41 years of age. They are of Cuban descent and are negroid. The proband has 4 older sibs, all normal. The oldest, a boy, is a balanced carrier of the chromosomal translocation. Fertility was apparently not reduced and the history was negative for spontaneous miscarriages. The father has 2 retarded nieces in Cuba, but government restrictions prevent obtaining blood for chromosome studies.

Blood grouping studies, kindly performed by Dr. Thomas Noto of our University, failed to reveal an informative cross.

In conclusion, we have reported a child who is trisomic for region q31 of chromosome number 2. Other than severe psychomotor retardation and abnormal dermatoglyphics, the physical deformities resulting from this trisomy are few.

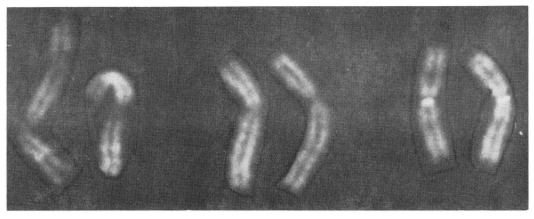

Fig. 5.

A New Recognizable Syndrome Associated with a Chromosomal Abnormality

Stanley D. Handmaker, M.D., D.Phil., Bryan D. Hall, M.D.
and Felix A. Conte, M.D.

A distinctive pattern of malformations was seen in a mother and her 2 sons. Their major findings include small ears; bilateral epicanthal folds; a broad nose with a high nasal bridge; malar hypoplasia; long philtrum; small mouth; pouting umbilical hernia; overriding scrotum; partial cutaneous syndactyly of digits 2 and 3 on both hands and feet; and bilateral transverse palmar creases.

Case Reports

Case 1

The proband, *M.D.*, was a 13½-year-old boy whose delayed development was first noted in infancy. He has never developed proper speech, and he has been variously described as moderately retarded and autistic. Observers have generally considered his behavior to be bizarre. Chromosome analysis done in 1963 was read as normal male, 46,XY. Family history was reported as negative for other persons with similar problems.

Except for decreased fetal movements, prenatal history was unremarkable. He was delivered vaginally following a full-term pregnancy, and he weighed 3090 gm at birth. Developmental milestones were delayed. He rolled over at 4 months, sat up at 9 months, walked without support at 21 months and has never talked in sentences.

Physical examination (Figs. 1-3) revealed height 150 cm, weight 32 kg and head circumference 54.5 cm (mean for age). Craniofacial features included low-set

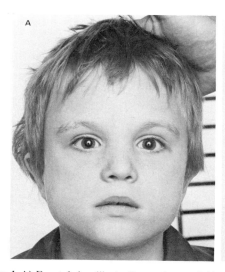
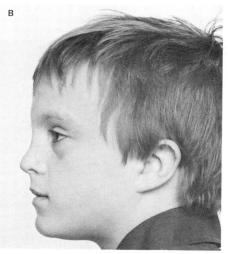

Fig. 1. *Case 1.* A) Frontal view illustrating antimongoloid eye slant, mild Brushfield spots, bilateral epicanthal folds, broad nasal bridge, long philtrum and small mouth. B) Lateral view illustrating high nasal bridge and low-set small ears.

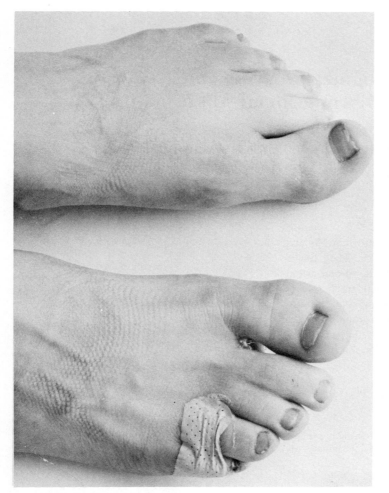

Fig. 3. View of feet of *Case 1* showing 2/3 cutaneous syndactyly.

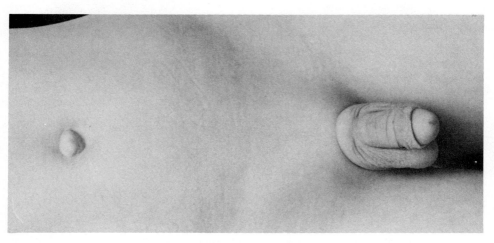

Fig. 2. Abdominal view of *Case 1* showing pouting umbilical hernia and overriding scrotum.

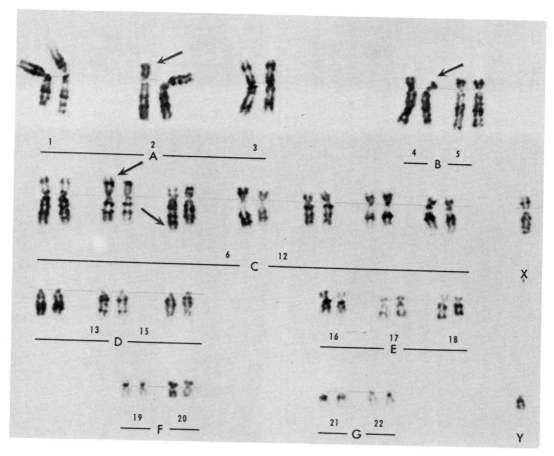

Fig. 4. Karyotype of *Case 1*. Arrows indicate sites of deletions of short arms of a No. 2 and a No. 4, and additions to short arm of a No. 7 and long arm of a No. 8.

small ears (left 4.5 cm, right 5.5 cm — more than 2 SD below mean); bilateral epicanthal folds; mild Brushfield spots; corneas 12 mm; antimongoloid eye slant; inner canthal distance 3 cm; interpupillary distance 5.25 cm; outer orbital distance 10.5 cm; mild malar hypoplasia; broad high nasal bridge; long philtrum; and small mouth with prominent frenulum of upper lip. Abdominal findings were pouting umbilical hernia and overriding scrotum. Abnormalities of the limbs included small broad hands; short nails; bilateral 2/3 finger syndactyly; bilateral 5th finger clinodactyly with single crease on right 5th finger; transverse palmar creases; and increased palmar markings. The dermal ridge patterns included 8 ulnar loops, 1 arch and 1 radial loop. The feet were short (19 cm), and there was 2/3 syndactyly — 80% on right and 60% on left.

Laboratory studies, including uric acid, serum calcium and phosphorus, and thyroid function, were all normal. Urine amino acid analysis by ion exchange chromatography showed no abnormalities, and combined gas chromatographic/mass spectrophotometric urine screen detected no abnormal organic acids.

Chromosome analysis of peripheral lymphocyte culture was performed using acid saline Giemsa banding. This revealed a 46,XY pattern, with deletions of the short arms on a No. 2 and a No. 4 chromosome, and additions on the short arm of a No. 7 and the long arm of a No. 8 (Fig. 4).

Case 2

S.D., the 7-month-old brother of the proband, was also noted to be developmentally slow. His birthweight was 2183 gm after a 36-week gestation. At birth, he was noted to be small-for-dates and to have a number of minor anomalies. During the neonatal period, he was treated with phototherapy for hyperbilirubinemia.

Physical examination (Figs. 5-8) revealed head circumference of 42 cm (2 SD below mean), anterior fontanel 4 × 4 cm, closed posterior fontanel and low-set small ears (3.25 cm — much more than 2 SD below mean) with a left helical pit. Facial features included bilateral epicanthal folds; small corneas (10 mm); inner canthal distance 2.5 cm; interpupillary distance 4.25 cm; outer orbital distance 7.5 cm; broad high nasal bridge; long philtrum; small mouth with prominent frenulum of upper lip; and nevus flammeus over glabellar area. Abnormalities of the limbs included mild bowing of forearm (left more than right); dimples at elbows and lateral wrists; small, broad and puffy hands; finger syndactyly of 2/3 and 3/4 on right and 2/3 on left; left thumb smaller and lower than right; hypoplastic flexion crease on left thumb; right simian crease; and left bridged simian crease. Dermal ridge patterns showed 6 ulnar loops and 4 whorls. His feet were short (7 cm) and puffy and were in an equinovarus position. The feet also showed dysplastic nails; excessive horizontal creases; borderline, laterally placed halluces; and bilateral 2/3 syndactyly (80% on left, 50% on right). In addition, he had pouting umbilical hernia, overriding scrotum, bilateral dislocated hips and pilonidal dimples.

Peripheral lymphocyte culture chromosome analysis revealed a 46,XY pattern with an addition to the long arm of a No. 8 (Fig. 9).

Case 3

E.D., the mother of the above children, had a history of severe emotional disturbance which required hospitalization for 3 months after *M.D.* was born. Her only other pregnancy resulted in an early trimester spontaneous abortion.

Physical examination (Figs. 10 and 11) revealed head circumference of 54 cm (25th%); low-set small ears (5.5 cm bilaterally); nevus flammeus over glabellar area; bilateral epicanthal folds; small corneas (10 mm); inner canthal distance 2.9 cm; interpupillary distance

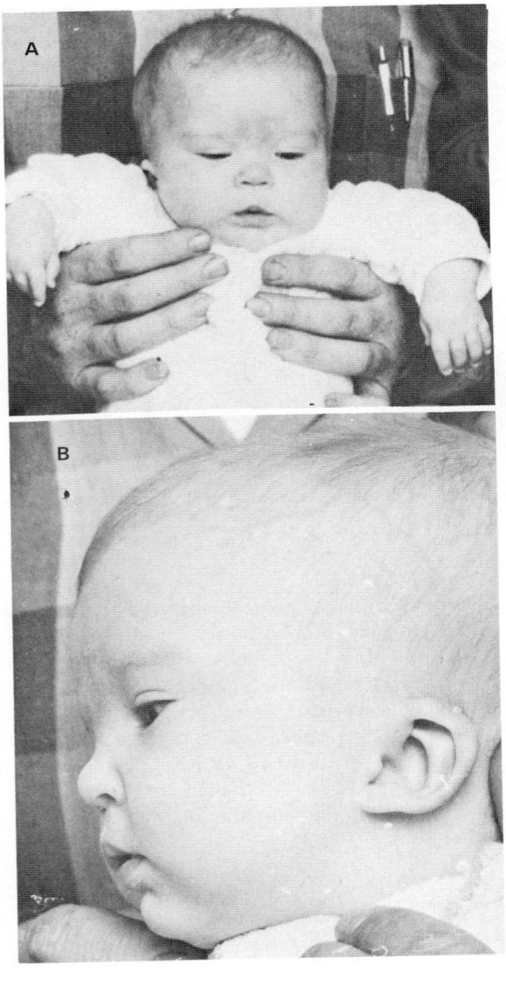

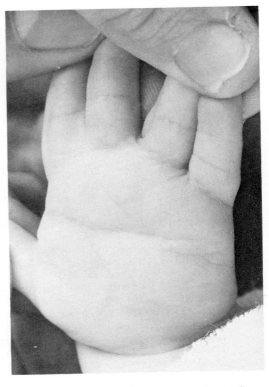

Fig. 5. *Case 2.* A) Frontal view illustrating wide nasal bridge, nevus flammeus, long philtrum and small mouth. B) Lateral view illustrating high nasal bridge, micrognathia and low-set small ear with helical pit.

Fig. 6. View of right hand of *Case 2* illustrating finger syndactyly of 2/3 and 3/4, and simian crease.

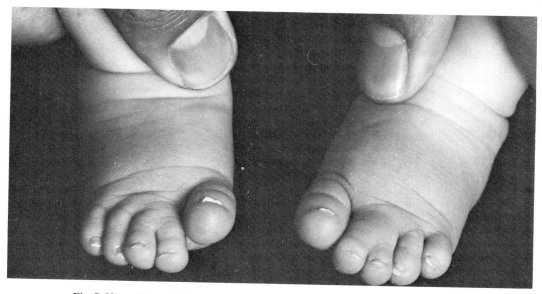

Fig. 7. View of feet of *Case 2* illustrating dysplastic nails and bilateral 2/3 syndactyly.

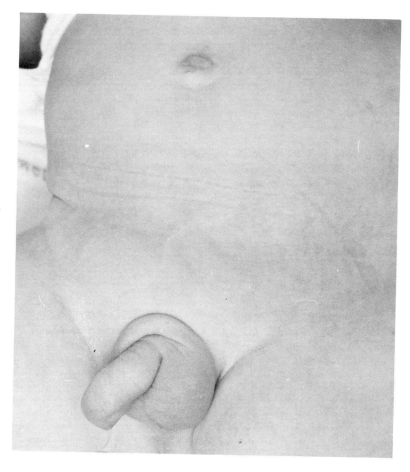

Fig. 8. View of abdomen of *Case 2* showing pouting umbilical hernia and over-riding scortum.

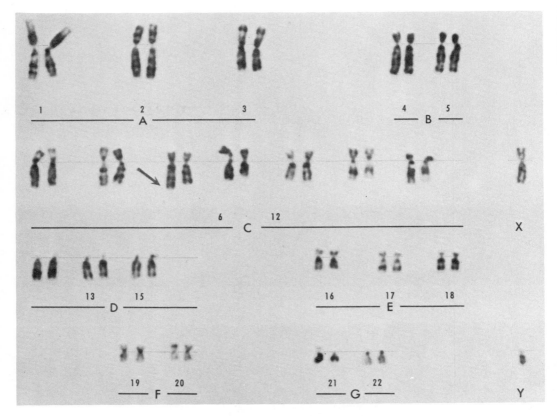

Fig. 9. Karyotype of *Case 2* illustrating addition to long arm of a No. 8.

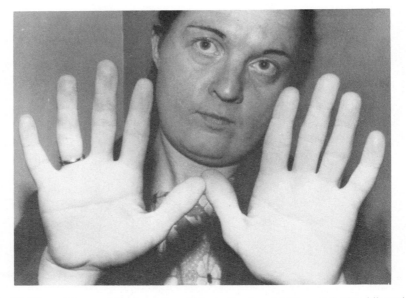

Fig. 10. View of face and hands of *Case 3* illustrating broad high nasal bridge, bilateral epicanthal folds, long philtrum, small mouth and bilateral simian lines.

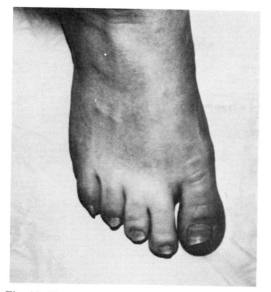

Fig. 11. View of right foot of *Case 3* illustrating 2/3 cutaneous syndactyly.

5.75 cm; outer orbital distance 11.0 cm; mild malar hypoplasia; broad high nasal bridge; long philtrum; and small mouth. Abnormalities of the limbs included short broad hands; mild 2/3 and 3/4 finger syndactyly; transverse palmar creases; and small feet (right 21.0 cm, left 20.5 cm) with bilateral 2/3 syndactyly (30%).

Chromosome analysis of peripheral lymphocyte culture revealed a 46,XY pattern with the same additions and deletions as found in *Case 1* (Fig. 12). The unaffected father of the boys (Fig. 13), as well as the mother's parents, had normal chromosomes.

Discussion

The pattern of malformations seen in this family constitutes a recognizable clinical syndrome which has not been previously reported. The occurrence of this distinctive pattern in a mother and both of her sons argues most strongly for a genetic etiology. Furthermore, to our knowledge, this represents the first description of humans having 4 separate chromosome abnormalities.

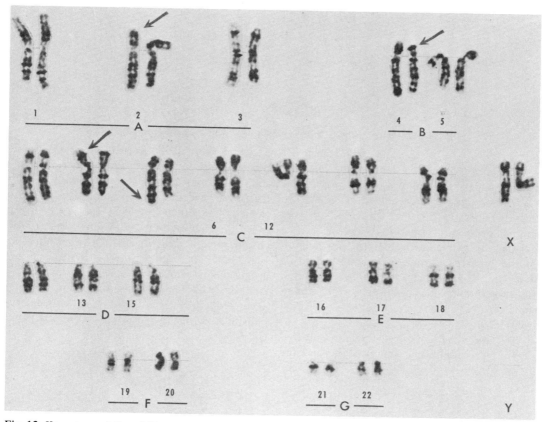

Fig. 12. Karyotype of *Case 3* illustrating deletions of short arms of a No. 2 and a No. 4, and additions to a short arm of a No. 7 and a long arm of a No. 8.

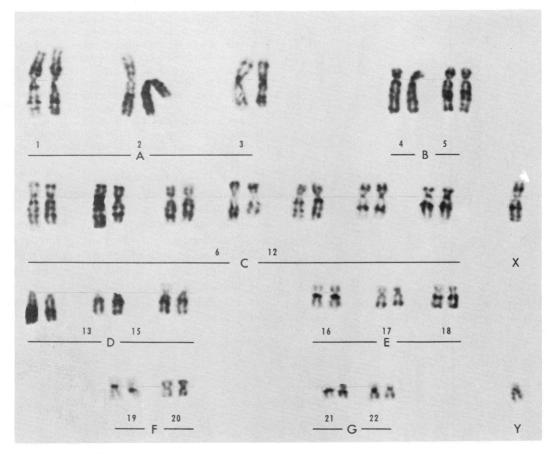

Fig. 13. Karyotype of the father of *Cases 1 and 2* illustrating no abnormalities.

The chromosomes of both of the mother's parents appear to be normal. This implies that the abnormalities arose either in the early zygotic divisions in the formation of the mother or in the formation of one or both of her parents' gametes. The simplest explanation of the observed chromosome abnormalities is that the 4 abnormal chromosomes resulted from the simultaneous occurrence of 4 chromosome breaks which gave rise to 2 separate translocations.

We are uncertain of the relationship between the chromosome abnormalities and the observed dysmorphology. The mother and one son, who appear to have balanced translocations, have the same pattern of malformations as the other son, who appears to have only the addition to the long arm of a chromosome No. 8 (Fig. 14). One possibility is that there are even further chromosome rearrangements which have escaped our detection, but which have resulted in genetic imbalance. Hopefully, identification of subsequent individuals with this pattern of dysmorphology will help to clarify the relationship.

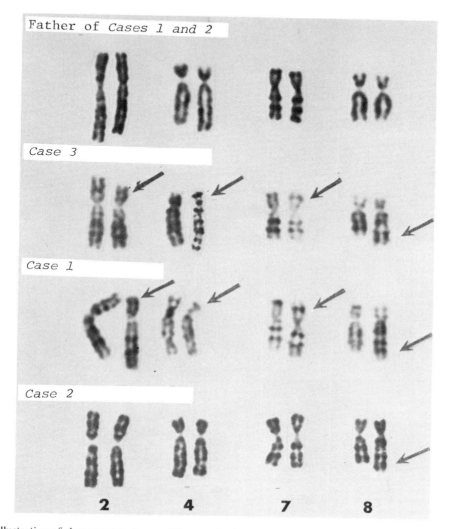

Fig. 14. Illustration of chromosome abnormalities seen in *Case 1, Case 2* and *Case 3* and no abnormalities seen in father of *Cases 1 and 2*.

A Partial Trisomy 5p Syndrome*

John M. Opitz, M.D.† and Klaus Patau, Ph.D.‡

A clearly defined (partial) trisomy 5p syndrome has not emerged from previously published reports.[1-5] We report here an infant girl with a multiple congenital anomaly/mental retardation (MCA/MR) syndrome presumably largely due to almost complete partial trisomy for the short arm of chromosome 5. A translocation between that chromosome and chromosome 12 was inherited in her family, and 4, or possibly 5, of her first and second degree relatives had a more or less severe expression of the same syndrome. This report is an attempt to define a syndrome associated with almost complete partial trisomy 5p. The history of multiple defective infants born over 2 generations to normal carriers suggested transmission of a chromosome abnormality in this family and was the reason for performing the clinical and cytogenetic studies reported below.

Case Reports

The *W/F Family* was ascertained through *III-6* (Fig. 1) who approached us in 1964 for a "genetic work-up" regarding recurrent infant deaths in her family. She and her mother (*II-3*) were interviewed before her third affected child (*IV-3*) was examined.

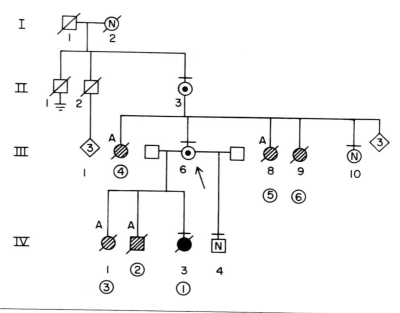

Fig. 1. Pedigree of the *W/F Family*. Bar over pedigree symbol: personally studied, cytogenetically or by PE. Diagonal line through pedigree symbol: Individual now dead. N within symbol: chromosomes apparently normal. Bull's-eye symbol: translocation heterozygotes. Solid black symbol: proved partial trisomy 5p. Cross-hatched individuals: suspected or presumed partial trisomy 5p. Arrow indicates proposita. Symbol grounded: no offspring during marriage. A above and to left of pedigree symbol: autopsy. Circled numbers: case numbers.

*Paper No. 1774 from the University of Wisconsin Genetics Laboratory; Studies of Malformation Syndromes of Man XXXV.

†Supported by NIH grants GM 15422, 5 KO4 HD 18982 and GM 20,130.

‡Supported by NIH grant GM 15422.

With the possible exception of this child's brother (*IV-2*), all of the deceased infants (*IV-1, III-4, 8 and 9*) had multiple congenital anomalies. The only defective individual in the family who was examined by us was *IV-3*; data concerning the 5 other deceased infants were collected from several Wisconsin physicians, hospitals and institutions and were more or less incomplete. *III-6*, her younger sister (*III-10*), her mother (*II-3*) and grandmother (*I-2*) were interviewed. These individuals were healthy and intelligent; they had no obvious anomalies. Since ascertainment of the family nearly 10 years ago, *III-6* has remarried and her son from that second marriage (born 7/24/72) is physically normal.

Case 1

J.M.F. (*IV-3*) was born on 10/5/66 after an unremarkable 40- to 43-week gestation, weighing 4026 gm and measuring 57 cm in length. She was hypotonic and her head was noted to be large (? 41 cm). At 2 months she was admitted to the Milwaukee Children's Hospital and was found to be reasonably alert. She was said to smile, follow and to turn her head. Her skull was long and narrow, measuring 46.75 cm in circumference; the occiput was prominent. The upper frontal region of the head was full, the anterior and posterior fontanels were large and full, and the sagittal suture appeared to be quite prominent. The pupils were relatively constricted. She had somewhat deformed external ears and a small umbilical hernia. Roentgenograms confirmed the clinical impression of premature closure of the sagittal suture, and thinning of the cranial vault suggested the diagnosis of hydrocephalus. Ventriculography demonstrated a Dandy-Walker malformation. The rest of the internal organs appeared normal on physical examination; pyelograms showed an apparently normal urinary tract. A ventriculoatrial shunt was created.

The infant was readmitted to the same hospital at 6 months with a head circumference of 48 cm for revision of a nonfunctioning Pudenz valve. Three days after discharge she had to be readmitted because of the onset of left-sided seizures. She had an infection of the right middle ear and fluid from the right ventricle was bloody. After antibiotic treatment and another revision of the valve, she improved and was discharged. She was treated with phenobarbital for her seizures.

The patient was examined by us at 7 months, after her discharge from the Milwaukee Children's Hospital and after a chromosome abnormality had been discovered in her mother and maternal grandmother. The baby appeared to be well-nourished and of normal length for her age (Fig. 2A); she was rather placid, hypotonic and apathetic, showing a paucity of spontaneous movements, but appearing otherwise healthy. Head circumference was 48.5 cm; the skull was long and narrow, the occiput was prominent (Fig. 2B) and she had marked frontal bossing (Fig. 2C). The anterior fontanel was large. The right and left ears were posteriorly angulated; the upper outer crus of the right

anthelix was absent and the fossa triangularis merged with an enlarged scapha. The left auricle showed indications of a similar developmental defect. The lower portion of both helices were hypoplastic (Figs. 2C and D). The inner canthal distance was 3 cm. She had bilateral external rectus weakness; mild micrognathia; rudimentary upper epicanthic folds; moderate mongoloid slanting of the palpebral fissures; and a faint, diffuse capillary hemangioma of the forehead. Her palate was somewhat narrow, she had a small umbilical hernia and her great toes were shorter than normal (Fig. 2E). She appeared markedly retarded; her muscle tone was greatly reduced, more so in the upper than in the lower limbs. She had a whorl pattern on both thumbs, ulnar loops on the rest of her fingers and distal loops in both hallucal areas of the sole. The rest of the physical examination was otherwise unremarkable.

During the succeeding years the child had multiple infections; she was profoundly retarded and died at home (on 2/12/71) at 4 4/12 years, possibly of renal failure; no autopsy was performed. Death certificate states death was due to atelectasis and probable bronchopneumonia.

Case 2

E.F. (*IV-2*) was born on 8/17/64 after an uneventful 43-week gestation, weighing 3345 gm and measuring 53.5 cm in length. Neither the attending physician nor the parents suspected any problems (although the birth certificate bears the notation: malformations – "yes"). In retrospect the mother states that he was relatively hypotonic and that he had a very poor cry. He died suddenly at home at 29 days. At the time of autopsy (report of the Milwaukee County Medical Examiner), he weighed 4536 gm and measured 56 cm in length; no external anomalies were noted and the fontanels were described as "patent and not bulging." The internal organs were apparently all unremarkable with the exception of the lungs: death was ascribed to "viral pneumonia." The central nervous system was not examined.

Case 3

M.F. (*IV-1*) was born on 6/6/63 after a 43-week gestation. Early during the pregnancy the mother's abdomen enlarged markedly. A roentgenogram at 5 months showed only one fetus. At birth the infant weighed 3119 gm and measured 48 cm in length; she was cyanotic and remained in an isolette for 3 days. Her head was described as large at birth (circumference 37.7 cm) and bilateral metatarsus varus deformities were corrected by casts. Ventriculograms during the first months of life did not show a hydrocephalus. Serial head measurements showed rather slow, although definite, enlargement. She manifested progressively greater psychomotor retardation; she sat at 10 months, pulled herself to a standing position at 12 months, said one or 2 words at 16 months. After her sixth month she fed poorly; this resulted in weight

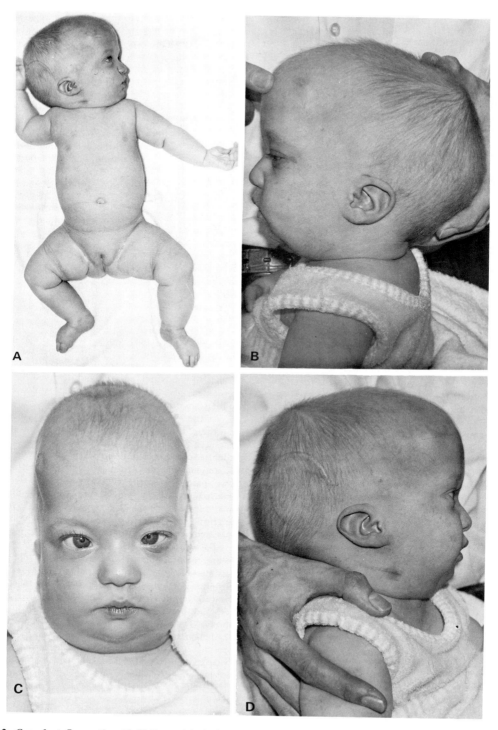

Fig. 2. *Case 1* at 7 months. A) Well-nourished, hypotonic, retarded infant; B) note long skull, micrognathia, position and shape of auricle; C) note narrow skull, lateral bifrontal bossing, apparent hypertelorism, slight mongoloid slant of palpebral fissures, upper epicanthic folds, apparent strabismus; D) scars of ventriculocaval shunt operation; E) short 1st toes.

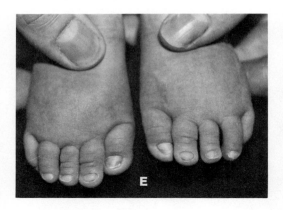

Fig. 2. Continued.

loss. At 6 months she was reexamined in the Milwaukee Children's Hospital and again was not found to have hydrocephaly. At that time she weighed 6435.5 gm (∿3rd%), she was 64.5 cm long (∿50th%) and her head circumference measured 45.5 cm (98th%). Six days before her death she developed a cold, but initially she was not particularly ill, and she had no fever until 2 days before death when she developed respiratory distress with severe coughing and moderate fever. She was readmitted to the Milwaukee Children's Hospital with a head circumference of 49 cm (∿90th%), a weight of 7881 gm and a right upper lobe pneumonia. Epinephrine did not relieve her severe wheezing and retraction. Distress increased, the respiratory rate varied from 50-60/minute, and she developed pin-point pupils, areflexia, flaccidity, unresponsiveness and extreme pyrexia (temperature 108°F rectally). She died suddenly on the following day at 17 months of age.

The immediate cause of death was congestive heart failure due to, or accompanied by, acute interstitial pneumonia, atelectasis and emphysema, and a chronic nonspecific laryngotracheobronchitis. The autopsy protocol also states that the infant had a pectus excavatum, residual clubfoot deformities, shortness of the great toe phalanges and of the first metatarsals, and an accessory spleen. The brain weighed 1460 gm (about 400 gm above average). The ventricles were not dilated, no gross brain abnormalities were found and the finding of marked widening of periglial, perineuronal and perivascular spaces was interpreted as evidence of cerebral edema, which may have been responsible for the 3.5 cm increase in head circumference which occurred between admission and death.

Case 4

K.L.W. (III-4) was born on 12/21/40 after an uneventful 40-week pregnancy, weighing 3203.5 gm and measuring 48.5 cm in length. The child had difficulty crying for about the first month after birth; she was said to go through all of the emotional manifesta-

tions of crying, but would become cyanotic without being able to make the noise of a cry. The mother stated that the child had always been weak and sickly, that she was a poor feeder and that she showed a paucity of body movements. Her head was not remembered as being unusually large. Her breathing had been very noisy since birth.

The infant appeared to be in good health until 2½ months when she began to cry "as if in pain." A mass appeared in the right groin and the child became feverish. She was admitted to the Milwaukee Children's Hospital and was noted to be dehydrated and ashen colored; her respirations were shallow, labored and very rapid, and were accompanied by definite lower costal retraction. "There seemed to be marked depression just right of the xiphoid." She had a lateral nystagmus and 11 days after the onset of the illness her temperature rose from 103.6°F to 106° after a bilateral myringotomy was performed for purulent otitis media. Heart and mediastinum appeared to be shifted to the right and the right portion of the diaphragm was elevated. Roentgenographic and fluoroscopic examinations of the chest showed infiltrates of the right upper lobe and middle portion of the right lung, poor expansion of the thorax and hypoventilation of the right lung which improved when the child was made to cry. There were no visible bone centers at the wrist. Anomalies of the little finger and radiographic signs of mongolism or of any other skeletal defects of hands and feet were not observed. The child developed increasingly severe respiratory distress and respirations ceased suddenly.

At the time of autopsy the infant was exactly 3 months old; she was described as very thin and she measured 56 cm in length (3rd%); there was a "mongoloid expression about the eyes and nose." She had an umbilical hernia and a right inguinal hernia. The lower part of the right chest was somewhat deformed and "pulled in." The pupils were 2.5 mm in diameter and round. The head was "somewhat long" and the anterior fontanel measured 3.5 × 2 cm. The bronchi appeared small; the left main stem bronchus measured 4 × 3 mm in diameter compared to a 7 × 5 mm measurement obtained in a 5-week-old child. There was marked atelectasis of the right upper lobe and the posterior portion of the right middle lobe. There were 2 small accessory spleens. The kidneys were normal and the brain (weight 750 gm) appeared grossly normal. There was bilateral purulent otitis media. The diaphragmatic and intercostal muscles were thick and considered hypertrophic. Cause of death was thought to be staphylococcal sepsis accompanied by bronchitis and bronchiolitis with "congenital atresia of bronchi."

Case 5

M.A.W.(a) (III-8) was born on 8/19/49 after a normal, full-term (40-week) gestation with a birthweight of 3430 gm. She was considered an apparently normal baby in the neonatal period, but "her breathing had always been of a stuffy nature." At the 6-week examination she was found to have very prominent veins on her chest and an apparent murmur indicating possible congenital heart disease. One week before death she developed a cold; on the day of death she developed diarrhea and vomiting; a temperature of 104°; and rapid, weak and shallow respirations. On admission to St. Michael's Hospital in Milwaukee she was found to be cyanotic and dehydrated, and she had a loud systolic murmur which was heard over the entire precordium. She died shortly after admission at the age of 4 months. The extremely brief postmortem protocol states that the infant appeared well-developed and well-nourished; the pupils were equal and measured 2 mm in diameter. The heart was twice the normal size. The patent ductus arteriosus was 2 times normal size and connected the pulmonary artery with the right subclavian artery. The left kidney was 3 times normal size; its pelvis and calyces were distended and its cortex measured 1-2 mm in thickness. The right kidney was twice normal in size and showed changes similar to those of the left kidney. The cause of death was stated as "congenital heart disease and bilateral hydronephrosis."

Case 6

M.A.W.(b) (III-9) was born at term on 12/6/50 and died on 1/17/56. The pregnancy was apparently unremarkable; at birth the infant weighed 3544 gm and she measured 49½ cm in length. She was cyanotic at birth and suffered intermittent apneic spells during the first month of life. She stayed in an incubator with oxygen for about one month after birth; improvement in respiratory efficiency coincided with irradiation of the thymus during the first month of life. Her head was noted to be large; however, a head circumference measurement was lacking for the first 6 months. After discharge from the hospital the infant fed poorly; she was lethargic, her head rolled uncontrollably, and her psychomotor maturation progressed at an extremely slow rate.

At 6 months she measured 67 cm in length (between 50th-75th%), she weighed 7257.6 gm (50th%) and her head circumference was 47 cm (>98th%). Shortly thereafter she was admitted to the Milwaukee Children's Hospital to be evaluated for hydrocephalus. On admission her head circumference was 48½ cm, the fontanels were wide and the head was flattened from side to side. Pyelograms showed a dilated right ureter. Chest roentgenograms showed "retraction of the heart to the right" and considerably increased density of the medial portion of the right lung and some emphysema at the base suggesting probable "massive atelectasis of the right lower lobe." Ventriculograms showed grade 1-2 dilatation of the lateral ventricles and some enlargement of the third ventricle with air being present subdurally. The fourth ventricle and aqueduct were seen and appeared normal. These findings were interpreted as evidence either for cerebral atrophy or for internal hydrocephalus. She was discharged to be observed and

managed conservatively; however, 2 months later her head measured 50 cm and she was readmitted to the Milwaukee Children's Hospital for a spinoureterostomy during which "the thickened, dilated and widened right ureter was isolated" and the right kidney was removed. Upon opening the dura mater the neurosurgeon noted that "the spinal cord seemed to be lower than normal" and he speculated that this apparent deformity may have led to the development of the hydrocephalus. The right kidney measured 5.2 × 3.7 × 2.5 cm; the surface was lobulated and the cortex and medulla measured 3 and 7 mm, respectively. Many tubules were dilated to a cystic degree, more prominently so in the medulla than in the cortex.

During the next 18 months she grew in length from 76 to 84 cm (25th%); her weight increased from 7938 to 9185 gm (<3rd%); her head circumference remained arrested at 49.5 cm (between 50th-98th%). She started to sit up at 18 months, but was noted to show a deformity of the spine. Orthopedic evaluation showed that the muscle tone of the upper limbs was below that for a child of her age. "Her chest cage was underdeveloped" and she had a lower dorsal-lumbar kyphoscoliosis, causing some prominence of the left chest posteriorly. Radiographically a 20° left dorsolumbar curve was found with an apex at D12, as well as a spina bifida occulta at L5. The vertebral deformity was attributed to hypotonia of the trunk muscles.

After 3½ years she developed numerous respiratory infections which were preceded or accompanied by unusually high fevers and stiffness of the neck. At 4 3/12 years she was hospitalized briefly at the Milwaukee Children's Hospital for convulsions lasting 2-3 hours, cyanosis, gurgling respirations, incontinence and petechiae around the head and face. Legs and feet were found to be hyperextended, the arms were flaccid, eyes were turned to the right and the left pupil was smaller than the right and failed to react to light. She was unresponsive and her temperature was 104°F. It was thought that this episode had been precipitated by a bout of pharyngitis and possible hyponatremia. She was treated with antibiotics, salt and phenobarbital, and she improved quickly. Her chest film at that time showed a triangular shadow in the right cardiophrenic angle which was interpreted either as a fat pad or as atelectasis of the lower lobe. Her head was grossly deformed and showed a large occiput; her face was flat. There was a slight anterior thoracic deformity.

Recurrent bouts of fever prompted an evaluation at the University of Wisconsin Children's Hospital; this showed that the left kidney was normal on the pyelogram; she had the above-mentioned scoliosis and in addition, spina bifida was noted of L1 and L2 (surgical ?). ECG showed sinus arrhythmia with incomplete right bundle branch block.

At 5½ years she was admitted to the Southern Wisconsin Colony and Training School because of

Table 1. Tabulation of Some of the Manifestations of the
Defective Infants in the W/F Family

Manifestation	Case No.					
	1	2	3	4	5	6
Gestation (wks)	40-43	43	43	40	40	40
Birthweight (gm)	4026	3345	3119	3203	3430	3544
Birth length (cm)	57	53.5	48	48.5	?	49.5
Birth head circumference (cm)	?41	?	37.7	?	?	?
Age of death	4 4/12	29d	1 5/12	3/12	4/12	5 6/12
Growth failure (length)	-(7/12)	?	?	+	?	+
"Large head" (CNS anomaly)	+	?	+	?	?	+
		Dandy-Walker				?Arnold-Chiari; int. hydrocephalus
Dolichocephaly, prominent occiput	+	?	?	+	?	+
Severe mental retardation	+	?	+	?	?	+
Pupillary constriction	+	?	+	+	+	+
Hypotonia (uppers > lowers)	+	+	+	+	?	+
Respiratory and/or crying difficulties	-	+	+	+	+	+
Seizures	+	-	-	-	-	+
Clubfeet	-	-	+	-	-	-
"Pectus excavatum"	-	-	+	+	?	+
Hernia (umbilical and/or inguinal)	+	?	?	+	-	-
Accessory spleen(s)	?	-	+	+	-	-
Renal/ureteral anomalies	-*	-	-	-	bilateral hydro-nephrosis	"small cystic right kidney; dilated right ureter"
Congenital heart disease	-	-	-	-	PDA	IRBBB
Short first toes	+	?	+	?	?	?

*Death due to renal failure?

mental retardation. At this time she was sitting alone and could walk with support, but she was unable to speak. She was then 101 cm tall (<3rd%); she weighed 19.5 kg (50th%); and her head measured 52 cm in circumference (between 50th-98th%), 20½ cm in length and 15 cm in width. The interpupillary distance was 5 cm; she had a highly arched palate, 20 teeth (8 incisors, 4 canines, 4 premolars and 4 molars) and a pilonidal "cyst." She died 7 days after admission following an episode of laryngitis with high fever, cyanosis, loose stools and progressive debilitation, unresponsiveness and preterminal coma. No autopsy was performed. Death certificate states cause of death: "Encephalopathy, spina bifida, hydrocephalus."

Phenotypic Analysis

The biologic nature of the condition in these 6 cases is primarily conveyed in the narrative clinical histories; Table 1 summarizes the available vital statistical data and the manifestations of these patients. The incompleteness of several of these case reports notwithstanding, we think that all 6 patients probably had the same condition. III-6 and her mother state

that all 6 of these infants resembled each other strikingly in appearance, their initially weak cry and "stuffy" respirations and the paucity and "weakness" of their movements. The pathologist of *Case 4* stated that the patient had "a mongoloid expression about the eyes and nose"; this suggests similarity to the appearance of *Case 1*.

With respect to malformations these cases can probably be graded in severity: *Cases 2 and 5* appear to have been the least obviously malformed, *Cases 1 and 6* the most severely affected, with *Cases 3 and 4* representing an intermediate degree of severity. The manifestations of the condition may be summarized and interpreted as follows:

A) Postnatal death occurred between 29 days and 5½ years. Respiratory disease was the most common cause of death; *Case 1* may have died of "renal failure."

B) Postnatal growth failure (following normal intrauterine growth) was documented in 2 cases and may have been present or become evident in others had they lived longer.

C) Severe mental retardation was evident in the 3 children who lived over 6 months.

D) In addition, they probably all shared an MCA syndrome which involves predominantly the 1) CNS, 2) tracheobronchial tree and 3) kidneys (possibly other viscera) and which includes 4) certain minor anomalies and changes of appearance.

1) CNS: "Large head," internal hydrocephalus (of unknown pathogenesis), Dandy-Walker malformation, possible spinal cord malformation, MR, unusual pupillary responses, hypotonia and its complication (clubfeet, micrognathia, high and narrowly arched palate, chest infections) can probably all be cited or regarded as manifestations of CNS involvement in this syndrome. This may also be true of seizures, or else they may represent the results of CNS surgery and/or infection.

2) Tracheobronchial involvement: Neonatal respiratory distress, cyanosis, stridor, later atelectasis, chest deformity and hypertrophy of diaphragmatic and intercostal muscles can all be explained on the basis of narrowing of the tracheobronchial tree which was actually demonstrated in one case. We think that it is much more likely that *Case 2* died of this cause rather than of the "sudden infant death syndrome" or of "viral pneumonia." Patency of the ductus arteriosus may also reflect pulmonary rather than primary cardiovascular involvement.

3) Renal involvement: "Death due to renal failure" (no autopsy data available), bilateral hydronephrosis and unilateral dilatation of a ureter associated with a hypoplastic polycystic kidney represent the known urologic manifestations of the partial trisomy 5p syndrome.

Accessory spleen(s) in *Cases 3 and 4* suggest that other viscera may also be affected.

4) Appearance and minor anomalies: The effect of this trisomy 5p syndrome on appearance and occurrence of minor anomalies is documented, in part, in the illustrations (Fig. 2) and includes presumed premature synostosis of the sagittal suture (to produce dolichocephaly), relative shortness of 1st toes and a possible increase in the number of ulnar loops on the fingertips. Upon careful dissection further anomalies would presumably have been found.

Cytogenetic Observations

With ordinary staining (mostly azure A), the chromosomes of the proposita were found to be normal except for the presence of considerable extra material at the long arm of a C chromosome (Fig. 3). The aberration turned out to have been inherited. The carrier was the proposita's mother, and, further back, her mother. These women had the chromosome Cq+

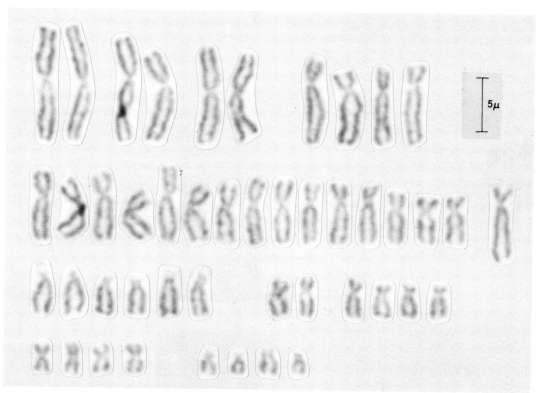

Fig. 3. Karyotype of *Case 1*. Note chromosome Cq+ at right of C group.

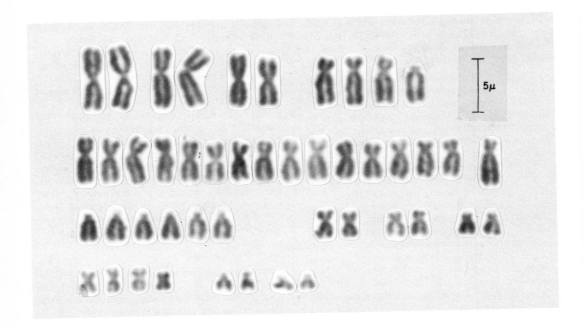

Fig. 4. Karyotype of maternal grandmother of *Case 1,* representative also of mother's karyotype. Note chromosomes Bp- and Cq+.

but also a deletion comprising almost the whole short arm of a B chromosome (Fig. 4). Fluorescent quinacrine staining (Fig. 5) showed the carriers to be classic examples of a reciprocal translocation of the type t(5p-;12q+). The proposita was trisomic for almost the whole arm 5p and, presumably, monosomic for a terminal segment of 12q, but this segment must have been very small. Individuals *IV-4, III-10 and I-2* have apparently normal chromosomes.

Cytogenetic Interpretation

The short arm of the present chromosome 5p-seems to be as minute as that of any cri-du-chat chromosome seen by us or reported elsewhere and is much shorter than that found in most such cases.

Furthermore, an unknown part of that short arm, conceivably even the whole arm, is likely to consist of a translocated terminal segment of 12q. Thus, our patients were trisomic probably not only for all genes that are deleted in most cri-du-chat children but also for a block of genes that are never, or at least usually not, included in cri-du-chat deletions. It is therefore hardly surprising that the partial 5p trisomy syndrome in this family was by far more severe than it was in the other cases reported to date (see below). However, it must not be forgotten that some of the anomalies of the present patients may have resulted from the terminal 12q deletion — small as it is, it may still be larger than any 12q deletion described previously (eg the 3q;12q translocation studied by Herrmann et al[6]).

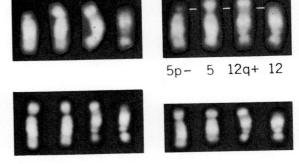

Fig. 5. Top: The reciprocal translocation chromosomes 5p- and 12q+ and their normal partners in grandmother (left) and mother (right) of *Case 1.* Bottom: The corresponding chromosomes from 2 cells of *Case 1* with partial trisomy for 5p. Quinacrine fluorescence.

5p− 5 12q+ 12

In view of the relatively large 5p segment for which our patients were trisomic, it is possible that the present 5p- chromosome, if not balanced by its reciprocal translocation partner, was prenatally lethal, which would explain the absence of the cri-du-chat syndrome in this family.

Discussion

In 1963 Lejeune and co-workers described the cat cry syndrome[7,8]; in 1964 they reported its "reciprocal" state in 2 sisters whose phenotypically normal 46,XX,t(5p-;Dq+) carrier mother also had 2 children with the cat cry syndrome.[1] One of these partial trisomy 5p girls had the appearance of a "normal newborn infant"; her 16½-year-old sister was profoundly retarded and short of stature, and had "small eyes without epicanthus," hypertelorism, normal ears, 10 ulnar loops, overlap of 5th over 4th toes, and normal menses and secondary sexual characteristics.

Laurent and Robert[2,3] published a 46,XX,t(5p-;?Cq+) mother who had 3 boys with the cat cry syndrome, and one boy with a presumed partial trisomy 5p syndrome consisting of mental retardation; full facies; slightly large tongue; scaphoplagiocephaly; bilateral ectopy of testes; slight hypertelorism and mongoloid slanting of palpebral fissures; ogival palate; clinodactyly of both 5th fingers; and 9 ulnar loops.

De Capoa et al[4] studied a 46,XX,t(5p-;Dq+) man who had a son with the cat cry syndrome and 2 children with partial trisomy 5p. One of these is cited as having "moderate mental retardation" and as being "physically quite normal"; the other as "slightly mentally retarded with no apparent malformations." These 2 children had 19 ulnar loops. Noel et al[5] reported a balanced 46,XX,t(5p-;Gp+) woman who had a cytogenetically normal girl, 2 cat cry syndrome children and a girl with partial trisomy 5p, who at 7 years was of normal height (127 cm) and weight; had a normal head circumference (52 cm); dolichocephaly; minor anomalies of the auricles; bilateral clinodactyly; 5 ulnar loops; and an IQ of 25.

The above reports on 6 cases of partial trisomy 5p from 4 families have not added up to a clearly defined 5p+ syndrome. Three of them are said to be "physically normal"; 2 of these 3 are retarded, but the "normal newborn infant" studied by Lejeune et al may have developed MR later. The only other manifestations which the other 3 cases share with each other and/or with our cases are hypertelorism (2 cases, ref. 1-3); dolichocephaly (patient of Noel et al and 3 of our cases); mongoloid slanting of palpebral fissures (ref. 2,3 and our *Case 1*); clinodactyly (ref. 2,3,5); shortness of stature (ref. 1 and our *Cases 4 and 6*); and minor anomalies of the auricles (ref. 5 and our *Case 1*). No dermatoglyphics are cited in one of the cases,[1] 5 others had each 10, 9, 5, 10, 9 and 8 (our *Case 1*) ulnar loops. This seems to be a significantly increased incidence of ulnar loops. Since some of the earlier reports lack sufficient clinical detail, the frequencies of these manifestations may actually be higher. Nevertheless, it seems evident that in the previously described instances of partial trisomy 5p the frequency and severity of component anomalies is too low to add up to a characteristic definable syndrome.

Our cases are not only more severely affected but also have a somewhat different syndrome from the previously reported cases. We have suggested above that these differences and the unusual severity of the present cases reflect at least in part the inclusion into the trisomic segment of additional important genetic material which was not included in the previously reported cases[1-5] and which is not usually included in cat cry deletions. There may also have been an effect of the terminal 12q deletion, which, although very small, may still be larger than any previously detected. It is interesting to note that in the present family the terminal 12q deletion may have been combined with as many as 4 different normal chromosomes No. 12 (ie those from the husbands of the 2 carrier women *II-3 and III-6*). This may have contributed to some of the clinical differences between the several affected children.

We do not think that the condition(s) due to partial trisomy 5p should be called the "anti-cat cry syndrome" or the "reciprocal" or "countertype" of the cat cry syndrome.

Addendum

The proposita's mother (*III-6*) is pregnant again; amniocentesis performed by Dr. G. E. Sarto of the University of Wisconsin, Department of Obstetrics and Gynecology, showed that she is carrying a 46,XY fetus with a balanced 5p-12q+ translocation. The mother has elected to carry the pregnancy to term.

References

1. Lejeune, J., Lafourcade, J., Berger, R. and Turpin, R.: Ségrégation familiale d'une translocation 5∿13 déterminant une monosomie et une trisomie partielles du bras court du chromosome 5: maladie du "cri du chat" et sa "réciproque." *CR Acad. Sci. (Paris) 258*:5767-5770, 1964.
2. Laurent, C. and Robert, J.-M.: Etude génétique et clinique d'une famille de 7 enfants dans laquelle trois sujets sont atteints de la "maladie du cri du chat." *Ann. Génét. 9*:113-122, 1966. (Same family is reported in ref. 5).
3. Robert, J.-M., Hugon, G., Laurent, C. et al: La maladie Cri du chat: à propos d'une fratrie avec trois observations et un syndrome réciproque. *Lyon Méd. 46*:1037-1132, 1966.
4. De Capoa, A., Warburton, D., Breg, W. R. et al: Translocation heterozygosis: A cause of 5 cases of the *cri du chat* syndrome and 2 cases with a duplication of chromosome number 5 in 3 families. *Am. J. Hum. Genet. 19*:586-603, 1967.
5. Noel, B., Quack, B. and Thiriet, M.: Ségrégation d'une translocation balancée t(5p-;(7p+). *Ann. Génét. 11*:247-252, 1968.
6. Herrmann, J., Ruffle, T., Meisner, L. F. et al: The partial trisomy 3q syndrome. (Abstract) This volume.
7. Lejeune, J., Lafourcade, J., de Grouchy, J. et al: Délétion partielle du bras court du chromosome 5. Individualisation d'un nouvel état morbide. *Sém. Hôp. 40*:1069-1079, 1964.
8. Lejeune, J., Gautier, M., Lafourcade, J. et al: Délétion partielle du bras court du chromosome 5. Cinquieme cas de syndrome du cri du chat. *Ann. Génét. 7*:7-12, 1964.

Discussion

Moderator: Can anybody be of help to Dr. Opitz in answering his request for additional information on similar cases?

Dr. Dixson: We have 2 patients who are partially trisomic for 5p. One is a male, 26 years old, who is mildly retarded; otherwise, physically normal. His sister, about 23 years of age, is physically normal, has an IQ of about 35. There are 2 other sibs. One is a 12-year-old normal male and the youngest sib is a 9-year-old boy with trisomy 21 and a balanced translocation which is also present in the father.

Dr. Alfi: Are photographs available of any of the family members who died early?

Dr. Opitz: Unfortunately, no. All we have is the hearsay evidence concerning their appearance.

Dr. Alfi: If we take all of these trisomy 5p cases, apart from the cases that we have just heard about now, this would be a very unusual situation, in which the 5p- monosomy (the cat cry syndrome) is surviving and the trisomic condition is lethal.

Dr. Opitz: I know of no a priori reason why this cannot occur, although in this case the explanation is made difficult by the presence of a terminal 12q deletion in the individuals who are trisomic for 5p.

Dr. Warren: I am wondering about the antithetical hypothesis, as with antimongolism. Can you relate what you see to the other side of the coin?

Dr. Opitz: No, in this syndrome I see no clinical "opposites" to the cat cry syndrome and I cannot think of any a priori biologic reason why the idea of countertypes or "reciprocal" or "antisyndrome" should be valid. I think that idea should be abandoned.

The 9p Trisomy Syndrome Due to Inherited Translocation*

Felice Weber, M.D., Helga Muller, M.D. and Robert Sparkes, M.D.

The recently developed differential chromosome stains are permitting the recognition and definition of new chromosomal syndromes. The trisomy 9p is one such syndrome and the case presented below, as well as others from the literature, demonstrates the utility of chromosome banding analysis in establishing this syndrome.

Case Report

T.B. born 11/7/68 was the 2440-gm product of a normal full-term pregnancy of a 25-year-old para 2, gravida 2 mother and a 25-year-old father. Her early appearance was not noted to be strikingly unusual, but her subsequent development was slow: sat without support at 9 months; crawled at 14 months; walked with support at 20 months; and said first words at 20 months. At 18 months, she had H. influenza meningitis and required myringotomy for otitis media.

At 20 months of age she was referred for evaluation of suspected Rubinstein-Taybi syndrome. At that time her physical features included open anterior fontanel (2.5 cm), parietal bossing, widely spaced eyes, left esotropia, low-set ears, widening of the bridge of the nose, epicanthal folds, right simian line, short broad thumbs, broad feet, height and weight at the 3rd percentile and head circumference at the 10th percentile. A skull x-ray film showed wormian bones. X-ray films of the hands and feet showed a 6-month bone age, broad appearance of the great toes and internal rotation of the talus. A developmental quotient was estimated at 53.

Evaluation at 5 years of age (Fig. 1) demonstrated a head circumference of 49.5 cm (normal) and the parietal bossing was less prominent. Height was 101 cm and weight was 16.4 kg (both below 3rd%). In addition to earlier described findings she was noted to have antimongoloid slant, down-curving mouth, deep crease between lower lip and chin, large anthelix, anthelical dimple, dysplastic nails, short thumbs with bulbous ends, single crease on the 3rd, 4th and 5th fingers bilaterally and 5th finger clinodactyly bilaterally.

Dermatoglyphics showed: on the right, 5 digital arches and absent *d* palmar digital triradius; on the left, 5 digital arches and absent *b, c* and *d* palmar digital triradii. Air conduction hearing was normal. On the Utah Test of Language Development she scored at the 2 5/12-year level and on the Assessment of Children's Language Comprehension Test she scored below the 3-year level. Based on the Peabody Picture

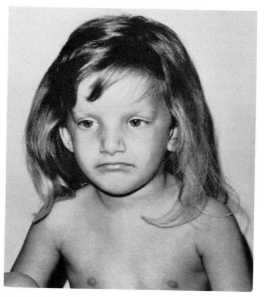

Fig. 1. *T.B.* at 5 years of age. Note the hypertelorism, antimongoloid slant, epicanthal folds, down-curving mouth and fleshy nose.

*Supported in part by grants HD-04612 and HD-05615 from the National Institute of Child Health and Human Development.

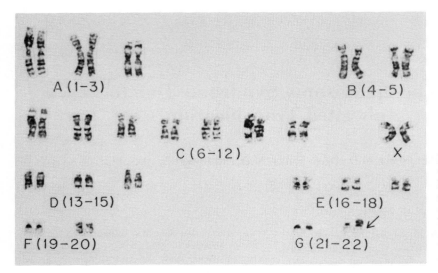

A (1-3)

B (4-5)

C (6-12)

X

D (13-15)

E (16-18)

F (19-20)

G (21-22)

Fig. 2. Trypsin-Giemsa banding karyotype on *T.B.* showing the 22p+ chromosome; the p+ banding pattern is compatible with it being 9p chromosome material.

Vocabulary Test she was estimated to have an IQ of 59.

Laboratory studies included normal routine urine and blood analyses. Serum protein electrophoresis, quantitative immunoglobulins and hemoglobin electrophoresis were all normal. Red cell galactose-l-phosphate uridyl transferase was elevated at 34.5 units (normal 18-28). She and her parents showed normal inheritance patterns for HL-A antigens, red blood cell antigens (ABO, Lewis, Rh, MNSs, Duffy, Lutheran, Kell, Kidd), Gm, Inv, phosphoglucomutase and haptoglobin.

The family history was negative for the occurrence of other similar problems. The patient had one older sister and the mother experienced no miscarriages. Shortly after initial referral the father died of acute lymphocytic leukemia, as had his mother at age 47.

Cytogenetic Studies

The routine blood chromosome analysis of the proband showed 46,XX,Gp+ which was also present in a skin biopsy. Trypsin-Giemsa banding analysis showed 46,XX,22p+ (Fig. 2). Chromosome analysis on her mother was normal. However, her father showed 46,XY,t(Gp+;Cp-) in blood, skin and bone marrow samples; he died before more definitive banding studies could be performed. The patient's sister (*R.B.*) showed a pattern similar to that of her father in blood and skin. Trypsin-Giemsa banding demonstrated an apparent balanced and reciprocal 46,XX,t(9p-;22p+) (Fig. 3); most of the short arms of the affected No. 9 chromosome were missing but satellites appeared to be present on the remaining short arms. C-banding analysis showed the characteristic heavy staining around the centromere of the No. 9 chromosome confirming the impression that the centromeres were probably not translocated. The father's brother and

father had normal chromosomes without evidence of the translocation. The final chromosome interpretations were: sister *R.B.* had 46,XX,t(9;22)(pl;pl)pat; proband *T.B.* had 46,XX,der(22),t(9;22)(pl;pl)pat.

Discussion

Based on routine chromosome studies in which the affected C group chromosome was identified as a No. 9 chromosome because of its prominent secondary constriction, Rethore and co-workers[1] formulated the concept of the 9p trisomy syndrome. There had been earlier cases with partial Cp trisomies[2-11] but only that of Butler et al,[9] utilizing the prominent secondary constriction of the No. 9 chromosome, suggested a 9p trisomy. Rethore et al[12] studied one new case and reevaluated 7 earlier reported cases[1,5,13,14] with chromosome banding analysis and demonstrated all had a 9p trisomy. Based on clinical phenotypes they determined that the 2 cases of Cantú et al[15] also had the same chromosome syndrome. Subsequently, 3 additional cases[16,17] have been found by banding analysis to have the same chromosome change. Evaluation of all 12 cases in which banding analysis has been performed (including present case) suggests the concurrence of a number of phenotypic features in common (Table 1). Our own case lacked only the deep-set eyes, microcephaly and brachycephaly.

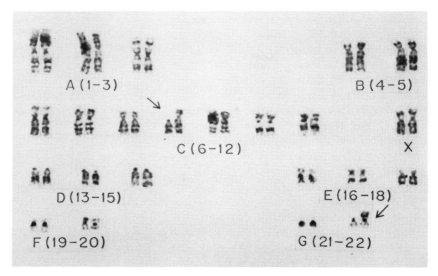

Fig. 3. Trypsin-Giemsa banding karyotype on *R.B.* showing the apparent balanced and reciprocal translocation with satellites from a No. 22 chromosome on the short arm of the affected No. 9 chromosome and most of the short arms of a No. 9 chromosome translocated to a No. 22 chromosome.

Of the 12 cases, 4 also had a short neck, 4 had clinodactyly, 3 had parietal prominence and 3 had hydronephrosis. As noted by Rethore et al,[12] the 2 cases of Cantú et al[15] also had many of the features listed in Table 1. The sexes appeared to be almost equally affected, with 5 males and 7 females. In general the birthweight among the term infants was within normal limits. When the degree of retardation had been estimated, it seemed to be of mild-to-moderate degree. Most of the cases (9 of 12) have resulted from an inherited translocation, 6 having come from the mother and 3 from the father. The trisomy appears to include most of the short arm of the No. 9 chromosome and the translocation has involved chromsomes 15, 18, 19 and 22. Since some, and perhaps all but 2, represent reciprocal translocations, the persons with the 9p trisomy also have some partial monosomy for another chromosome. To what extent the monosomy contributes to the variability of the clinical phenotype remains to be determined.

As with other chromosomal syndromes, there does not appear to be a single pathognomonic finding and the anomalies which are found are also present in many of the other chromosomal syndromes. In addition to varying genetic and environmental backgrounds, there are possible variabilities due to differences in the extent of the trisomy, the possible position effects depending on where the 9p material is translocated, as well as the above noted different monosomies resulting from the translocation.

Another aspect of the problem is why so many of the Cp trisomies appear to be 9p trisomies. Does this reflect some special character-

Table 1. Phenotypes in Cases with Trisomy 9p*

Phenotype	Proportion Affected
Mental retardation	9/9
Hypertelorism	12/12
Fleshy nose	10/10
Simian crease	11/12
Phalangeal hypoplasia	10/12
Deep-set eyes	9/11
Absent digital palmar triradii (*b* and/or *c*)	8/10
Brachycephaly	8/10
Antimongoloid slant	8/10
Microcephaly	8/11
Unusual flexion creases on fingers	8/11
Down-curving mouth	7/10
Protruding ears	6/10
Epicanthal folds	4/10
Anomalous anthelix	4/10

*Based only on cases on whom chromosome banding studies have been done, including present case. Cases with a specific phenotype are included only if report notes its presence or absence.

istic of the No. 9 chromosome or some selective factor against survival of other Cp trisomies or some unrecognized factors?

Finally, in the family reported here, there was the unusual occurrence of acute lymphocytic leukemia in the proband's father and his mother; the father was a carrier of the translocation, but it is not known whether his mother also had the translocation. The leukemic aspect of the problem was the subject of a previous report[18] in which earlier quinacrine fluorescent studies indicated a 12p trisomy, which is inconsistent by the present trypsin-Giemsa banding analysis in his daughters. The apparent lack of occurrence of leukemia in other 9p trisomic translocation families suggests that the occurrence of leukemia in the present family probably is not related to the chromosome change, although this possibility cannot be definitely excluded.

References

1. Rethore, M. O., Larget-Piet, L., Abonyi, D. et al: Sur quatre cas de trisomie pour le fras court du chromosome 9. Individualisation d'une nouvelle entite morbide. *Ann. Genet. (Paris) 13*:217, 1970.
2. Edwards, J. H., Fraccaro, M., Davies, P. and Young, R. B.: Structural heterozygosis in man: Analysis of two families. *Ann. Hum. Genet. 26*:163, 1962.
3. Gray, J. E., Dartnall, J. A., Creery, R. D. A. and Croudace, J.: Congenital anomalies due to transmission of a chromosome translocation. *J. Med. Genet. 3*:59, 1966.
4. Gray, J. E., Darnall, J. A. and MacNamara, B.: A family showing transmission of a translocation between a 6-12 chromosome and a 21-22 chromosome. *J. Med. Genet. 3*:62, 1966.
5. Lejeune, J., Berger, R., Rethore, M. O. et al: Translocation Cc/F familiale, determinant une trisomie pour le bras court du chromosome 12. *Ann. Genet. (Paris) 9*:12, 1966.
6. de Grouchy, J., Roy, C., Lachance, R. et al: Trisomie partielle C par translocation t(Cp-;Bq+). *Arch. Fr. Pediatr. 24*:849, 1967.
7. Lord, P. M., Casey, M. D. and Laurence, B. M.: A new translocation between chromosomes in the 6-12 and 21-22 groups. *J. Med. Genet. 4*:169, 1967.
8. Insley, J., Rushton, D. I. and Jones, H. W.: An intersexual infant with an extra chromosome. *Ann. Genet. (Paris) 11*:88, 1968.
9. Butler, L. J., Eades, S. M. and France, W. E.: Transmission of translocation t(Cp+;Dq-) through three generations. Including an example of probable trisomy for the short arm of the C group No. 9. *Ann. Genet. (Paris) 12*:36, 1969.
10. Deminatti, M., Maillard, E., Gosselin, B. et al: Trisomic partielle C par translocation t(Cp-;Gp+). *Ann. Genet. (Paris) 12*:36, 1969.
11. Lozzio, C. B. and Kattini, A. A.: Familial transmission of a chromosomal translocation t(2q+;Cp-). *J. Med. Genet. 6*:174, 1969.
12. Rethore, M. O., Hoehn, H., Rott, H. D. et al: Analyse de la trisomie 9p par denaturation menagee. A propos d'un nouveau cas. *Humangenetik 18*:129, 1973.
13. Hoehn, H., Engel, W. and Reinwein, H.: Presumed trisomy for the short arm of No. 9 chromosome not due to inherited translocation. *Humangenetik 12*:175, 1971.
14. Rott, H. D., Schwanitz, G. and Grosse, K. P.: Partielle Trisomie Cq bei balancierter B4/C9 Translokation bei der Mutter. *Z. Kinderheilkd. 109*:293, 1971.
15. Cantú, J. M., Buentello, L. and Armendares, S.: Trisomie Cp: Un nouveau syndrome. *Ann. Genet. (Paris) 14*:177, 1971.
16. Baccichetti, C. and Tenconi, R.: A new case of trisomy for the short arm of No. 9 chromosome. *J. Med. Genet. 10*:296, 1973.
17. Ebbin, A. J., Wilson, M. G., Towner, J. W. and Slaughter, J. P.: Prenatal diagnosis of an inherited translocation between chromosomes No. 9 and 18. *J. Med. Genet. 10*:65, 1973.
18. Hinkes, E., Crandall, B. F., Weber, F. and Craddock, C. G.: Acute leukemia with C-G chromosome translocation. *Blood 41*:259, 1973.

Discussion

Dr. Centerwall: We have also seen a case (see Abstracts, p. 326). I would like to make the point that the first cases were discovered and reported in 1970 by Marie Rethore from Lejeune's lab in Paris, France; then, in 1973, she summarized the 10 cases which were known up to that time. I think that this will now make 15 cases known. I think that the clinical findings are adequate enough to make the diagnosis or at least to strongly suspect it, from the clinical morphology.

Dr. Poznanski: Is there phalangeal hypoplasia? Which phalanges are affected, and how?

Dr. Weber: There was no actual phalangeal hypoplasia, but the thumbs were short with soft tissue swelling which gave them a broad appearance.

Dr. Cantú: We described 2 cases in 1971 with the regular nonbanding methods. Now we have confirmed those findings with the Giemsa banding. We found that it was a 9p syndrome. This case is almost the same as the case reported. I would like to ask you if you have found delayed bone age, because it was a finding that we observed in 2 cases? We reviewed the cases some months ago and found that they started with convulsions at 9 years of age. They are 2 children. I understand that Dr. Loesch in Warsaw has found another family with 2 cases of 9p trisomy, in which the translocation involved another acrocentric. I think that this is important to differentiate, to exclude partial micro-monosomies, as in the case presented by Dr. Opitz.

Dr. Weber: I think that this would be very difficult. Her bone age was delayed. At 21 months of age her bone age was 6 months.

Dr. Feingold: There have been quite a few cases reported now with 9p trisomy. We described a trisomy 9. I was wondering whether anyone had ever seen a trisomy 9. The only one of which I am aware is the one that we described. Has anybody else seen it? If not, why not?

Moderator: No one seems to have seen such a patient.

10p-: A New Autosomal Deletion Syndrome?*

Uta Francke, M.D., George M. Mahan, M.D.,
Barbara K. Dixson, R.N., M.N. and Oliver W. Jones, M.D.

Case Report

K.H., a 5-year-old girl with mental and growth retardation; brachy- and trigonocephaly; antimongoloid slants; hypotelorism; epicanthal folds; ptosis; strabismus; dysplastic nose; high-arched palate; microdontia and dental crowding; small, low-set and posteriorly rotated ears; asymmetric thorax; wide-spaced nipples; and minor abnormalities of hands and feet, was found to have partial deletion of the short arm of a chromosome 10.

Genetic Background. Both parents were American blacks, unrelated, healthy and of normal height and intelligence. They were 25 years old at the patient's birth. There was a 7-year-old normal brother. Father and brother had bronchial asthma. The mother's fingers showed significant distal tapering, a sign which was also present in the patient, but not in the brother.

Potentially Dysmorphogenetic Environmental Influences during Gestation. The mother received several series of active immunizations against poliomyelitis, typhus, typhoid, cholera and influenza during the time period from approximately 3 weeks before to 6 weeks after the estimated time of conception.

Patient's History. After 9 months of uncomplicated gestation, the patient was delivered spontaneously from occipitoposterior position. Apgar rating at 1 minute was 7. Birthweight was 3300 gm. The newborn was feeding poorly and had a weak cry. She was hospitalized after one tonic-clonic seizure at 6 months of age. The work-up was entirely normal, and no seizures have occurred since then. The child had a history of continuous nasal discharge. Growth and motor development had been moderately retarded. She sat at 7 months and walked at 2 years. She started to talk and became toilet-trained at 5 years of age.

Patient Evaluation

Growth Retardation. Height was 104 cm (between 3rd and 10th%) and weight 17.5 kg (10th%). Bone

*Supported in part by The National Foundation-March of Dimes.

age, according to the standards of Greulich and Pyle, was 5 years at a chronologic age of 5 4/12 years when height age was 4 years. The short stature appeared proportionate (Fig. 1).

Developmental Retardation. At 3 4/12 years her IQ score was 47 on the Cattell Infant Intelligence Scale. When tested with the Stanford-Binet Intelligence Test at 5 3/12 years, she scored in the severely retarded range with 33. Her behavior was hyperactive and she was reportedly very slow to respond in classroom situations. Speech was significantly delayed. Her voice was hoarse and she had a habit of tongue thrusting. A hearing test was normal.

Craniofacial Abnormalities. The head was symmetric and of normal circumference (51.5 cm, 50th%), but brachycephalic and mildly trigonocephalic with a narrow, slightly prominent forehead and a wide biparietal diameter. Radiographs of the skull showed the metopic suture to be fused and the presence of prominent digital markings on the lateral aspects. The striking narrowness of the face was further manifested by hypotelorism, dysplastic nose and narrow, high-arched palate (Fig. 2). The nasal bridge was wide with prominent epicanthal folds, and there were bilateral antimongoloid slants. Orbital dimensions were as follows: inner canthal distance 2.5 cm (close to mean), outer orbital distance 8.5 cm (2 SD below mean), interpupillary distance 4.75 cm (below mean). Eye abnormalities included bilateral ptosis, more severe on the left; esotropia and amblyopia of the left eye; and bilateral astigmatism (Fig. 3). The left optic disk revealed irregularity of the temporal margin. The external ears were short with well-formed helices and prominent anthelices. They were symmetrically low-set and slightly posteriorly rotated (Fig. 4). The teeth were small, irregular and poorly spaced in the upper and lower anterior segments. The lateral upper incisors were peg-shaped (Fig. 5).

Thorax Abnormalities. The thorax was asymmetric with left anterior prominence. The nipples were wide-spaced (IND 15.5 cm, chest circumference 54.5 cm). There was flaring of the lower ribs.

Limb Abnormalities. The palms could not be flattened out fully, and the thumbs remained in

207

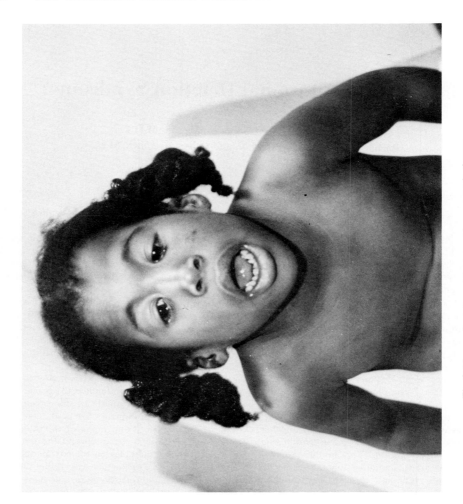

Fig. 2. Narrow face, hypotelorism and asymmetric thorax.

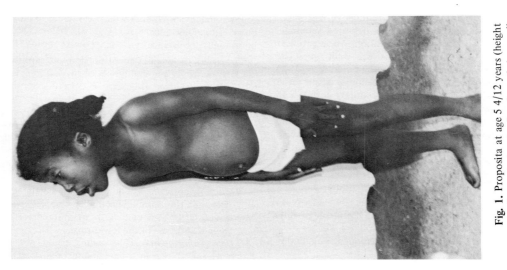

Fig. 1. Proposita at age 5 4/12 years (height age 4 years) showing brachycephaly, small low-set ears, flat nose and pes planus.

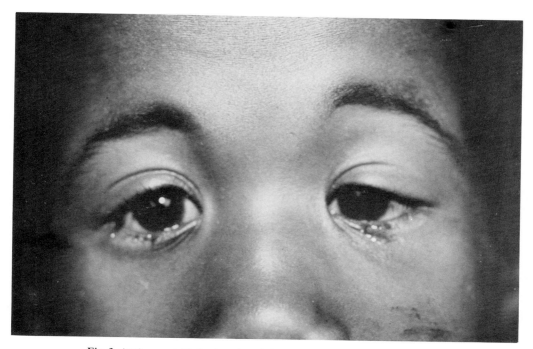

Fig. 3. Antimongoloid slants, epicanthal folds, bilateral ptosis and left esotropia.

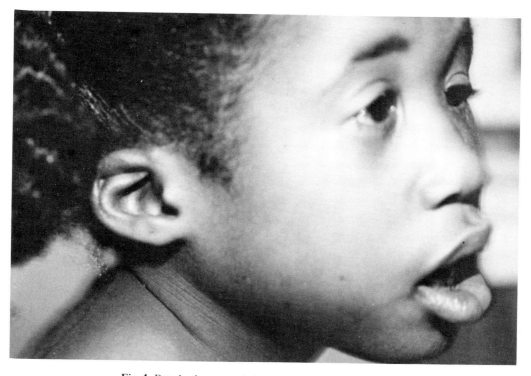

Fig. 4. Dysplastic nose and short, low-set, posteriorly rotated ear.

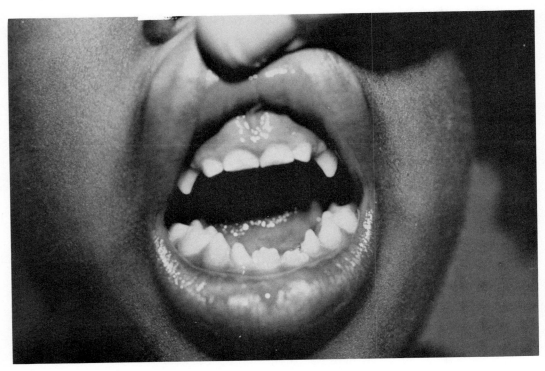

Fig. 5. Microdontia and poor spacing.

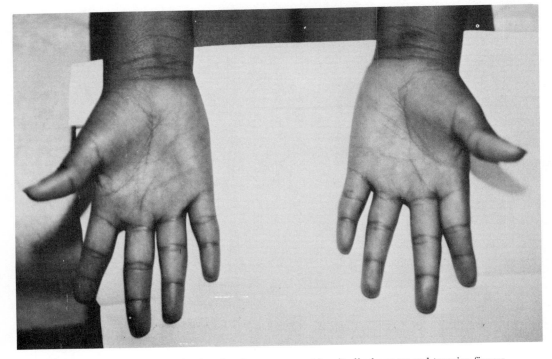

Fig. 6. Incompletely flattened palms showing pronounced longitudinal creases and tapering fingers.

slightly opposed position. There were abnormal longitudinal creases. The fingers were hyperextensible and showed tapering of the terminal phalanges (Fig. 6). This abnormality was also found in the patient's mother, and probably represented an independent genetic trait. Both 5th fingers showed mild clinodactyly. The dermatoglyphic patterns were very similar to the findings in the other family members. The child walked with a wide-based gait and legs in external rotation. Her feet were narrow and completely flat. The 3rd toes were slightly longer than the 2nd toes, and the 5th toes were slightly curved outward. Radiographs of the feet showed pseudoepiphyses in the proximal parts of both 2nd metatarsals.

Laboratory Examinations. Tests which yielded normal results included EEG, radiographs of chest and hands, IVP, routine blood counts and urinalysis, and metabolic screening on urine.

Cytogenetic Findings. A chromosome study performed in 1971 without banding techniques for chromosome identification was reported as normal. Recently, peripheral blood lymphocytes and skin fibroblasts were cultured for a repeat study. In all of 22 trypsin-Giemsa banded and 20 quinacrine mustard stained metaphases from blood and 8 from skin, a

partial deletion of the short arm of one chromosome 10 was apparent. There was no evidence of translocation of the missing piece onto another chromosome. The breakpoint appeared to be located in band 10p13; the intensely staining band p14 was clearly absent (Figs. 7 and 8). Whether the deletion was terminal or interstitial could not be determined with certainty. The patient's karyotype was designated 46,XX,del(10)p13. The parents' and brother's karyotypes were normal.

Comments

The usefulness of banding techniques for identification of structural chromosomal abnormalities has once again been demonstrated. In the earlier unbanded karyotype, the 10p- chromosome was apparently interpreted to represent a chromosome No. 12, which has the lowest short-arm/long-arm ratio in the C group, and thus it had escaped detection.

To our knowledge, this is the first report of a patient with a del(10)p chromosomal abnor-

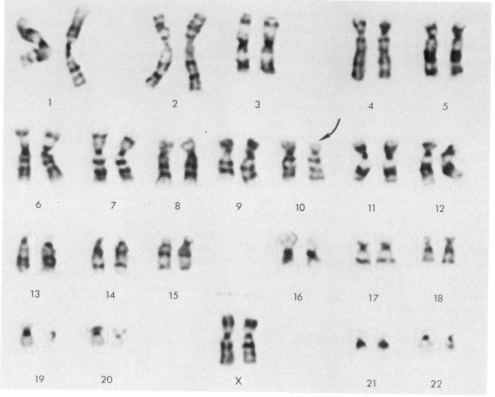

Fig. 7. Karyotype of proposita: 46,XX,del(10)p13. G-banding pattern produced by Giemsa staining after trypsin treatment of air-dried metaphase spreads from peripheral lymphocyte culture, in modification of the method described by Seabright.[1]

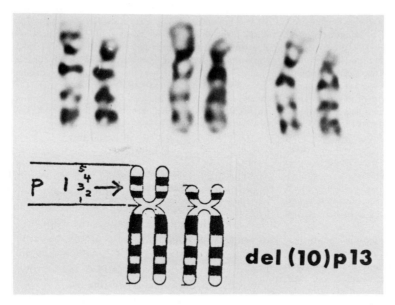

del (10) p13

Fig. 8. Chromosome pair 10 from different cells with G-banding and ideogram demonstrating breakpoint in region p13.

mality. It represents the fourth short-arm deletion of a C-group chromosome shown to be compatible with life. One single case each, with a ?6p- and a 12p- deletion and 3 cases with 9p-syndrome have been reported.[2-4] All these patients displayed dysmorphogenetic features distinctly different from our patient.

The significance of the different live vaccines that were given to the mother around the time of conception for the origin of chromosome deletion, retardation or dysmorphogenetic features cannot be determined. Although one could speculate that a deleterious effect on the zygote or the early embryo would have most likely led to spontaneous termination of the pregnancy, a virus-induced chromosomal break in the last stages of oocyte meiosis remains a possibility. Certain viruses have been shown to be capable of inducing chromosomal breaks, some of them specifically in well-defined regions of human chromosomes, eg adenovirus 12 in band 17q21/22.[5]

The combination of abnormalities encountered in this case, in particular the facial dysmorphia, appears to be unique and does not resemble a known syndrome. At this point, we can only assume that it results from the 10p-chromosomal abnormality. Further observations will be necessary for the definition of a 10p- syndrome.

Acknowledgments

We gratefully acknowledge the expert technical assistance of Ms. Christy Bradshaw and Ms. Carol Kernahan. We thank Drs. S. Stella for ophthalmologic and K. E. Miller for radiologic evaluation, A. L. Anderson for dental examination and Mrs. B. Crupi for psychologic testing.

References

1. Seabright, M.: A rapid banding technique for human chromosomes. *Lancet* 2:971-972, 1971.
2. deGrouchy, J., Veslot, J., Bonnette, J. and Roidot, M.: A case of ?6p- chromosomal aberration. *Am. J. Dis. Child. 115*:93-99, 1968.
3. Mayeda, K., Weiss, L., Lindahl, R. and Dully, M.: Localization of the human lactate dehydrogenase B gene on the short arm of chromosome 12. *Am. J. Hum. Genet. 26*:59-64, 1974.
4. Alfi, O. S., Sanger, R. G., Sweeny, A. E. and Donnell, G. N.: 46,del(9)(22:) a new deletion syndrome. In Bergsma, D. (ed.): *Clinical Cytogenetics and Genetics*, Birth Defects: Orig. Art. Ser., vol. X, no. 8. Miami:Symposia Specialists for The National Foundation-March of Dimes, 1974, pp. 27-34.
5. McDougall, J. K., Kucherlapati, R. and Ruddle, F. H.: Localization and induction of the human thymidine kinase gene by adenovirus 12. *Nature (New Biol.) 245*:172-175, 1973.

Familial Chromosomal Translocation with Distinctive Phenotype Due to Effective Trisomy of No. 9p*

Havelock Thompson, M.D.

Two of three female sibs, 4½ years and 16 months of age, were found to have similar and distinctive clinical features associated with identical chromosomal abnormalities. Both girls have mild-to-moderate psychomotor retardation with developmental quotients of 50 to 60. Both have mild microcephaly with head circumferences well below the 3rd percentile, while the heights are on the 3rd percentile and between the 10th and 25th percentiles, respectively. Distinctive facial features (Figs. 1 and 2) include a dull appearance; deep-set eyes; alternating strabismus; large, low-set, protruding ears; prominent nasal root; and mild micrognathia. The hands (Fig. 3) show brachydactyly, ulnar deviation of the distal phalanges of

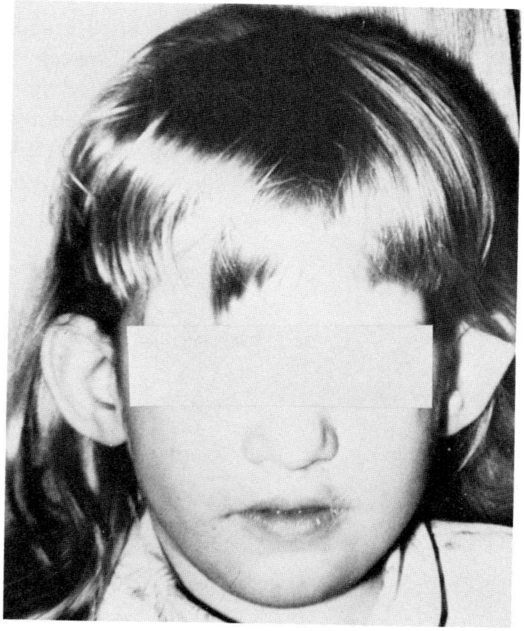

Fig. 1. Older affected sib showing facial features.

*The original abstract of this paper was in error in identifying the No. 9 chromosome as a No. 11 chromosome. The clinical features of these patients and subsequent C-banding studies correspond with data reported by others.

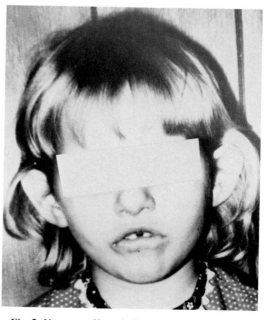

Fig. 2. Younger affected sib showing facial features.

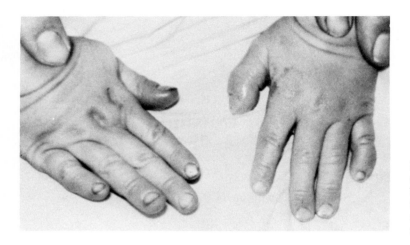

Fig. 3. Hands of the younger affected sib showing brachydactyly, clinodactyly of 5th fingers and ulnar deviation of the thumbs.

the thumbs and clinodactyly of the little fingers. Both girls have bilateral transverse palmar creases. The fingernails are short and soft but not dysplastic. The feet (Fig. 4) are small and the toenails are hypoplastic. Both girls had equinovarus deformity in infancy. This required casting in the older sib. The affected girls have complex thenar-first interdigital patterns, not seen in the parents or normal sib. The dermal prints are otherwise unremarkable, except for a t'' axial triradius in the older affected sib. The older girl had congenital hydronephrosis due to a left ureterocele, right ureteropelvic adhesions and aberrant vessels, and urethral obstruction. These abnormalities were surgically repaired at 9 days of age. Both affected girls have had recurrent urinary tract infections, and the younger sib is said to have had an abnormal IVP during the neonatal period.

The parents are physically and intellectually normal. They have been able to produce only 3 pregnancies in 8 years of marriage, despite desire for children and lack of contraceptive use. Two of the mother's 5 sibs are infertile (Fig. 5). A third sib has fathered 2 phenotypi-

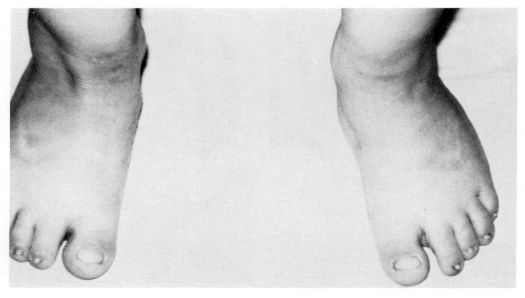

Fig. 4. Feet of the older affected sib showing brachydactyly and nail hypoplasia.

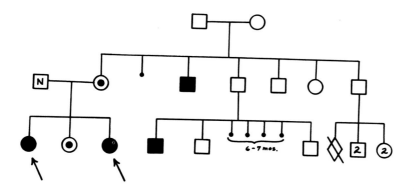

Fig. 5. Pedigree of the family.

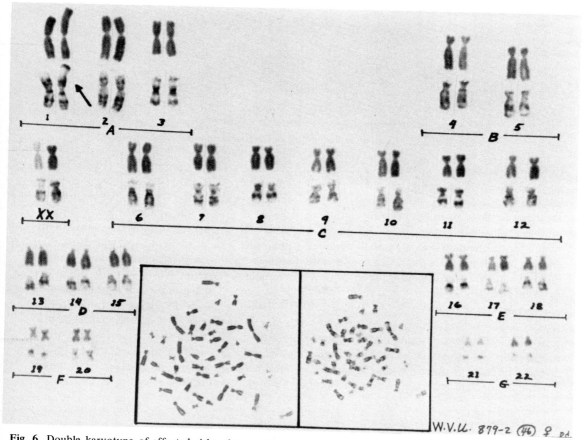

Fig. 6. Double karyotype of affected girls using standard preparation on top and trypsin G-banding on bottom. The arrow indicates the 1p+ chromosome.

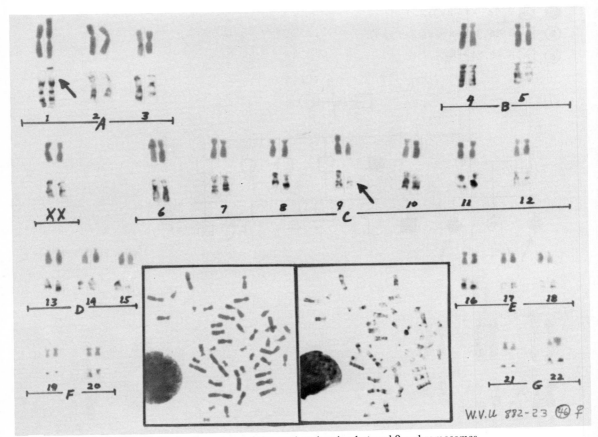

Fig. 7. Similar karyotype of the mother showing 1p+ and 9p- chromosomes.

cally normal sons, 4 late spontaneous abortions, and a 13-year-old mentally retarded son with chronic hydronephrosis and physical features identical to those seen in the propositi. The mother's 27-year-old brother is said to have the same physical features. He is mentally retarded and has had recurrent urinary tract infections said to be due to a neurogenic bladder.

The affected sibs have the same structural chromosome abnormality (Fig. 6), which consists of additional material on the short arm of a No. 1 chromosome. Trypsin G-banding shows a terminal Giemsa-staining band. Their mother and the normal sib show the same structurally abnormal No. 1 chromosome plus a structurally abnormal No. 9 chromosome (Fig. 7). The entire short arm of the abnormal No. 9 chromosome appears to be translocated terminally to the short arm of the abnormal No. 1 chromosome. All preparations show the structurally abnormal No. 9 to be telocentric. C-banding studies on the mother's chromosomes confirm the identity of the No. 9 chromosome. The karyotype of the mother and normal sib is as follows: 46,XX,t(1:9)(1qter→1pter::9p11→9pter;9qter→9cen). That of the unbalanced propositi is: 46,XX,der(1)mat. They appear to be effectively trisomic for the short arm of a No. 9 chromosome. There is no evidence for reciprocity of the translocation.

Partial Trisomy for Different Segments of Chromosome 13 in Several Individuals of the Same Family*

Robert S. Wilroy, Jr., M.D., Robert L. Summitt, M.D., and Paula R. Martens, B.S.

We wish to present a family in whom 3 members have partial trisomy for chromosome 13. Two of the 3 have partial trisomy for the long arm of chromosome 13 and the third member is trisomic for the proximal portion of chromosome 13.

Case Reports

The proband, *IV-3*, of this black kindred (Fig. 1) was the third illegitimate offspring in the sibship. She was seen in consultation at age one day because of multiple congenital anomalies. She weighed 3000 gm and was 51½ cm long. The cranial bones were sepa-

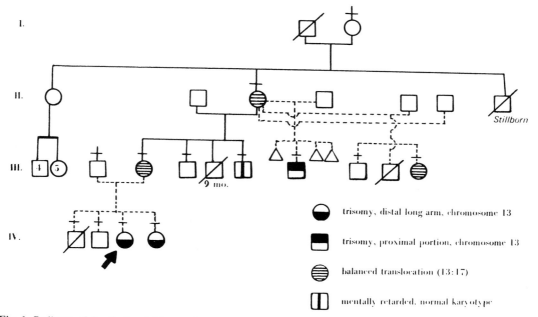

Fig. 1. Pedigree of family in which members are partially trisomic for different segments of chromosome 13. A horizontal mark above a symbol denotes a chromosomal analysis has been performed.

trisomy, distal long arm, chromosome 13

trisomy, proximal portion, chromosome 13

balanced translocation (13:17)

mentally retarded, normal karyotype

Stillborn

9 mo.

*Supported in part by Special Project No. 900, Division of Health Service, MCHS, HSMHA, DHEW, and a grant from The National Foundation-March of Dimes.

217

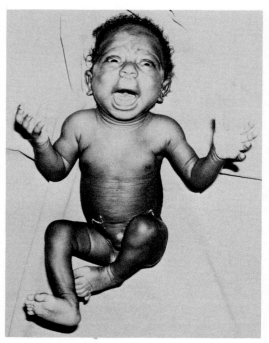

Fig. 2. Proband, *IV-3*, age 3 weeks.

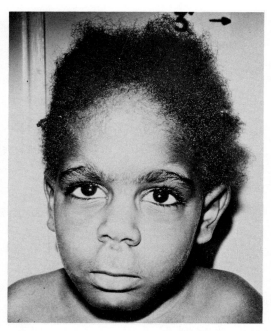

Fig. 3. Proband, *IV-3*, age 3 years. Note the abnormal long, broad, indented philtrum.

rated and large mastoids protruded from the skull. The philtrum was long, broad and 2 indented areas were present beneath each nostril (Fig. 2). This abnormality persisted and was evident at age 3 years (Fig. 3). The frenulum of the upper lip was short. Additional phenotypic findings included a narrow palate, micrognathia, long fingers and toes. Postaxial hexadactyly was present and all digits possessed an arch pattern. Growth rate had been adequate but at age 3 years she was mildly mentally retarded with a mental age of 15.6 months.

Her karyotype is illustrated on Figure 4. Forty-six chromosomes are present with 6 chromosomes in the D group. Only one chromosome 17 could be identified. An extra large submetacentric chromosome was evident in each cell.

The karyotype of the proband's mother, *III-11*, is shown in Figure 5. Forty-six chromosomes are present with only one identifiable chromosome 13 and only one chromosome 17. A large submetacentric chromosome was found in each cell as was a small acrocentric chromosome. This balanced reciprocal translocation was interpreted as follows. The large submetacentric chromosome resulted from a translocation of the major portion of the distal long arm of chromosome 13 to the short arm of chromosome 17. The small acrocentric chromosome was the proximal portion of chromosome 13.

The proband was, therefore, partially trisomic for the long arm of chromosome 13. The maternal grand-

mother, *II-3*, and maternal half-aunt, *III-21*, were also balanced translocation carriers.

Two years after the birth of the proband, a younger sister, *IV-4*, was born who possessed a similar phenotype (Fig. 6) and an identical karyotype. She was moderately mentally retarded.

The proband's oldest brother had previously been examined. He had multiple anomalies but a normal karyotype. He died at age one year of pneumonia which developed following surgical correction of esophageal stenosis.

Two maternal uncles, *III-12 and III-14*, had normal karyotypes although *III-14* was severely mentally retarded due to unknown causes. A third uncle, *III-13*, died at age 9 months of pneumonia. He had postaxial polydactyly of both hands and feet. Chromosomal analysis was not performed.

The maternal grandmother's sixth pregnancy terminated in the birth of a son (*III-16*) who is now 18 years old. He was severely mentally retarded, had scalp and skull defects and a large bulbous nose (Figs. 7 and 8). His karyotype (Fig. 9) contained the small extra acrocentric chromosome. He was trisomic for the proximal portion of chromosome 13.

Neutrophilic polymorphonuclear leukocytes were evaluated for the presence of nuclear projections in one patient with proximal 13 trisomy, one patient with distal 13 trisomy, a normal control, and a known complete 13 trisomic child. The evaluation was conducted in a blind coded fashion. The frequency of

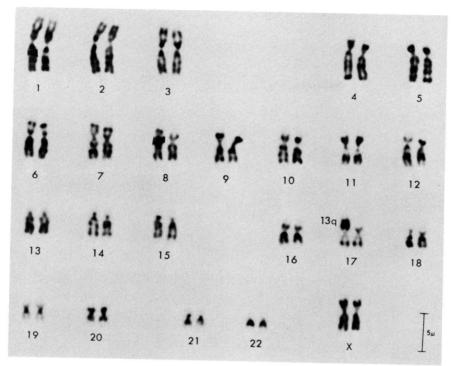

Fig. 4. Karyotype of the proband, *IV-3*: 46,XX,der(17),rcp(13;17)(q14;p13)mat. Forty-six chromosomes are present with only one identifiable chromosome 17 and an extra large submetacentric chromosome. *IV-3* is trisomic for the distal portion of chromosome 13.

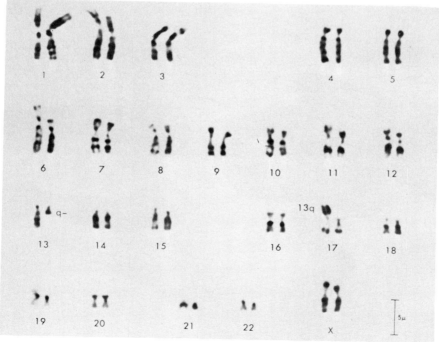

Fig. 5. Karyotype of proband's mother, *III-11*: 46,XX,rcp(13;17)(q14;p13). The small acrocentric chromosome is the proximal portion of chromosome 13 while the distal long arm of chromosome 13 has been translocated to the short arm of 17. This balanced reciprocal translocation was also found in *II-3 and III-21*.

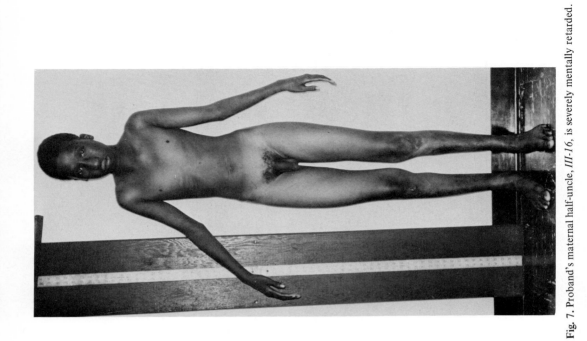

Fig. 7. Proband's maternal half-uncle, *III-16*, is severely mentally retarded.

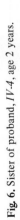

Fig. 6. Sister of proband, *IV-4*, age 2 years.

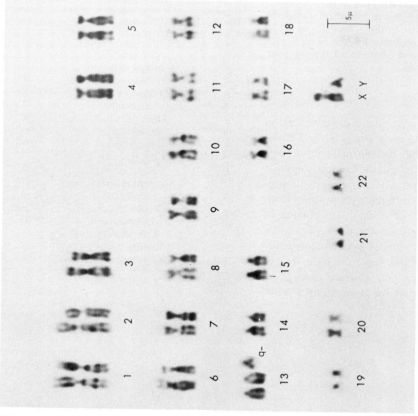

Fig. 9. Karyotype of *III-16*: 47,XY,+der(13),rcp(13;17)(q14;p13)mat. Forty-seven chromosomes are present with an extra small acrocentric chromosome, the proximal portion of chromosome 13. *III-16* is trisomic for the proximal portion of chromosome 13.

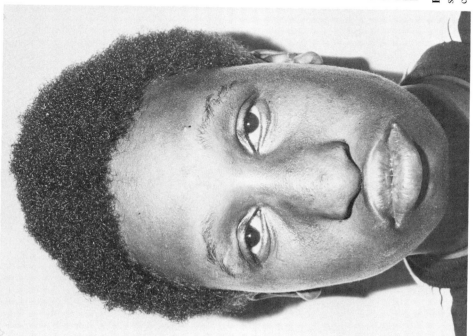

Fig. 8. Proband's maternal half-uncle, *III-16*, illustrating his large bulbous nose.

nuclear projections in cells from the patient with proximal 13 trisomy was 4X that in the patient with distal
13 trisomy and 3X that in the normal control. The
frequency of nuclear projections in the patients with
proximal 13 trisomy and complete 13 trisomy were
not significantly different.

Discussion

In this family 2 balanced translocation
mothers have had 15 pregnancies. Only 3 children were normal and had normal karyotypes.
Two points deserve emphasis. First, trisomy for
the proximal portion of chromosome 13 produces a distinctly different phenotype from
that of trisomy for the distal major portion of
the long arm of chromosome 13 (Table 1).
Second, balanced female heterozygotes for
reciprocal translocations may have a greater risk
of producing unbalanced gametes than those
who are heterozygotes for Robertsonian translocations.

Table 1. Abnormalities of 13 Trisomy

Distal	Complete	Proximal
0	Short stature	0
0	Microcephaly	0
+	Mental retardation	+
0	Seizures	0
0	Telecanthus	+
0	Eye abnormalities	0
+	Malformed ears	+
0	Bulbous nose	+
+	Long philtrum	0
0	Cleft lip-palate	0
0	Short neck	0
+	Umbilical hernia	0
+	Polydactyly	0
+	Digital arches	0
0	Arch fibular	0
0	Scalp defects	+
0	Hemangioma	0
0	Increased nuclear projections	+

Trisomy 14q-*

Lt. William A. Fawcett, MC, USNR, Lt. Commander William K. McCord, MC, USN
and Uta Francke, M.D.

V.J., a 2220-gm white female, was born 11/20/73 to a 21-year-old gravida 2, para 2 mother, blood type AB negative, VDRL negative. During the last trimester, the pregancy was complicated by preeclampsia, which resulted in hospitalization and induction of labor at 38-weeks' gestation. The fetal membranes were ruptured and the baby was spontaneously delivered 2 hours and 22 minutes later. Prior to delivery, there were no signs of fetal distress. The infant was born depressed, with Apgar scores of 2 and 3 at 1 and 5 minutes, respectively. Respiratory assistance was initially required in the form of endotracheal intubation and manual ventilation. Thirty minutes after delivery, the infant's respiratory status stabilized and she was extubated, but continued to require a high ambient oxygen environment for the next 7 hours. At approximately 8 hours of age, the infant was on room air and doing well.

The infant's maternal grandmother had 2 spontaneous abortions during the first trimester of pregnancy. The cause of abortion was undetermined. The patient's mother is one of 5 sibs; all are alive and in good health. The growth and development of the infant's 20-month-old brother has been within normal limits. The patient's 23-year-old father had camptodactyly as an infant, and had a single simian crease. Other paternal family members have also exhibited these features.

Clinical findings revealed weight 2220 gm (<10th%), length 44 3/4 cm (approximately the 10th%), head circumference 33 cm (between the 25th and 50th%). The infant was hypertonic with mottled skin. The subcutaneous tissue was decreased. Additional findings included: brachycephaly; long, fine blonde hair; low and posterior-set ears; malformed pinnas; low anterior and posterior hairline; long philtrum; peculiar facies; hypotelorism; small palpebral fissures; a globular nose with anteverted nostrils; large halluces; camptodactyly; a left simian crease; clinodactyly; short neck; and high-arched palate (Figs. 1-4). A nonsignificant cardiac murmur was also noted. In the course of her hospital stay, intermittent episodes of acrocyanosis, circumoral cyanosis and opisthotonos were observed. These were usually associated with feeding or physical contact. The serum bilirubin rose to a maximum level of 11.0 mg% the fourth day of life, then gradually declined without treatment. Periumbilical cellulitis was noted during the first week and was successfully treated with oxacillin. Due to inadequate dermatoglyphics of the patient, no conclusions could be made. These will be repeated at a later date. Roentgenograms of the limbs revealed a small bony

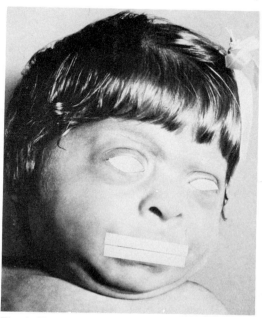

Fig. 1. Note the long blonde hair, globular nose with anteverted nostrils, long philtrum, and hypotelorism. (Figs. 1-4 are Official U. S. Navy Photographs.)

*The opinions or assertions contained herein are those of the authors and are not to be construed as official or as reflecting the views of the Navy Department.

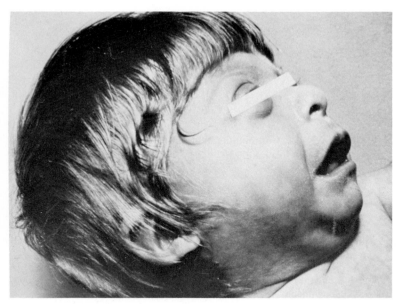

Fig. 2. Note the low posteriorly set ears.

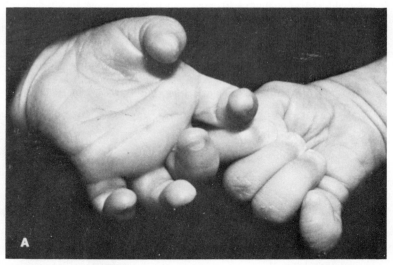

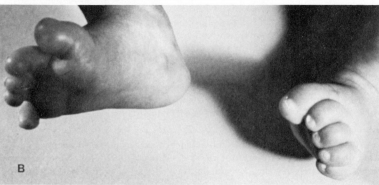

Fig. 3. Hands and feet of the patient demonstrating A) clinodactyly and camptodactyly and B) large halluces.

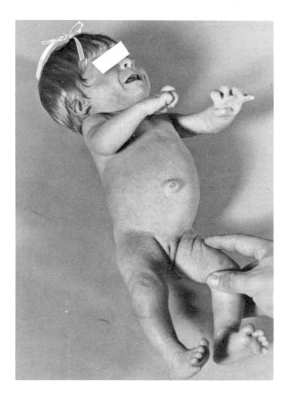

cyst of the styloid process of the right radius. Films of the skull, spine, chest and abdomen showed no abnormalities.

The patient's length, weight and head circumference have continued to increase parallel, but just below the 3rd percentile. At 6½ months of age, her developmental milestones were normal to marginal.

Chromosome analysis of the patient's peripheral lymphocytes revealed a karyotype of 47 chromosomes. Initially, the extra chromosome was thought to be a 21, 22 or Y. However, these possibilities were excluded by differential staining with trypsin-Giemsa and quinacrine mustard. Analysis of chromosomes from the patient's mother and 20-month-old sib (Figs. 5 and 6) demonstrated what appeared to be a reciprocal translocation involving chromosomes 14 and 20, t(14;20)(q22;q13).

The patient's derivative chromosome der(14) was assumed to be due to a meiotic nondisjunction. The resulting chromosome consisted of the proximal portion of chromosome 14 plus the terminal q13 segment of chromosome 20. The karyotype was designated 47,XX,+der(14),t(14;20)(q22;q13)mat (Fig. 7). No other studied family members carried the balanced translocation (Fig. 8). The patient's 23-year-old uncle and maternal grandmother have not yet been studied.

Summary

Trisomy 14q- syndrome is relatively new and needs further delineation. In comparing our case with other reported cases (Table 1), some similarities are seen. Although the comparison of our case of partial trisomy 14 with the other

Fig. 4. Appearance of the patient shortly before being discharged from the hospital.

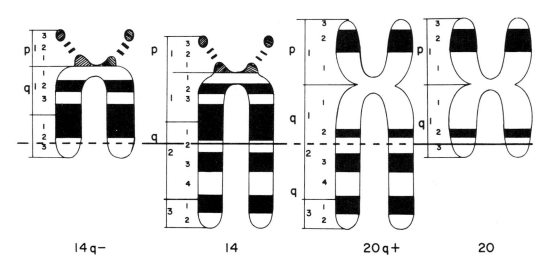

14q-   14   20q+   20

Fig. 5. A diagrammatic representation of the reciprocal translocation of patient's mother and brother.

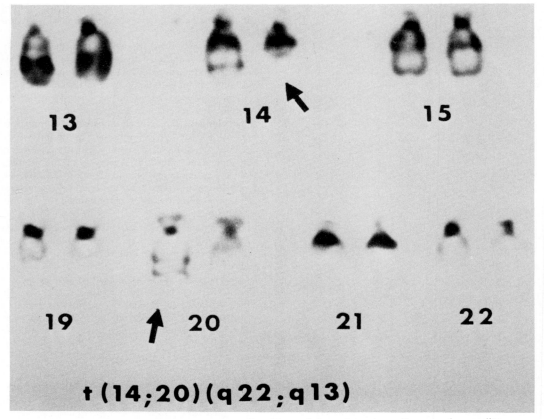

t (14;20)(q22;q13)

Fig. 6. Partial karyotype of the patient's mother. Her son's karyotype shows the same abnormality.

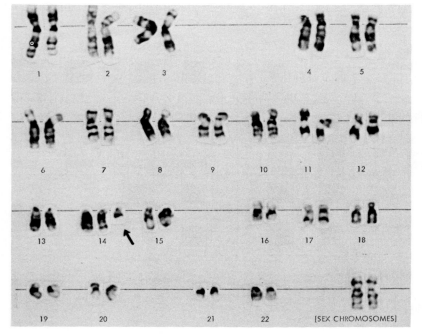

Fig. 7. The patient's karyotype [47,XX,+ der(14),t(14;20)(q22; 13)mat]. The derivative chromosome der(14) is indicated by the arrow.

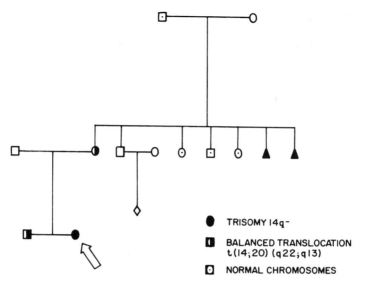

TRISOMY 14q⁻ → TRISOMY 14q-

● TRISOMY 14q-

▣ BALANCED TRANSLOCATION
   t(14;20) (q22;q13)

▢ NORMAL CHROMOSOMES

Fig. 8. Patient's pedigree.

Table 1. Clinical Features of Partial Trisomy 14

	Present Case	14 Trisomy (Short et al[3])	14 Trisomy (Allerdice et al[1])	14 Trisomy (Muldal et al[2])	Trisomy 14 (Surana et al[4])
Brachycephaly	+	N	N	N	N
Low anterior-posterior/hairline	+	N	N	N	N
Hypotelorism	+	N	N	O	N
Globus nose with anteverted nostrils	+	+	N	O	N
Long philtrum	+	N	N	+	N
Micrognathia	+	+	+	O	N
Low posteriorly set ears	+	+	+	+	N
Hypertonia	+	+	N	O	N
Loose mottled skin	+	N	N	O	N
↓Subcutaneous tissue	+	N	N	O	N
Long fine hair	+	N	N	N	N
Umbilical hernia	+	N	N	N	N
Camptodactyly	+	+	N	N	N
Simian creases	+	+	N	N	N
Small palpebral fissures	+	N	N	N	N
Malformed pinnae	+	+	N	N	N
Clinodactyly	+	+	N	+	N
Talipes equinovarus	O	+	+	N	+
Microcephaly	O	+	N	N	N
Microphthalmus	O	+	+	N	N
Short neck	+	+	N	O	N
Congenital heart disease(PDA, ASD, other)	O	+	+	?	+
Failure to thrive	?	+	+	+	+
Mental retardation	?	?	+	+	N
Death in early infancy	O	+	+	O	N
High-arched palate	+	+	+	+	N
High-pitched cry	O	+	+	O	N
Undescended testis	O	+	+	O	N
Seizures	O	+	O	+	N

+ = present; O = absent; N = Not observed or no comment; ? = too early

cases reported in the literature may not be entirely justified (in that the reciprocal translocations are not always identical), it is hoped that by doing so, we can further delineate the common features and prognosis of such individuals.

References

1. Allerdice, P. W., Miller, O. J., Miller, D. A. et al: Familial translocation involving chromosomes 6, 14, and 20 identified by quinacrine fluorescence. *Humangenetik 13*:205-209, 1971.

2. Muldal, S., Enoch, B. A., Ahned, A. and Harris, R.: Partial trisomy 14q- and pseudoxanthoma elasticum. *Clin. Genet. 4*:480-489, 1973.

3. Short, E. M., Solitare, G. B. and Breg, W. R.: A case of 14 trisomy. 47,XX,(14q-)+ and translocation t(9p+;14q-) in mother and brother. *J. Med. Genet. 9*:367-373, 1972.

4. Surana, R. B., Conen, P. E., Braudo, M. and Keith, J. D.: Familial t(14q-;1+?). Meiotic nondisjunction marker C chromosome. *Pediatr. Res. 5*:278, 1971.

5. Taylor, M. B., Juberg, R. C., Jones, B. and Johnson, W. A.: Chromosomal variability in the D_1 trisomy syndrome. *Am. J. Dis. Child. 120*:374-381, 1970.

16q Trisomy in a Family with a Balanced 15/16 Translocation

Roy Schmickel, M.D., Andrew Poznanski, M.D.C.M. and Janet Himebaugh, B.A.

Case Report

An infant born at Mott Children's Hospital was trisomic for the long arm of the 16 chromosome. The family of this infant contained 3 members with a balanced translocation between the 15 and 16 chromosomes.

The infant was born to a 25-year-old mother who was in good health and had previously had a normal child. There was no history of previous abortions. The pregnancy was uneventful until the last trimester of pregnancy when slow fetal growth was detected by the obstetrician. At 40 weeks because of falling estriols and oligohydramnios, a C section was performed.

At birth the infant had an Apgar of 8 and was noted to have an unusual appearance (Fig. 1). His weight was 1.86 kg, length was 44 cm and head circumference 30.5 cm. The child had an asymmetric skull as seen in Figures 2 and 3. The left frontal area transilluminated. The palpebral fissures were small with an antimongoloid slant. The left cornea was larger than the right. There were enlarged optic cups and some peripapillary pigmentation was noted in the left fundus. The vessels and macula were normal. The ears were small, round and had little cartilage. The mandible was hypoplastic. A grade 2/6 systolic murmur was present at the left sternal border with no evidence of heart enlargement or failure. A testicle was present in the left inguinal canal and the right testicle was not palpated. The penis was small. As seen in Figure 4, the hands had an abnormal appearance.

There was marked clinodactyly of the 5th finger which was associated with a very short middle phalanx (Fig. 5). There was marked alteration of the length of all of the hand bones as seen in the pattern profile (Fig. 6). With this technique the amount of deviation from the mean for age and sex is plotted against the location in the hand.[1] Very unusual areas of sclerosis were seen in the tufts of the distal phalanges of the hand (Fig. 5) and similar changes were seen in the feet (Fig. 7). There was some metatarsus adductus defor-

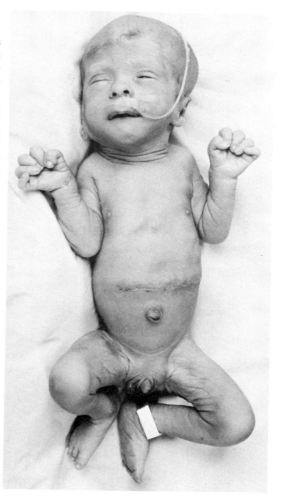

Fig. 1. Clinical photograph of the infant at 3 weeks of age.

229

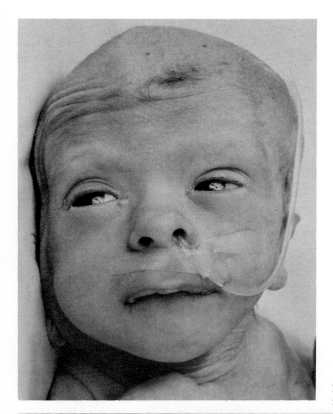

Fig. 2. Photograph demonstrating the facial features and unusual palpebral fissures.

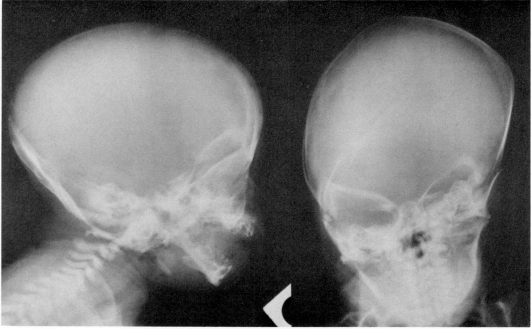

Fig. 3. Skull radiograph. There is flattening of the occipital bone and marked asymmetry of the skull is apparent. The mandibular angle is increased. Both molars are present which is indicative of term maturity.

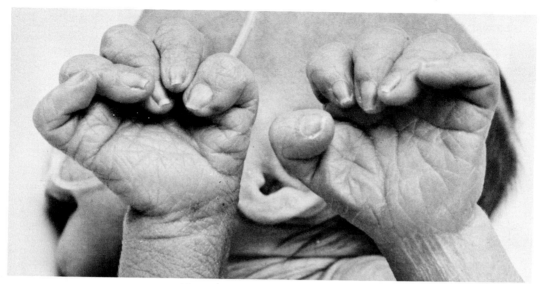

Fig. 4. Hand photograph of the infant.

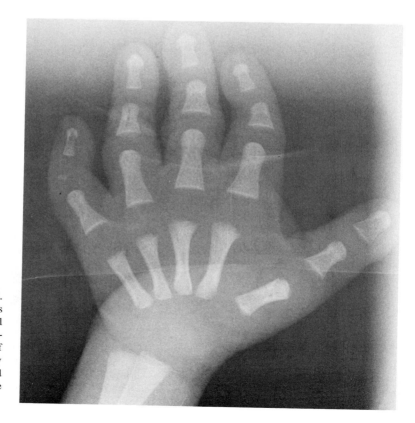

Fig. 5. Hand radiograph. There is an unusual sclerosis of the tufts of the distal phalanges, marked shortening of the middle phalanx of the 5th finger, which is only a very small ossicle; and some clinodactyly of the 2nd and 5th fingers.

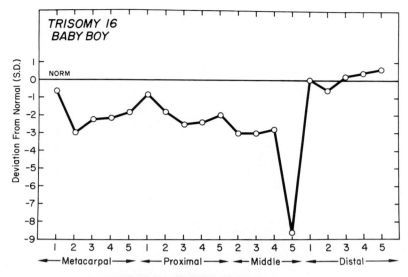

Deviation From Normal (S.D.)

TRISOMY 16
BABY BOY

NORM

Metacarpal — Proximal — Middle — Distal

Fig. 6. Pattern profile. The distal phalanges are relatively long, as compared to the proximal phalanges and metacarpals. The thumb is relatively long due to a relatively long 1st metacarpal and 1st proximal phalanx.

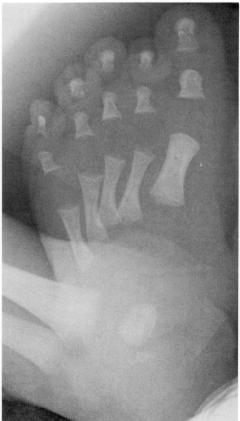

Fig. 7. Foot radiograph. There is some metatarsus adductus deformity. The calcaneus is markedly retarded. There are sclerotic tufts of the distal phalanges.

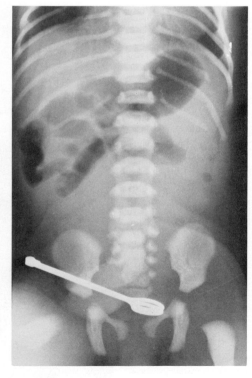

Fig. 8. There is an anomaly of the sacrum with fusion of several sacral vertebral bodies. The ribs are very slender. The 10th left rib is unusually short. The pelvic wings are somewhat anteriorly rotated. The proximal small bowel appears to be on the right, suggesting some degree of malrotation.

mity of the feet. Minimal anomalies were seen in the spine and ribs (Fig. 8). The sternum was very slender. Delayed maturation was noted in several regions. The fat thickness was decreased and was more than 2 SD below the mean for 40 weeks' gestation.[2] The knee maturation was retarded considerably since only a small femoral ossicle was noted, and the calcaneus had only a small ossicle present. However, maturation of teeth was normal using the Kuhns standards.[3]

There was a normal Moro reflex but no suck reflex was present. The child was fed with a nasogastric tube. On the second day of life the child became lethargic. By the fifth day the infant was jaundiced (bilirubin 12.9) and vomited frequently. IV feeding was begun. An upper GI series showed malrotation of the duodenum and there was also malrotation of the colon (Fig. 9). Abdominal distention at 16 days of age led to discovery of pneumotosis intestinalis and air was evident in the portal venous system. Exploratory surgery demonstrated a midilial perforation. Bowel resection and anastomosis led to improvement of the patient's condition. At 25 days of age, the IV alimentation was supplemented with nasogastric feedings. However, he failed to retain his weight, progressively weakened and died at 7 weeks of age.

Numerous biochemical, bacteriologic and hematologic tests did not add any further understanding of

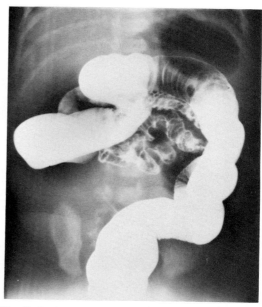

Fig. 9. Barium enema. There is malrotation of the colon with a high position of the cecum.

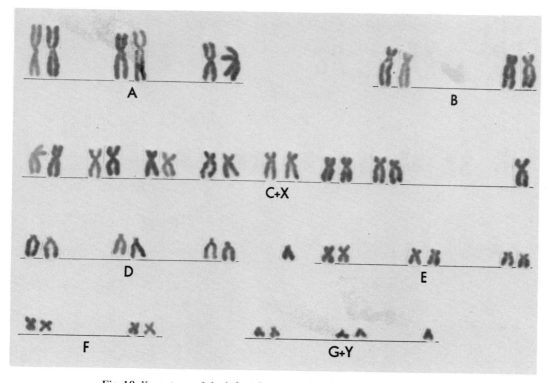

Fig. 10. Karyotype of the infant demonstrating the extra chromosome.

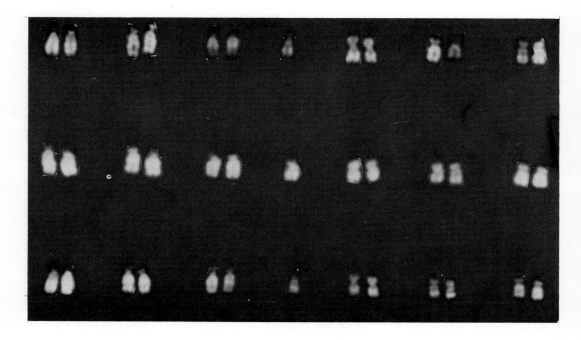

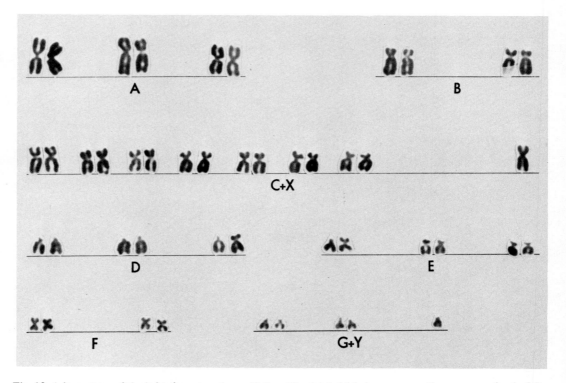

Fig. 12. A karyotype of the infant's maternal grandfather. The deleted 16 chromosome, the presence of only 5 D chromosomes, and an extra C-type chromosome can be seen.

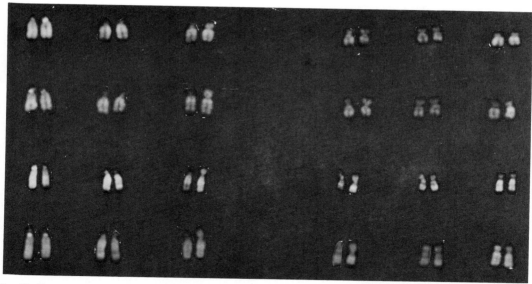

Fig. 13. Four partial karyotypes with fluorescent staining of the 2 abnormal chromosomes, the D- and E-group chromosomes, in the infant's mother. The analysis shows that the deleted chromosome is a 16 and that the deleted portion of the 16 is translocated to the number 15 chromosome.

the patient's problems. At necropsy, a 3 cm cystic lesion was present in the left frontal lobe. The ventricles were symmetric and not dilated. Microscopic examination of the brain showed poor myelination. A 4 mm ventricular septal defect was present in the heart. The duodenum was malrotated and elongated. The thymus showed depletion of lymphocytes with a loss of distinction of cortex and medulla.

Chromosomal studies of the infant's leukocytes and fibroblasts revealed a 47,XY,+16q karyotype. Figures 10 and 11 show the infant's karyotype. Chromosomal examination of other members of the family

identified 3 members of the family with a balanced translocation involving the 15 and 16 chromosomes. The karyotype of the mother, the maternal uncle and maternal grandfather demonstrated a 46,t(15p+;16p-) karyotype as seen in Figures 12 and 13.

Examination of the fluorescent staining of the chromosomes indicated that the short arm of the 16 chromosome was translocated to the short arm of the 15 chromosome. We were unable to karyotype the great-grandparents. The members of the family who were karyotyped and found to be normal are indicated in the family pedigree by the letter "N" (Fig. 14).

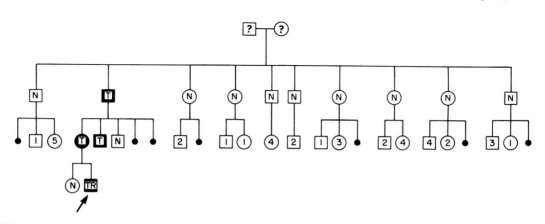

Fig. 14. A family pedigree for the propositus. The 3 persons with translocation are indicated by the letter "T" and those proved normal are indicated with "N." The number of children and their sex is indicated for each of the normal persons.

Discussion

This case illustrates the rather severe changes associated with partial trisomy of chromosome 16. Although trisomy 16 is frequently found among abortuses, this defect has not been documented in a live infant. In Carr's and Bouie's series of cultured tissue from spontaneous abortions, trisomy 16 was the most common autosomal trisomy.[4,5] A case reported by Hamerton[6] indicates that trisomy of 16p may be responsible for the lethality. A mother with a translocated chromosome t(Dp+;16q-) had 10 consecutive spontaneous abortions. The last abortus was studied and found to have a 47,XY,+16p karyotype. In this case trisomy of the short arm of 16 was lethal.

The balanced translocation does not seem to impart any abnormalities to its carriers. However, the meiotic pairing of the translocated chromosomes could permit discordant orientation and lead to an aneuploid gamete. In retrospect, this case illustrates the clinical rule that parents of partially trisomic infants should be studied for the presence of a balanced translocation. Genetic studies have placed the adenine phosphoribosyltransferase enzyme and the alpha haptoglobin loci on chromosome 16.[7,8] In the balanced translocation state illustrated in our case, the short and long arm of the chromosome 16 are not linked. Detailed analysis of the balanced carriers will permit the localization of genes for these proteins to specific arms of the chromosome.

References

1. Poznanski, A. K.: *The Hand in Radiologic Diagnosis*, Philadelphia:W. B. Saunders Co., 1974.
2. Kuhns, L. R., Berger, P. E., Roloff, D. W. et al: Fat thickness in the newborn infant of a diabetic mother. *Radiology 111*:665-671, 1974.
3. Kuhns, L. R., Sherman, M. P. and Poznanski, A. K.: Determination of neonatal maturation on the chest radiograph. *Radiology 102*:597-603, 1972.
4. Carr, D. H.: Chromosome studies as a cause of spontaneous abortions. *Am. J. Obstet. Gynecol. 97*:283-293, 1967.
5. Bouie, A. and Bouie, J. G.: Chromosomal aberrations in human spontaneous abortions. *Mammalian Chromosomes Newsletter 9*:246-248, 1968.
6. Hamerton, J. L.: *Human Cytogenetics*. New York: Academic Press, 1971, vol. 2, pp. 292-293.
7. Tischfield, J. A. and Ruddle, F. H.: Assignment of APRT locus to chromosome 16 in humans. *Proc. Natl. Acad. Sci. 71*:45-49, 1974.
8. Robson, E. B., Polani, P. E., Dart, S. J. et al: Probable assignment of the alpha locus of haptoglobin to chromosome 16 in man. *Nature 223*:1163-65, 1969.

Identification of a 19/20 Translocation by G-, Q- and C-Banding

Gurbax S. Sekhon, Ph.D., Laura S. Hillman, M.D. and Robert L. Kaufman, M.D.*

A stable dicentric chromosome has rarely been described. This is expected, since such chromosomes are unstable and are pulled in opposite directions during mitosis or meiosis leading to chromosome breakage, rearrangement and loss.

We describe here a chromosomal abnormality which is of special interest for 3 reasons. 1) It is a stable dicentric chromosomal abnormality involving 2 nonacrocentric autosomes. 2) It is a 19/20 translocation. 3) More than one banding technique was required to elucidate the structure of this chromosome.

Case Report

The patient was the 2090 gm (small for gestational age) product of a full-term pregnancy born to a healthy 26-year-old gravida 4, para 2 woman who had had one previous miscarriage at 8 weeks' gestation. The 28-year-old father had diabetes mellitus and a family history of diabetes mellitus. The infant was noted to have a number of dysmorphic features: low-set, posteriorly rotated ears; high-arched palate; long fingers; and congenital dislocation of the right hip (Fig. 1). The infant developed congestive heart failure at 2 days of age and cardiac catheterization revealed a large patent ductus arteriosus (PDA) and a secundum atrial septal defect, both shunting from left to right. The child was digitalized and improved with clinical closure of the PDA by age 6 months. At 24 months her weight remained far below the 3rd percentile but her height and head circumference were 15th per-

centile and 50th percentile, respectively. Development at 24 months was at the 6-month level; however, she has spent 16 of 24 months in a spica cast for correction of the congenitally dislocated hip and the majority of milestones have been attained over 2 months since removal of the cast. Sight and hearing appeared to be intact. Neurologic examination showed generalized hypotonia and mild athetoid motions

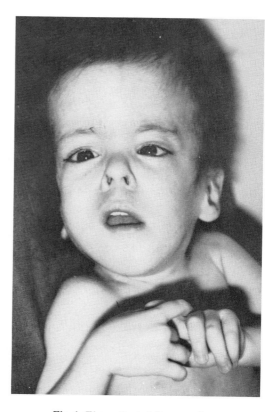

Fig. 1. The patient at 2 years of age.

*Dr. Robert L. Kaufman was supported in part by USPHS postgraduate training grant T01-GM 0511, the Ranken Jordan Trust Fund and the James H. Woods Foundation.

which were accentuated by a marked hyperextensibility of joints, especially in the hands.

Materials and Methods

Short-term lymphocyte cultures of the patient and her parents were made according to a modification of the Moorhead technique. Lymphocytes were cultured in Gibco McCoys 5A medium for 65 hours; colcemid was added for 2 hours prior to harvesting. Cells were treated with .075 M KCl for 12 minutes, fixed with fresh methanol-acetic acid (3:1), spread on wet slides and heat dried on a hot plate for 1½ to 2 minutes. Slides were stained by the ASG technique[1] for G-band identification of each chromosome. A total of 323 cells were counted and photographed using high contrast copy film. Each slide was destained, then restained with Atabrine for Q-banding.[2] The cells were relocated, photographed on a Zeiss photomicroscope with transmitted dark field illumination. The slides were destained and restained for C-banding.[3] Skin fibroblasts were cultured by the methods of Harnden and Brunton.[4]

Results

Conventional karyotype analysis had been carried out in this patient at 3 days of age. All cells studied from peripheral blood lymphocyte culture had 45 chromosomes, with 2 chromosomes missing from the F group and an extra chromosome in the C group. At 5 months of age repeat chromosomal analyses were carried out on peripheral blood lymphocytes and skin culture fibroblasts. G-, Q- and C-banding techniques were used sequentially on the same cells for the purpose of determining the translocation precisely (Figs. 2 and 3). In 323 cells examined from lymphocytes, 94.4% had 45 chromosomes including the translocation and 5.6% had a normal female karyotype. No normal cells were found in 30 skin fibroblasts. The karyotypes of both parents revealed neither structural nor numeric abnormality. According to Giemsa and fluorescent patterns, the translocation would result from a 19/20 translocation without any visible chromosomal loss; and one would expect to find 2 heterochromatic regions. Indeed, the C-staining revealed heterochromatic regions not only at the 19 centromere but also at the site where the centromere of the translocated chromosome No. 20 should be located (Fig. 4). It should be pointed out that the presence of heterochromatic regions does not necessarily mean that the centromeres are present. With G-banding the centromeric region of the trans-

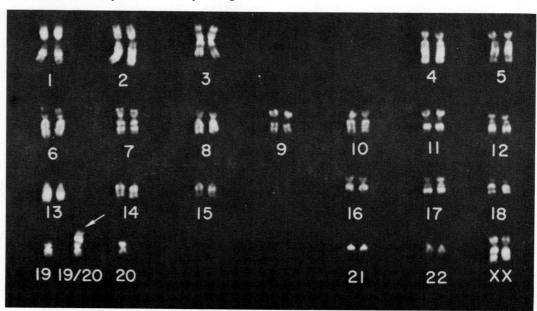

Fig. 2. Karyotype of Q-banded chromosomes showing 19/20 translocation (arrow).

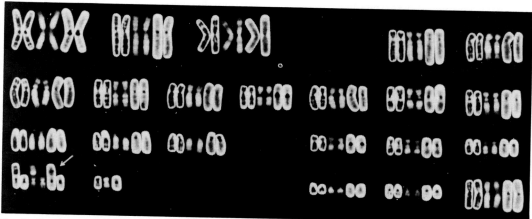

Fig. 3. G-, Q- and C-banded triple karyotype with 45 chromosomes. G-banded chromosomes are on the left, Q-banded chromosomes in the center and C-banded chromosomes on the right for each pair. The arrow indicates the C-banded dicentric chromosome.

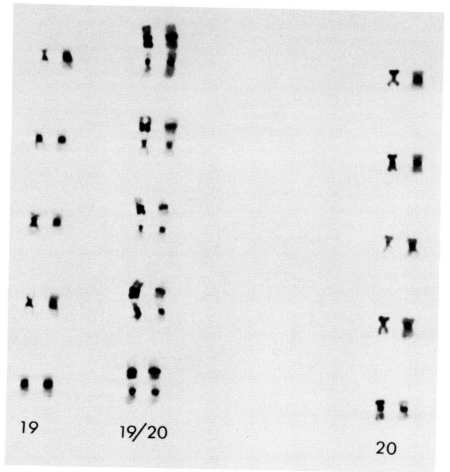

19   19/20   20

Fig. 4. Partial karyotype of chromosomes 19, 19/20 translocation and 20 from 5 different cells. G-banded chromosomes are on the left and C-banded chromosomes on the right.

located chromosome No. 20 shows 2 separate distinct dots or spheres instead of one as in a normal chromosome 20 (Fig. 4). However, the 2 dots or spheres seem to be fused together when C-banding is used, which could be attributed to the swelling of the chromosomes, typical of that technique.

Discussion

Our observations demonstrate that the translocation chromosome resulted from a short arm to short arm fusion between chromosomes 19 and 20, without any visible chromosomal loss and with both heterochromatic regions intact. The translocation chromosome behaved as a normal monocentric; since it was present in all the skin cells and in 94.4% of the lymphocytes. It is of interest that 5.6% of the lymphocytes had a normal female karyotype.

Dicentric chromosomes have been described in common wheat,[5] in Agropyron,[6] in narcissus[7] and in man.[8-12]

There are 3 explanations of the stability of a dicentric chromosome in the cytologic literature. Therman et al have discussed submicroscopic deletion versus inactivation of one of the centromeres and have concluded that one of the centromeres becomes inactivated rather than deleted.[11] Hair described the stability of a dicentric chromosome of *Agropyron scabrum* and postulated that the stability was due to the closeness of the 2 centromeres.[6] The same might be true in dicentric Y chromosomes and dicentric Robertsonian translocations.

Sears and Camara attributed stability of a dicentric chromosome in wheat to dominance of one centromere over the other.[5] They introduced the terms "primary" and "secondary" centromeres. In mitosis, the dicentric divided normally, with the 2 centromeres of each chromatid directed to the same pole. In meiosis, the dicentric was actually transmitted preferentially.

In the present case, the distance between the 2 centromeres is not as small as in a dicentric Y; therefore, the explanation of stability due to the closeness of centromeres does not hold true. We conclude that the translocation chromosome is a heterodicentric, with

dominant behavior of the 19 centromere over the 20 centromere. It appears less likely that a submicroscopic deletion of the 20 centromere occurred.

It is difficult to relate the patient's phenotype to the chromosome abnormality. However, a relationship between clinical abnormalities and a positional effect of the translocation cannot be ruled out.

References

1. Sumner, A. T., Evans, H. J. and Buckland, R. A.: A new technique for distinguishing between human chromosomes. *Nature (New Biol.)* 232:821-822, 1971.
2. Caspersson, T., Zech, L. and Johansson, C.: Analysis of human metaphase chromosome set by aid of DNA-binding fluorescent agents. *Exp. Cell Res.* 62:490-492, 1970.
3. McKenzie, W. H. and Lubs, H. A.: An analysis of the technical variables in the production of C bands. *Chromosoma (Berlin)* 41:175-182, 1973.
4. Harnden, D. G. and Brunton, S.: The skin culture technique. In Yunis, J. J. (ed.): *Human Chromosome Methodology*, New York:Academic Press, 1965, pp. 57-73.
5. Sears, E. R. and Camara, A.: A transmissible dicentric chromosome. *Genetics* 37:125-135, 1952.
6. Hair, J. B.: The origin of new chromosomes in *Agropyron. Hereditas (Suppl.)* 6:215-233, 1952.
7. Darlington, C. D and Wylie, A. P.: A dicentric cycle in narcissus. *Heredity (Suppl.)* 6:197-213, 1953.
8. Niebuhr, E.: A 45,XX,5-,13-,dic+ karyotype in a case of cri-du-chat syndrome. *Cytogenetics* 11:165-177, 1972.
9. Disteche, C., Hagemeijer, H., Frederic, J. and Progneaux, D.: An abnormal large human chromosome identified as an end to end fusion of two X's by combined techniques and microdensitometry. *Clin Genet.* 3:388-395, 1972.
10. Warburton, D., Henderson, A. S., Shapiro, L. R. and Hsu, L. Y. F.: A stable human dicentric chromosome, tdic(12;14)(p13;p13) including an intercalary satellite region between centromeres. *Am. J. Hum. Genet.* 25:439-445, 1973.
11. Therman, E., Sarto, G. E. and Patau, K.: Apparently isodicentric but functionally monocentric X chromosome in man. *Am. J. Hum. Genet.* 26:83-92, 1974.
12. Pallister, P. D., Patau, K., Inhorn, S. L. and Opitz, J. M.: A woman with multiple congenital anomalies, mental retardation and mosaicism for an unusual translocation chromosome t(6;19). *Clin. Genet.* 5:188-195, 1974.

Trisomy 22: A Clinically Identifiable Syndrome*

Omar S. Alfi, M.D., Roger G. Sanger, D.D.S. and George M. Donnell, M.D.

Trisomy 22 has not yet been documented as a clinically identifiable syndrome. Some reports suggest that the syndrome may actually exist as a clinical entity, but the cytogenetic documentation is uncertain since current banding techniques were not available. Other reports suggest that the syndrome may only exist as a cytogenetic entity but with no characteristic clinical features.

This present communication reports a child with trisomy 22 documented by Q-, G- and R-banding techniques; she was previously reported as trisomy G without Down syndrome.[1] On reviewing the clinical findings in other cases reported as either nonmongoloid trisomy G or trisomy 22 in the literature, at least 8 such cases had clinical features and craniofacial morphology similar to our proband.[2-5] The similarities were so striking that a clinical identification of this syndrome seems feasible.

Case Report

Our proband, L.C., was a 9-year-old, profoundly retarded white female born to a 20-year-old gravida 5, para 2, ab 3 female and a 30-year-old male. She was the product of a full-term uncomplicated pregnancy with normal delivery. Mother, father and older female sib were without obvious congenital anomalies.

Upon presentation at our Genetics Clinic, the child appeared very thin and exhibited profound mental retardation with inability to walk, stand or achieve any self-care activities. She possessed no discernible speech and was functioning below the 2-year level. She demonstrated intermittent choreoathetoid movements of her upper limbs.

Shortly after birth the infant experienced feeding problems, difficulty in swallowing and jaundice. Examination at one year revealed the following abnormalities: microcephaly, unusual facial appearance and asymmetry, dilated suprasternal vessels, tracheomalacia, heart murmur, limitation of abduction of the hips and a short perineal body.

Cardiac evaluation revealed pulmonary stenosis, atrial septal defect and anterior positioning of the superior vena cava. She failed to thrive, had gross motor retardation, and significant hypotonia.

The fingers were long, slender and hyperextensible. The thumbs were similarly long and finger-like.

Examination of the craniofacial morphology at one year of age (Fig. 1, top left) revealed the proband to have turricephaly with microcephalic measurements; frontal prominence; peculiar orbital morphology; long philtrum; downturned commissures of the mouth; facial asymmetry; large, low-set ears; and small lower face with apparent micrognathia.

Chromosomal analysis using Q-, G- and R-banding revealed the proband to have a karyotype of 47,XX,+del(22)(q13) which indicated the presence of trisomy 22, two of the No. 22 chromosomes appearing normal and the third having a deletion near the telomeric end of the long arm at band q13 (Fig. 2). The mother was found to have trisomy X and a deletion of one of her No. 22 chromosomes similar to that of the proband. Her karyotype was 47,XXX,del(22)(q13). The older female sib also had a similar deletion of a 22 chromosome with a karyotype of 46,XX,del(22)(q13). The karyotype of the father was 46,XY and apparently normal. Close study of the karyotypes of the mother and older daughter failed to detect translocation of the deleted telomeric end of this No. 22 chromosome or any other chromosome.

*Supported in part by Department of HEW Maternal and Child Health Service projects 422 and 914.

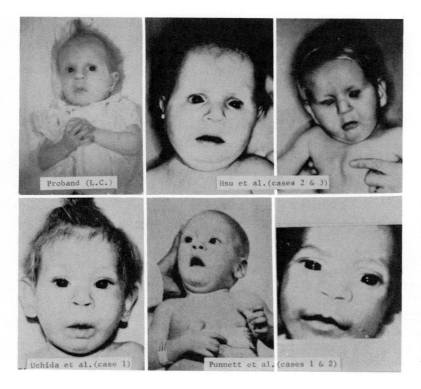

Fig. 1. Comparison of the facial morphology of the proband (top left) with other trisomy 22 patients showing the similarities. (From Hsu et al, *J. Pediatr.* 79:12-19, 1971; Uchida et al, *Am. J. Hum. Genet.* 20:107, Copyright 1968 by the American Society of Human Genetics, University of Chicago Press; and Punnett et al, *Theoret. Appl. Genetics 43*:134-138, 1973, with permission.)

Discussion

On reviewing cases of nonmongoloid trisomy G or trisomy 22 in the literature, 8 probands were found to have similar clinical features and craniofacial morphology compared with our proband. Table 1 represents these similarities. Our proband (*L.C.*) appears in the far right-hand column. To the left of this appear the 3 cases reported by Punnett et al[5] to have trisomy 22, confirmed also by Q- and G-banding. Note the similarities in both craniofacial morphology (top half of Table) and clinical features (bottom half of Table).

An attempt has been made to further compare the craniofacial morphology at ap-

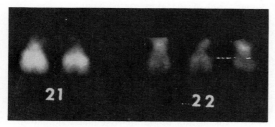

Fig. 2. Partial karyotype from the proband.

proximately one year of age. A collage has been made which represents frontal facial photographs of our proband and the other probands described in the Table (Fig. 1). Please note again the similarities in craniofacial morphology.

A medical artist's conception of the pertinent craniofacial features is represented in Figure 3. Note the following features: turricephaly with apparent increased vertical skull dimensions; frontal prominence; decreased bifrontal-temporal dimension; semicircular eyebrows merging with the lateral nasal borders; palpebral fissures with decreased transverse and increased vertical dimensions; superior lateral and inferior medial ocular skin folds; increased philtral length; downturned commissures of the mouth; small lower face with retruded chin; low-set ears with large lobules; and apparent facial asymmetry most notable in right ear being more medially positioned.

It is our feeling that the syndrome of trisomy 22 can have an identifiable phenotype. In the evaluation of a mentally retarded child the presence of these craniofacial features,

Table 1. Comparison of the Clinical Features in the Proband (*L.C.*) with 8 Other Probands in Literature

	Uchida et al[2]		Hsu et al[3]			Goodman et al[4]	Punnett et al[5]			L.C.
	Case 1	Case 2	Case 1	Case 2	Case 3		Case 1	Case 2	Case 3	
Sex	F	M	F	F	F	M	M	F	M	F
Craniofacial Morphology:										
Microcephaly	+	?	+	+	+	?	+	+	-	+
Frontal prominence	obs.	-	obs.	obs.	obs.	+	obs.	obs.	obs.	+
Narrow bitemporal width	obs.	?	obs.	obs.	obs.	?	obs.	obs.	?	+
Semicircular eyebrows	obs.	?	obs.	obs.	obs.	?	obs.	obs.	?	+
Depressed nasal bridge	obs.	+	obs.	obs.	+	?	obs.	obs.	obs.	+
Eyelid folds	obs.	?	obs.	obs.	obs.	?	obs.	obs.	?	+
Large external ears	obs.	obs.	+	+	+	+	+	?	?	+
Low-set ears	+	+	-	+	-	?	+	?	+	+
Preauricular anomalies	+	-	+	+	+	+	+	+	+	-
Long philtrum	obs.	obs.	obs.	obs.	obs.	+	obs.	obs.	?	+
Downturned mouth commissure	-	?	obs.	obs.	obs.	?	obs.	obs.	obs.	+
Micrognathia	+	+	+	+	obs.	+	obs.	?	+	+
Palatal morphology	cleft	high	cleft	cleft	cleft	high	high	?	cleft	high
Epiglottis Abnormality	?	?	?	?	?	?	+	?	?	+
Anomalies of Great Vessels	+	-	?	?	?	?	+	+	+	+
Cardiac Anomaly	+	+	+	+	?	?	+	+	?	+
Finger-Like Thumbs	+	-	+	+	+	+	+	+	?	+
Long Slender Fingers	+	?	obs.	obs.	obs.	+	obs.	?	?	+
Undescended Testicle		?				+	+		+	
Hypotonia	+	?	+	?	?	+	?	?	+	+
Mental Retardation	+	?	+	+	+	+	+	+	+	+
Feeding Difficulty	+	?	?	?	?	?	?	?	?	+
Failure to Thrive	+	?	+	+	+	+	+	+	+	+

obs. = Observed in photographs of patient.

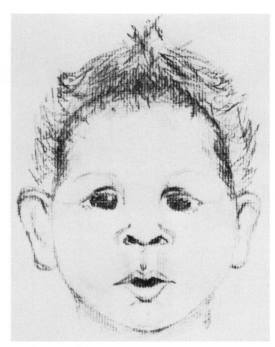

Fig. 3. A medical artist's conception of the pertinent craniofacial features in trisomy.

especially if associated with abnormalities in the epiglottis, great vessels and heart, could be suggestive of trisomy 22.

Acknowledgments

We are grateful to Ms. Carol Johnson for the drawing of Figure 3. We also thank Mrs. Helen Hamaguchi, Mrs. Anna Derecsenyi and the personnel of the Cytogenetics Laboratory, Childrens Hospital of Los Angeles, for their help.

References

1. Sparkes, R. S., Veomett, I. C. and Wright, S. W.: Trisomy G without Down's syndrome. *Lancet* *1*:270, 1966.
2. Uchida, I. A., Ray, M., McRae, K. N. and Besant, D. F.: Familial occurrence of trisomy 22. *Am. J. Hum. Genet. 20*:107, 1968.
3. Hsu, L. Y. F., Shapiro, L. R., Gertner, M., Lieber, E. and Hirschhorn, K.: Trisomy 22: A clinical entity. *J. Pediatr. 79*:12-19, 1971.
4. Goodman, R. M., Ratznelson, M. B., Spero, M. et al: The question of trisomy 22 syndrome. *J. Pediatr. 79*:174, 1971.
5. Punnett, H. H., Kistenmacher, M. L., Toro-Sola, M. A. and Kohn, G.: Quinacrine fluorescence and giemsa banding in trisomy 22. *Theoret. Appl. Genetics 43*:134-138, 1973.

Discussion

Dr. Brenner: We also have a case identified by banding of this syndrome. So I think that a specific syndrome will definitely emerge.

Dr. Kaufman: We have seen one case of trisomy 22 which we were asked to see as a potential Rubinstein-Taybi, which did not really clinically fit. We have another case, a 14-year-old girl in Missouri, who is well-known because her case is now before the Supreme Court of Missouri, as to whether or not a mentally retarded minor can be sterilized. I think that you will be hearing a lot more about such chromosomal anomalies in years to come. Just as an informal poll, I wonder how many people have documented trisomy 22 cases that they have seen? Would you raise your hands? I would imagine that it is a large number.

Moderator: You are quite right, it is a good size group.

Dr. Sanger: I did not previously mention that the only previously reported cases of documented trisomy 22 before our report today were the 3 cases reported by Punnett et al. The other cases reported were not definite.

Dr. Di Liberti: I worked with Dr. Punnett, and, as I recall, the 3 cases that we had all had dimples at the junction of the ear and the skull. Were you aware of these in your case?

Dr. Sanger: No, there were no preauricular pits, sinuses or tags in our patient.

Dr. Carnevale: We have 2 cases with an extra G chromosome that has been shown to be a 22. I want to ask if your case has some anorectal anomaly because our 2 have an anorectal anomaly; we thought we could see the cat-eye syndrome in one of them. I think that there may be some confusion in the literature about the cat-eye and the 22 syndrome.

Dr. Sanger: Our patient did have a prominent coccyx and a short perineal body with posterior displacement of the vulva and anterior displacement of the anus.

Dr. Temtamy: We have some interest in the description. You describe the fingers as long and the thumb as long and finger-like. A finger-like thumb reminds me of a thumb with three phalanges like other fingers, and long meta-carpals. Would this be the same abnormality as your case?

Dr. Sanger: No. Unfortunately, we took that description from what other authors had reported the thumbs to be like in their patients, which were finger-like, hyperextensible, more proximally placed, and so forth. There were no bony abnormalities of the thumb. The thumb has the apparent slenderness as the fingers do but does not exhibit three phalanges.

X-Autosome Translocation with a 47,XXYqs,t(9p-;Xq+) Karyotype[*]

Kenneth W. Dumars, M.D., Pamela Reed, M.A. and Helen J. Lawce, B.S.

Prior to 1971 and the development of banding techniques, C-group aberrations were difficult to accurately identify cytogenetically. The cytogenetic interpretation of X-chromosome abnormalities was dependent upon buccal smears and autoradiography.[1] In 1968, a patient came to our attention presenting multiple anomalies associated with a chromatin-positive buccal smear (23%) and an apparent 47,XXY karyotype. The diagnosis of Klinefelter syndrome was reluctantly entertained, but in view of the small testicular size, a positive buccal smear, lowered volar ridge count, and 47,XXY karyotype, this seemed most likely. Other investigators such as Grand et al[2] and Becker et al[3] had reported cases of Klinefelter syndrome with multiple birth defects and a variety of other clinical findings. With the advent of banding and in light of the atypical clinical manifestation, the patient was recently reevaluated.

Case Report

B.R., the proband, a male born 12/12/63, was the product of an uneventful 36-week pregnancy. His mother, at the time of the proband's birth, was 33 years old, gravida 7, para 5. The birthweight was 3006 gm with no immediate neonatal problems. Deformities of the hands and feet were noted at birth. Developmental milestones reveal that the proband sat alone at 18 months and walked at 3 years. Speech at 10½ years was minimal; comprehension of verbal and gestural communication was good. Examination of the proband at 10 years of age revealed a white male, obviously small for chronologic age; weight 25.6 Kg, height 128.9 cm and head circumference 50.45 cm (Figs. 1 and 2). He walked with a stiff-legged gait and slightly anteflexed at the waist. The forehead was narrow with marked bitemporal bossing. The ears were normally placed but the pinnas were prominent and cup-shaped. There was slight hypertelorism. The penis was small, the right testis was not palpable, and the left testis was in the scrotum and measured less than 1 cm in greatest diameter. The 3rd, 4th and 5th fingers of the right hand had a flexion deformity at the distal interphalangeal joint. There was a middle phalanx present on the 5th finger; however, only a single flexion crease. Clinodactyly was present in the 5th finger bilaterally. The 2nd, 3rd, 4th and 5th interphalangeal joints on the left hand were bulky with a slight flexion deformity and definite limitation of motion at these joints. The feet had very tiny nails with limitation of motion at the ankles. The 5th toe was displaced medially and overrode the 4th toe. The 4th toe was plantar-flexed at the proximal interphalangeal joint. He had a mild S-shaped scoliosis.

Laboratory Studies

Dermatoglyphic analysis revealed a volar ridge count of 28 (Table 1). Sex-chromatin analysis was positive for single Barr bodies in the buccal mucosa (23%), skin (28%) and testis (42%) (Fig. 3). Quinacrine fluorescence of the metaphase figures revealed a normally fluorescing Y with lightly fluorescing satellites at the distal end. Urine screen for inborn errors was negative. At 10½ years urine 17-ketogenic steroids were 1.5 mg for 24 hours and 17-KS, 1.2 mg for 24 hours. An EEG showed a grossly abnormal tracing. There was evidence of abnormal spike wave activity from the central and posterior hemispheres appearing at maximal intensity over the right occipital area.

*Supported in part by grant C-110 from The National Foundation-March of Dimes and grant 59-P-45211/9-02 from the Department of HEW Social and Rehabilitative Services.

247

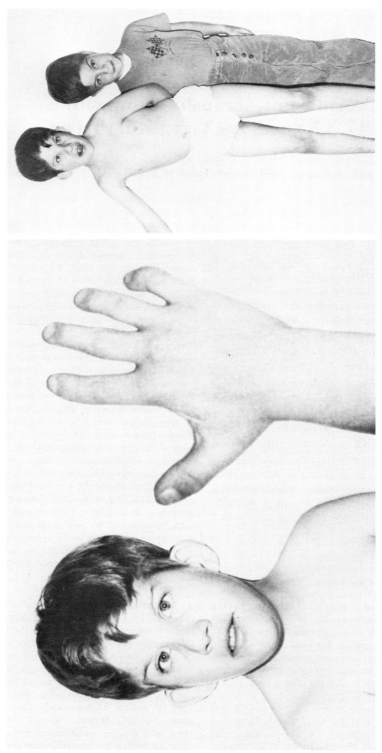

Fig. 2. *B.R.* at age 10½ with normal 6-year-old sib.

Fig. 1. *B.R.*, the proband, at age 10½ and left hand showing clinodactyly and slight flexion deformity.

Table 1.

DERMATOGLYPHIC ANALYSIS													

Digits

	Left					L	Total	R	Right				
	5	4	3	2	1				1	2	3	4	5
Patterns	U	U	U	A	TA				TA	A	U	U	U
Ridge Count	2	4	4	0	0	10	28	18	0	0	9	5	4

Palms

	D	C	B	A	Axial Triradius Height	ATD Angle	HT	T·I$_1$	I$_2$	I$_3$	I$_4$
Left	+	o	o	+	+	45°	L$_R$	L$_L$	0	0	0
Right	o	o	o	+	+	45°	%	%	0	0	0

Soles

	D	C	B	A	HaL	HT	CAL	TH	Th/I	I$_2$	I$_3$	I$_4$	Big Toe
Left	+	o	o	+	Ap	—	—	—	0	0	0	W	—
Right	o	o	o	+	Ap	—	—	—	0	L$_D$	0	0	—

Partial Simian Crease   Single Crease 5th Digit
Left +   Right +   Left +   Right +

KEY
A : Arch   U : Ulnar Loop
TA: Tented Arch   W: Simple Whorl
Ap: Arch proximal   L : Loop (L)Left (R)Right (D)Double

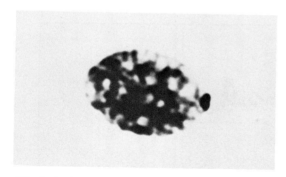

Fig. 3. An interphase nucleus from the buccal mucosa of the proband showing a single Barr body.

Cytogenetics

Analysis of 100 metaphase figures obtained from peripheral leukocytes revealed a modal chromosome number of 47. Analysis of 15 metaphase figures from skin fibroblasts and 15 figures from testicular fibroblasts also revealed a modal number of 47. ASG-banding after the method of Sumner et al,[4] revealed all cells with a complement of 47 chromosomes to

have a karyotype of 47,XXYqs,t(9p-;Xq+) (Fig. 4). Both the mother and father have been banded and karyotyped. Each presented a normal karyotype of 46 chromosomes with the exception of the satellited Y which appeared in the father (Fig. 5). Two of the proband's 5 brothers, a paternal uncle and the paternal grandfather have been karyotyped and presented normal complements of 46,XY with the satellited Y.

Discussion

The 47,XXYqs,t(9p-;Xq+) karyotype structurally produces a translocation between 9q and Xq with a loss of 9p, resulting in a 9p monosomy Xp disomy, a trisomy for Xq as well as satellites attached to the distal ends of the long arms of the Y. A review of the literature revealed this to be the first reported case of (9p-;Xq+) unbalanced translocation. Cohen[5] reported a balanced 46,X,t(Xq-;9p+) karyotype with no gross somatic phenotypic effect. Clinical descriptions of a 9p monosomy by Alfi[6]

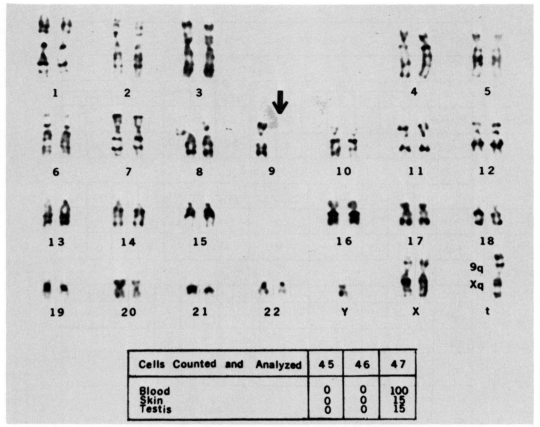

Cells Counted and Analyzed	45	46	47
Blood	0	0	100
Skin	0	0	15
Testis	0	0	15

Fig. 4. Karyotype from lymphocyte cultures of the proband utilizing ASG-banding, showing the t9p-;Xq+.

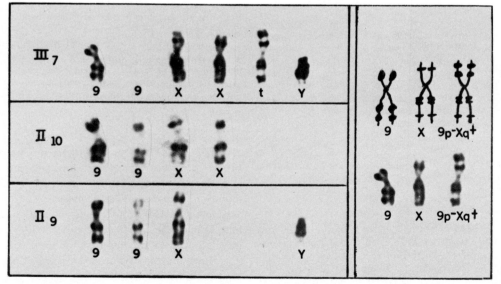

Fig. 5. Partial karyotype from the proband, mother (*II-10*) and father (*II-9*) comparing autosomes 9, and sex chromosomes X and satellited Y.

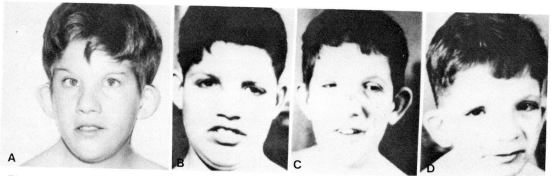

Fig. 6. A) Facial photograph of the proband, a 9p monosomy. B-D) Three reported cases of 9p trisomy. (Figs. 6B-D from Rethore, M. O. et al: Analyse de la trisomie 9p par dénaturation ménagée. *Humangenetik* *18*:129-138, 1973, with permission.)

and 9p trisomy by Rethore,[7] Baccichetti[8] and Cantú[9] reveal clinical findings similar to our patient with a 9p monosomy, ie flat nasal bridge, mild hypertelorism, external ear malformations, lowered volar ridge count and mental retardation. In this instance there is a rather similar facial configuration with those cases exhibiting trisomy 9p (Fig. 6).

Although our patient was disomic for the X and had a small penis and testis, he did not otherwise suggest the phenotype of Klinefelter syndrome. His height, weight and head circumference were more than 2 SD below the norm. He had a positive buccal smear (23% Barr bodies), and the volar ridge count and 17-KS were lowered as one would expect.

Kurschat[10] has described a patient trisomic for the X and associated anomalies such as scoliosis and bossing, but also a micropenis and anomalies of the eye which are not manifested in our patient. Clinically our patient more closely resembled those with monosomy or

trisomy for the 9p rather than a polysomy for the X.

X-autosome translocations have often been ascertained in studies of primary amenorrhea[11-13] and few males have been described with the aberration.[14-16] The issue presently under study is the determination of the late replicating of the X or the Xt chromosome. Autoradiographic studies on this case are not complete and will be reported at a later date. At present we see no cell nucleus with 2 Barr bodies and it would seem a priori that the (9p-;Xq+) would not be late replicating in view of Hamerton's thesis[1] that the final inactivation pattern is usually such that the genetic imbalance in the cell is minimal.

The satellited Y provided us with an intriguing aspect of the case. This chromosome appeared to be an extremely stable marker with no deleterious phenotypic effects. A family with a similar satellited Y has been traced by Genest[17,18] through 12 generations with a

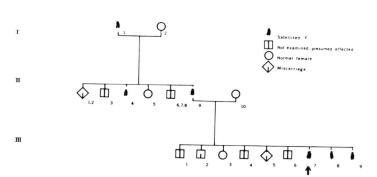

Fig. 7. Pedigree of *Family R* showing the satellited Y appearing in the males of 3 generations.

common ancestor of all those who exhibit the marker. Through personal communication with Dr. Genest, it is believed that this proband and his male relatives are indeed a part of this extensive pedigree (Fig. 7).

Summary

A male with a karyotype 47,XXYqs,t(9p-;Xq+) was ascertained utilizing ASG-banding. The karyotype was repeated because the original diagnosis of Klinefelter syndrome (47,XXY) was inconsistent with many of the stigmata present. It is suggested that many karyotypes completed prior to the advent of banding techniques will be repeated in an attempt to provide more accurate diagnosis, describe more aberrations, and possibly establish new syndromes.

Acknowledgments

The technical assistance of Gayle Fialko, Janet Burwell and Larry Shockey is gratefully acknowledged. The cooperation established with Dr. Paul Genest is greatly appreciated.

References

1. Hamerton, J. L.: *Human Cytogenetics.* New York:Academic Press, 1971, vols. 1 and 2.
2. Grand, R. J., Rosen, S. W., Di Sant'Agnese, P. A. and Kirkham, W. R.: Unusual case of XXY Klinefelter's syndrome with pancreatic insufficiency, hypothyroidism, deafness, chronic lung disease, dwarfism and microcephaly. *Am. J. Med.* *41*:478-485, 1966.
3. Becker, K. L., Hoffman, D. L., Albert, A. et al: Klinefelter's syndrome. *Arch. Intern. Med.* *118*:314-321, 1966.
4. Sumner, A. T., Evans, H. J. and Buckland, R. A.: A new technique for distinguishing between human chromosomes. *Nature (New Biol.)* *232*:31-32, 1971.
5. Cohen, M. M., Lin, C., Sybert, V. and Orecchio, E. J.: Two human X-autosome translocations identified by autoradiography and fluorescence. *Am. J. Hum. Genet.* 24:583-597, 1972.
6. Alfi, O., Donnell, G. N., Crandall, B. F. et al: Deletion of the short arm of chromosome #9(46,9p-): A new deletion syndrome. *Ann. Genet. (Paris)* 16:17-22, 1973.
7. Rethore, M. O., Hoehn, H., Rott, H. D. et al: Analyse de la trisomie 9p par dénaturation ménagée. *Humangenetik 18*:129-138, 1973.
8. Baccichetti, C. and Tenconi, R.: A new case of trisomy for the short arm of No. 9 chromosome. *J. Med. Genet. 10*:296-298, 1973.
9. Cantú, J. M., Buentello, L. and Armendares, S.: Trisomie Cp: Un Nouveau Syndrome. *Ann. Genet. (Paris) 14*:177-186, 1971.
10. Kurschat, G., Leyh, F. and Tolksdorf, M.: Atypisches Klinefelter-Syndrom mit XXXY-geschlechs chromosomen. *Andrologie 4*:269-275, 1972.
11. Sarto, G. E., Therman, E. and Patau, K.: X inactivation in man: A woman with t(Xq-;12q+). *Am. J. Hum. Genet. 25*:262-270, 1973.
12. Mann, J. D., Valdmanis, A., Capps, S. C. and Puite, R. H.: A case of primary amenorrhea with a translocation involving chromosomes of groups B and C. *Am. J. Hum. Genet. 17*:377, 1965.
13. Thorburn, M. J., Martin, P. A. and Pathak, U. N.: Case report: Possible X/autosomal translocation in a girl with gonadal dysgenesis. *J. Med. Genet. 7*:402-406, 1970.
14. Summitt, R. L., Martens, P. R. and Wilroy, R. S., Jr.: X-autosome translocation in normal mother and effectively 21-monosomic daughter. *J. Pediatr. 84*:539-546, 1974.
15. Allerdice, P. W., Miller, O. J., Klinger, H. P. et al: Demonstration of a spreading effect in an X-autosome translocation by combined autoradiographic and quinacrine-fluorescence studies. In de Grouchy, J., Ebling, F. J. G., Henderson, I. and Francois, J. (eds.): *Fourth International Congress on Human Genetics.* Amsterdam:Excerpta Medica, 1965, pp. 14-15.
16. Buckton, K. E., Jacobs, P. A., Rae, L. A. et al: An inherited X-autosome translocation in man. *Ann. Hum. Genet. 35*:171-178, 1971.
17. Genest, P.: A human satellited Y chromosome with a probably illegitimate paternal origin. *Can. Med. Assoc. J. 107*:1205-1206, 1972.
18. Genest, P.: Origine Probable D'un Chromosome Y à Satellites Trouvé dans une Famille Canadienne-Francais. *L'Union Medicale du Canada 102*:2470-2472, 1973.

Discussion

Dr. Summitt: If this is a 9-X translocation, and if this involves most or all of the long arm of X, why do you not see a second X-chromatin there?

Dr. Dumars: At the present time we are trying to resolve this with autoradiography. I believe that the translocated X is not inactivated; that, in keeping with Hamerton's thesis, inactivation is going to follow the course that disturbs the genotype the least. We have looked vigorously for a second X-chromatin but we have not found it.

Dr. Summitt: The reason I ask the question is that I wonder if this banding pattern would be compatible with another design, which would be that the band which appears to be the major G-positive band in what would appear to be the long arm of the X might be the short arm of 9, and that the negative band and the distal G-positive band be something else besides an X.

Dr. Dumars: I cannot deny that. It is just that the length of that translocated segment is so large that it did not seem to be the short arm of the 9, plus the fact that we could not find the source of any other translocated segment.

Dr. Francke: From looking at your karyotype, I had a similar impression. Would it not be possible that this long chromosome represents a full No. 9 which has a duplication of part of No. 9 added on to the No. 9? Therefore, you have an effective trisomy for No. 9, and this would explain the phenotype.

Dr. Dumars: I cannot deny that. I hope that our future autoradiography will clear up the matter.

Dr. Pallister: I think that in a case that we reported, one by Reynolds and Miller, plus other cases, the heterochromatization will follow the line that will protect the patient. We had a familial translocation in a boy with Klinefelter disorder who had a very large Barr body, with an autosome translocation to the long arm of the X, that involved almost the entire 14 chromosome. This heterochromotype is in such a fashion that the X turned off the entire effect of the trisomy of the D and formed the large Barr body. But the patient was only trisomic for the long arm of the X and still was Klinefelter, showing that the short arm of the X has no bearing upon whether a person becomes Klinefelter or not. He is a clear Klinefelter and nothing else.

Dr. Dumars: I think that, if we take the long arm of the X and the long arm of the 9, and superimpose them, next to the translocated chromosome, they are identical.

Dr. Warren: I think that all of us here would agree that the banding technique has increased the resolution of our art tremendously, but what I hear here today is the trap that we all seem to fall into, and that is, a significant amount of overinterpretation. I would like to publicly ask for some restraint in this regard, before we really do get bogged down and start calling a lot of things that are not what they seem to be.

Dr. Dumars: I think that is part of what we were saying about the similarity between the 9 monosomy and a 9 trisomy. I think that we are going to need a lot more information about the gene loci on the chromosome before we can make much in the way of deductions from this sort of information. I agree with you.

Sex Chromosome Mosaicism of X/XY or X/XY/XYY*

Miriam G. Wilson, M.D., Allan J. Ebbin, M.D., Nancy W. Shinno, M.D.
and Joseph W. Towner, Ph.D.

Sex chromosomal mosaicism of X/XY, first described by Hirschhorn et al[1] is recognized to be an infrequent but not a rare event. In a recent review, 78 cases of X/XY were noted.[2] The majority of these patients were phenotypically female, although frequently masculinized, and usually had mixed gonadal dysgenesis with a dysplastic testis on one side and a gonadal streak on the other. Genital ambiguity occasionally led to a clinical problem in selecting the appropriate sex of rearing. A further clinical consideration is that a gonadal tumor, usually a gonadoblastoma, was found in about one quarter of these patients.

We have had the opportunity over a 7-year period to study 7 patients with X/XY or X/XY/XYY mosaicism. These cases illustrate the range of presenting phenotype and gonadal

pathology in this disorder, and further emphasize the importance of making the diagnosis of a mosaic Y-line because of the possibility of a gonadal tumor. The cytogenetic results suggest that the Y chromosome is structurally modified in at least some patients with X/XY mosaicism.

Case Reports

Patient 1

D.B. (061273) was the third child of a gravida 3 para 3, 23-year-old Mexican-American mother and a 21-year-old white father of German descent. At term birth the child weighed 3500 gm and measured 51 cm in length. The pregnancy was uneventful.

At birth the patient was noted to have a third degree hypospadias, left cryptorchidism, and a common urogenital sinus into which the vagina opened (Fig. 1). The scrotum was bifid and of normal size. A

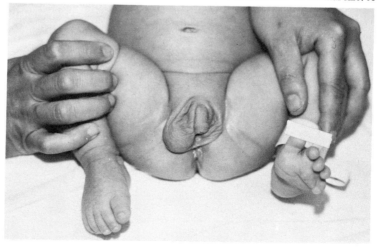

Fig. 1. Patient 1 (D.B.) at 1 month of age: The external genitalia appeared primarily male.

*Supported by grant 286 from Maternal and Child Health Services, USPHS.

gonad was palpable in the right scrotum. No gonad was palpable on the left. The phallus was small with a chordee in the opening at the junction of the shaft and the scrotum. A small sacral dimple was present. There was a 1½ × 1 cm café-au-lait spot on the right anterior chest. The physical examination was otherwise unremarkable.

The patient had a normal brother and sister. The father had an uncle with mental retardation which was thought to result from a febrile illness. The father had a brother and a cousin with speech defects. The mother's family history was unremarkable.

A buccal smear for sex chromatin was negative (100 cells examined). Chromosome analysis of peripheral blood revealed 45,X/46,XY and analysis of fibroblasts from skin culture revealed 45,X in all cells. Chromosome analyses of peripheral blood from the parents were normal. The Y chromosomes from child and father were the same size. Serum testosterone, urinary 17-KS and ketogenic steroids were normal. Radiographic studies revealed a hypoplastic vagina. An IVP showed normal kidneys, ureters and bladder.

Since there was uncertainty whether the external genitalia would develop adequately for adult male sexual function, the decision was made in conjunction with the parents to assign the female gender to this child. At 3 months, an exploratory laparotomy revealed a very small uterus and vagina, a fallopian tube and gonadal streak on the left side and a vas deferens and epididymis on the right side where the testis was found. The child had a bilateral gonadectomy and reconstructive surgery of the external genitalia consisting of removal of the excess scrotal skin and a clitoral recession (Fig. 2). A small (1.2 × 0.7 × 0.4 cm) testis was removed from the right scrotal sac. Microscopic examination of this gonad showed a disorganized appearance with testicular tubules separated by large amounts of primitive mesenchymal stroma. The epididymis and spermatic cord were normal. Tissue culture of the right gonad for chromosome analysis revealed 45,X/46,XY.

Tissue removed from the left gonadal streak on microscopic examination showed connective tissue stroma. No primordial follicles were identified. This tissue was in continuity with a small but microscopically normal fallopian tube. Tissue culture for chromosome analysis from the left side revealed 45,X/46,XY. No gonadal tumor was found.

The vagina and uterus were rudimentary, and plastic surgery for vaginal reconstruction was planned for a later date.

At 5 months of age this child was growing and developing normally. Her height was at the 50th percentile for age.

Patient 2

G.M. (040372) was the first child born to a 21-year-old, gravida 1 mother and a 33-year-old, unrelated father. Both parents were black. Following a 38-week uneventful pregnancy, the child was born weighing 2835 gm and measuring 49 cm in length. The pregnancy and family history were unremarkable.

The infant appeared normal at birth except for ambiguous genitalia. The phallus was 3 cm long and was fused at the corona to the scrotal sac. The labioscrotal folds were fused. The urethra opened at the base of the phallus. There was no palpable right gonad. A gonad was felt in the left inguinal canal.

Analysis of 100 cells from a buccal smear showed a negative X-chromatin result. Chromosome analysis of peripheral blood from the child demonstrated 45,X/46,XY mosaicism. Chromosome analyses of peripheral blood from both parents were normal, and the father's Y and child's Y were similar in length. Urinary 17-KS and pregnanetriol were normal.

At 3 months of age the child had a clitoral resection and bilateral gonadectomy. The left gonad (1.2 × 0.5 × 0.5 cm) was connected to a tubular structure and a hernia sac. Microscopically, this gonad was an abnormal testis consisting of small tubules composed of primitive germ cells separated by connec-

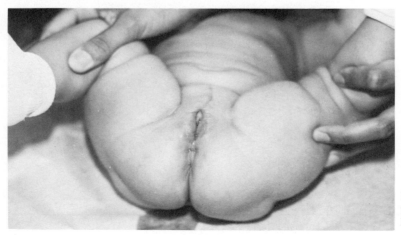

Fig. 2. Postoperative appearance of external genitalia of *Patient 1.*

tive tissue stroma. In addition, rete testis, epididymis, vas deferens and hernial sac were identified. Tissue culture obtained from the left gonad revealed both cell lines of 45,X and 46,XY.

The right gonad measured 1.2 × 0.2 × 0.2 cm and was attached to a tubular structure identified as a fallopian tube. Microscopic examination of the gonad revealed connective tissue stroma with a few undifferentiated primitive germ cells. No follicles or oocytes were identified. Chromosome analysis from tissue culture from this gonad revealed 45,X/46,XY. A small vagina and uterus were present.

At 2 years of age, this child was at the 50th percentile for height and was reportedly normal in development.

Patient 3

L.W. (111072), a Mexican-American female, was the first child born to a 30-year-old, gravida 1 mother and a 32-year-old father. Their union was nonconsanguineous. The infant was the product of a 38-week gestation, weighed 3515 gm and was 50.5 cm long. The only congenital abnormality was a large clitoris (Fig. 3).

The parents had attempted a pregnancy for 5 years. One month prior to conception the mother had radiographic studies of her fallopian tubes. The mother took 120 mg of thyroid daily for 2 years prior to the pregnancy and used marijuana and LSD occasionally before the pregnancy. The mother had an aunt with syndactyly and a cousin with syndactyly and polydactyly.

Buccal smear was negative for sex chromatin (100 cells examined). A fluorescent stain from cultured peripheral blood showed a fluorescing Y body. Chromosome analysis from peripheral blood culture revealed 45,X/46,XY. A skin fibroblast culture also showed both cell lines. Chromosome analyses of

peripheral blood from the parents were normal. The child's and father's Y chromosomes were similar in length. Serum testosterone was normal.

At 16 months of age, bilateral gonadectomy and clitoral recession were performed. Microscopic examination of the left gonad (measuring 1 × 0.5 × 0.5 cm) showed a well-differentiated fetal testis. Chromosome analysis from this gonad revealed 45,X/46,XY. The tubal structure on the left side had portions which resembled fallopian tube and areas which appeared to be epididymis and vas deferens. The right gonad was a thin strip of pinkish-tan tissue measuring 1 × 3 cm. A small tubular structure measuring 2 mm in diameter traversed through the specimen and on microscopic examination was a well-developed fallopian tube with fimbriated end. The gonad tissue was identified as ovarian stroma. No primordial ova or germinal cells were seen. There was no evidence of tumor. A tissue culture from the right gonad failed to grow.

The vagina was normal in length. The uterus, which was in a normal anatomic position, was small.

The child's height was between the 50th and 75th percentiles and her development was apparently normal at 18 months of age.

Patient 4

L.L. (180768) was born at 39 weeks' gestation, weighing 2550 gm and measuring 47 cm long. The mother was 16 years old and gravida 1. The father was 18 years old. The parents were black, healthy and consanguineous. The pregnancy and family history were not remarkable.

At birth the infant was noted to have a flat hemangioma over the brow, nose and upper lip; a medial epicanthus of the left eye; webbing of the neck; increased distance between inverted nipples; coarctation of the aorta; and bilateral simian lines (Fig. 4). A diagnosis of Turner syndrome was made.

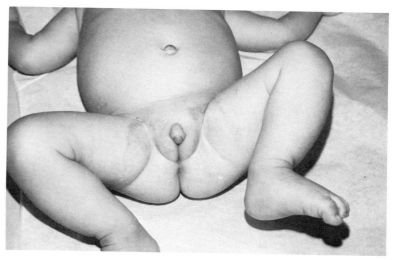

Fig. 3. *Patient 3 (L.W.):* The only external abnormality was a large clitoris.

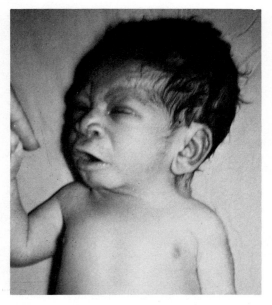

Fig. 4. *Patient 4 (L.L.)* at birth: Coarctation of the aorta was present in addition to the stigmata of Turner syndrome observed here.

A buccal smear was negative for X-chromatin bodies. Chromosome analysis from peripheral blood demonstrated the cell lines of 45,X and 46,XY. Analysis from a skin biopsy culture showed predominately the 45,X line.

A cardiac catheterization demonstrated coarctation in the descending portion of the transverse aorta. An IVP, a serum T_4 determination and thyroid antibody studies gave normal results. A radiogram of the hands showed short 4th and 5th metacarpals.

At 2½ years of age, the child had a bilateral gonadectomy. A normal appearing uterus and fallopian tubes, a fibrous streak of 1.8 cm replacing the left gonad, and a right gonad of 1.0 cm diameter also grossly appearing to be connective tissue were noted. These streaks were in the normal anatomic position for ovaries. On microscopic examination, the right gonad was found to have dysplastic testicular tissue and gonadoblastoma (Fig. 5). After careful sectioning of the left streak, gonadoblastoma was found on this side also. Chromosome analysis from the tissue on the left showed primarily the 45,X line, while the tissue on the right side showed only the 45,X line. No X-chromatin body was found in 600 cells examined from fibroblast cultures from the skin and left streak.

At 5½ years of age, this child was developing normally. Her height was less than the third percentile for age. A bone age at 5 years was consistent with the chronologic age.

Patient 5

M.H. (130756) was born at 40 weeks' gestation, weighing 2495 gm and measuring 48.5 cm in length, to a gravida 2, 21-year-old mother and a 24-year-old father. Six normal sibs were subsequently born. The parents were black, healthy and not related. The pregnancy and family history were not remarkable.

The infant was born by a breech delivery and had transient respiratory distress at birth. She was considered normal up to about 10 years of age when her short stature was apparent. At 14 years of age she was noted to have no secondary sexual characteristics and no menarche. She had a normal facial appearance, widely spaced and hypoplastic nipples, no breast development, slight cubitus valgus, and normal external genitalia, vagina and cervix. A buccal smear was negative for X-chromatin bodies.

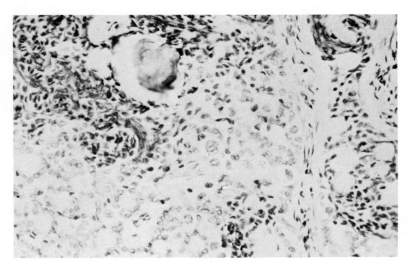

Fig. 5. Gonadoblastoma found in *Patient 4*. Note the characteristic appearance of nests of cells and hyaline bodies (high power).

At 16 years of age, following a trial of androgen therapy to stimulate height, she was noted to have sparse pubic and axillary hair. Height and weight were less than the third percentile. Height and arm span were each 136 cm. Bone age was 13 years. Radiographs of the chest and skull and an IVP were normal. Intelligence appeared normal.

A chromosome analysis from peripheral blood showed both cell lines: 46,XY (the predominant line) and 45,X.

Additional laboratory studies at 16 years included the following: elevated plasma FSH and LH, elevated urinary gonadotropic hormones, normal plasma testosterone, low urinary estrogens and normal serum T_4.

A bilateral gonadectomy was done at 16 years. The uterus and fallopian tubes appeared normal. Dense fibrous stroma without follicles replaced the gonads. There was no testicular tissue nor tumor found. Chromosome analysis from each gonad demonstrated 45,X/46,XY mosaicism.

She was placed on estrogen therapy. Height and weight remained less than the third percentile.

Patient 6

S.C. (180753) was the fifth child born to Chinese parents, both 35 years of age, healthy and not related. The pregnancy was uncomplicated except for premature delivery at 32 weeks' gestation. Birthweight was 2100 gm. The mother was gravida 5. Family history was noncontributory. Two older sisters had normal menstrual histories.

This patient presented for genetic work-up at 18 years of age because of amenorrhea and failure to develop sexually. She was a very attractive, but short girl, only 147 cm tall. She weighed 41 kg and had an arm span of 152 cm. The following were noted: a high-arched palate, low posterior hairline, widely spaced nipples, no breast development, a small amount of pubic hair, no facial or axillary hair, normal external genitalia, a small vagina, small cervix, and a palpable uterus.

Buccal smear showed no X-chromatin body and no Y-fluorescing body in 200 cells examined. Chromosome analysis from blood culture demonstrated 2 cell lines: 45,X and 46,XY. The karyotypes were studied by trypsin-Giemsa banding and quinacrine fluorescence. The Y was small and did not fluoresce. Chromosome analyses from the parents showed normal results. The father's Y compared in size to that of his child and showed bright fluorescence over the distal long arm.

FSH was elevated, LH was elevated, and estrogen (E_2) was low. Thyroid function tests (T_3, T_4 PBI) were normal. Bone age was 13 years. Skull radiographs and visual fields were normal.

The patient had a bilateral gonadectomy. The gonads were represented by fibrous streaks in which no ovarian follicles, testicular tissue or tumor were identified. A small uterus and normal fallopian tubes were present.

At 18 years of age this patient had hormone-induced menses and breast development. She was attending college.

Patient 7

D.H. (130163), previously reported,[3] was born at home after a term pregnancy and weighed 2290 gm. The mother was an 18-year-old primigravida of German descent. There is no information whatsoever about the father except that he was said not to be related.

The child first presented at 2 years of age because of a minor infection. The physical examination disclosed a large obese child with a clitoris measuring 2 cm in length. The clitoris had been enlarged since birth according to the mother. A small vaginal orifice and normal labia were noted. Urinary pregnanetriol and 17-KS determinations were normal. The bone age corresponded to the chronologic age. The child did not return for completion of diagnostic studies and was next seen at 5 years of age, at which time the physical findings were the same. Urinary pregnanetriol and 17-KS were again normal. The bone age approximated the chronological age. An IVP showed a ureteropelvic constriction.

A buccal smear was negative for X-chromatin bodies (600 cells examined). A chromosome analysis from blood culture demonstrated 2 cell lines of 46,XY and 47,XYY. Chromosome analysis from skin showed additionally a 45,X line, thus constituting a 3-cell line mosaicism.

Abdominal surgery at 6 years of age demonstrated a normal uterus, fallopian tubes, a right fibrous gonadal streak and a small left gonad measuring 0.8 cm in length. Bilateral gonadectomy and a clitoral resection were done.

Histopathologic examination of the removed gonad tissue demonstrated connective tissue stroma without follicles on the right side and dysplastic, immature testicular tubular tissue in the left gonad. Chromosome analysis from each gonad demonstrated the 3-cell line mosaicism: 45,X/46,XY/47,XYY.

At 8 years of age, this child was of normal height (50th%) and obese (>90th%). Intellectual abilities were considered normal.

Summary of Cytogenetic Results

Chromosome studies from blood and both gonads were obtained from all 7 patients, and from skin in 4 patients, and from blood of all parents with one exception (father of *Patient 7*). The results are found in Table 1. The Y line was detected in the blood in all patients, and predominated in analyses from blood culture in 4 patients. This finding, consistent with the

Table 1. Cytogenetic Results

Patient	Tissue	% of cells with 45,X	% of cells with 46,XY	% of cells with 47,XYY	No. of Cells Analyzed
1 (D.B.)	Blood	(25%)*	75%		64
	Skin	100%			50
	Rt. testis	94%	(6%)		50
	Lt. streak	72%	(28%)		25
2 (G.M.)	Blood	(35%)	65%		31
	Rt. streak	92%	(8%)		25
	Lt. testis	88%	(12%)		25
3 (L.W.)	Blood	76%	(24%)		50
	Skin	61%	(39%)		23
	Rt. streak	culture failure			
	Lt. testis	58%	(42%)		24
4 (L.L.)	Blood	91%	(9%)		105
	Skin	94%	(6%)		50
	Rt. testis	100%			50
	Lt. streak	97%	(3%)		38
5 (M.H.)	Blood	(26%)	74%		47
	Rt. streak	79%	(21%)		24
	Lt. streak	68%	(32%)		22
6 (S.C.)	Blood	88%	(12%)		75
	Rt. streak	83%	(17%)		24
	Lt. streak	100%			25
7 (D.H.)	Blood	0	75%	(25%)	100
	Skin	34%	(18%)	48%	50
	Rt. streak	47%	50%	(3%)	100
	Lt. gonad	68%	28%	(4%)	50

*Minor cell line is inclosed in ( ).

report of Ferrier et al,[4] is important since it suggests that examination of karyotypes from blood are most informative in the detection of Y mosaicism. The predominant cell line in the majority of other tissues was 45,X. In *Patients 1, 4 and 6,* no cell line with a Y chromosome was found in 3 tissues (gonads and skin), which showed only the nonmosaic 45,X constitution. There was no relationship between the degree of masculinization of the phenotype and the proportion of cell lines with a Y chromosome.

All patients showed negative X-chromatin from buccal smear or fibroblast culture, as expected.

The G-group of chromosomes and the Y chromosomes from these patients and their fathers are illustrated in Figure 6. The paired Y chromosomes from *Patients 1-6* and fathers resembled each other morphologically. The

unusual Y chromosome found in *Patient 7* is illustrated in partial karyotypes from her XY and XYY cell lines (Fig. 7). Her father was not available for examination.

The fluorescence patterns of the G-group chromosomes and Y chromosomes from the patients are presented in Figures 8 and 9. In *Patient 6,* the Y chromosome, although slightly larger than a member of the G-group, showed no brightly fluorescing band over the long arm. The father's Y chromosome was about the same size but demonstrated bright fluorescence over the distal portion of the long arm (Fig. 9).

In *Patient 7,* the fluorescing segment of the long arm did not extend to the end of the arm (Fig. 9). To date, our experience with other Y chromosomes of this size (all show fluorescence to the end of the arm) suggests that the Y chromosome observed in *Patient 7* may be a

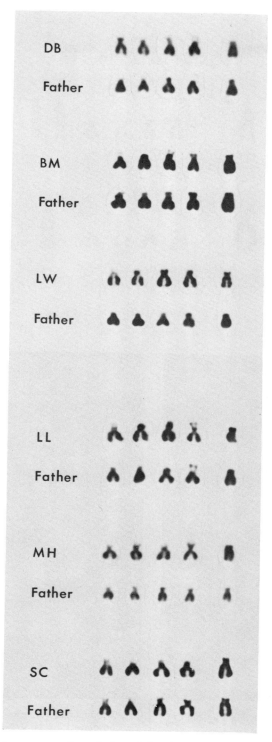

Fig. 6. G-group and Y chromosomes from *Patients 1-6* and their fathers. The morphology of the Ys of the patients is similar to that of the fathers.

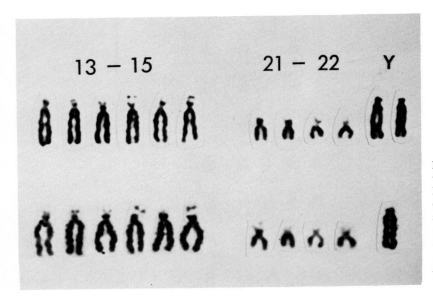

Fig. 7. Partial karyotypes from the XYY and XY lines from *Patient 7*. (From Wilson, M. G. et al: Identification of an unusual Y chromosome in YY mosaicism by quinacrine fluorescence. *Nature* 231:388-389, 1971, with permission.)

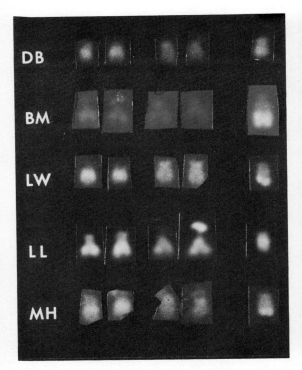

Fig. 8. Quinacrine fluorescence of the G-group and the Y chromosomes from *Patients 1-5*.

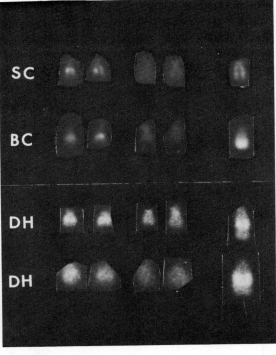

Fig. 9. Quinacrine fluorescence of the G-group and the Y chromosomes from *Patient 6, S.C.* (top), and her father, *B.C.* (second line); and from the XY and XYY cell lines of *Patient 7, D.H.* (two bottom lines).

structural rearrangement. Since the father was not available, we were not able to determine whether this Y was a structural abnormality or a normal variant.

In other patients, the quinacrine fluorescence pattern of the Y chromosomes was related to the length of the long arm (Fig. 8). The small Y in *Patient 4* (and father) showed no bright fluorescence, as expected for a Y chromosome of comparable size to a G chromosome.

Discussion

Four of these 7 patients were referred at birth because of abnormalities of the external genitalia (*Patients 1-3*) or Turner syndrome with severe somatic defects (*Patient 4*).

Although strikingly short, *Patients 5 and 6* did not present for a genetic work-up until after the expected age of puberty when the failure of sexual maturation was apparent. Only minor stigmata of Turner syndrome other than short stature were present. In another instance (*Patient 7*), work-up was initiated when a routine pediatric examination at 4 years of age disclosed clitoromegaly. Because of the family's failure to keep appointments, the genetic work-up on this patient was delayed for several

years. Clinical findings from these 7 patients are summarized in Table 2.

All children were assigned the female gender at birth, with the one exception of *Patient 1* whose external genitalia appeared primarily male. The female sex was assigned to this child at one month of age following the genetic work-up.

The patients were of relatively low birthweight for gestation, which was usually term in length (Table 2). Parental ages were not unusual in this group of patients, and various racialethnic groups were represented. The family history was not informative in any case.

Gonadectomies were done in all 7 patients, as early as 3 months of age in 2 instances (Table 3). The 4 patients with masculinization (*Patients 1-3, 7*) had plastic repair of the clitoromegaly. Mixed gonadal dysgenesis, characterized by a dysplastic or immature testis on one side and a gonadal streak on the other, was found in these 4 masculinized patients. *Patients 1, 2 and 3* showed asymmetric development of the müllerian and wolffian systems.

Of the 3 patients (*4-6*) presenting with nonmasculinized Turner syndrome, 2 had streak gonads in which no testicular tissue or tumor was identified (*Patients 5 and 6*). *Patient 4* was explored at 2½ years of age and was

Table 2. **Summary of Clinical Data**

Patient	Birth-weight	G.A.	Mat. Age	Pat. Age	Ethnicity	Assigned Gender (birth)	Age at Referral	Reason for Referral
1 (D.B.)	3500 gm	term	23	21	White/Mexican	Male at birth; female at 1 month	1 mo	Incomplete male development
2 (G.M.)	2835 gm	term	21	33	Black	male/female at birth; female at one week	birth	Ambiguous genitalia
3 (L.W.)	3515 gm	term	30	32	Mexican	female	birth	Ambiguous genitalia
4 (L.L.)	2550 gm	term	16	18	Black	female	birth	Turner syndrome
5 (M.H.)	2495 gm	term	21	24	Black	female	16 yrs.	Delayed puberty
6 (S.C.)	2100 gm	32 wks	35	35	Chinese	female	18 yrs.	Delayed sexual maturation
7 (D.H.)	2290 gm	term	18	unk.	White	female	5 yrs.	Masculinization

Table 3. Summary of Findings at Surgery

Patient	Age at Surgery	Surgical Procedure	Gonads Left	Gonads Right	Müllerian	Wolffian System
1 (D.B.)	3 mos.	gonadectomy and clitoral recession	streak	testis	hypoplastic uterus and vagina, left fallopian tube	right vas deferens and epididymis
2 (G.M.)	3 mos.	gonadectomy and clitoral resection	testis	streak	normal on right	left vas deferens and epididymis
3 (L.W.)	16 mos.	gonadectomy and clitoral recession	testis	streak	normal on right, small fallopian tube on left	remnants vas deferens and epididymis on left
4 (L.L.)	2½ yrs.	gonadectomy	streak grossly, gonado-blastoma (bilat.)	testis	normal	not present
5 (M.H.)	16 yrs.	gonadectomy	streak	streak	normal	not present
6 (S.C.)	18 yrs.	gonadectomy	streak	streak	normal	not present
7 (D.H.)	6 yrs.	gonadectomy and clitoral resection	testis	streak	normal	not present

found to have a left gonadal streak, a right dysplastic testis and bilateral gonadoblastoma. No wolffian remnants were found in this patient.

The growth and development of the 7 patients are summarized in Table 4. The stature of the masculinized patients (*Patients 1-3,7*) is between the 50th and 75th percentiles. The patients who presented as Turner syndrome (*Patients 4-6*) were less than the third percentile in height. All patients were apparently normal in intellectual development. One patient (*Patient 1*) appeared to be normal at 5 months of age, but later intellectual development could not be predicted for certain.

The cytogenetic finding of an unusual Y chromosome in *Patients 6 and 7* suggests the possibility of an abnormal Y chromosome in at least some cases of X/XY mosaicism, and is consistent with the experience of others.[5-9]

Table 4. Growth and Development

Patient	Age at Latest Examination	Stature	Mental Development
1 (D.B.)	5 mos.	50%	normal (apparently)
2 (G.M.)	2 yrs.	50%	normal (apparently)
3 (L.W.)	18½ mos.	>50%	normal
4 (L.L.)	5½ yrs.	< 3%	normal
5 (M.H.)	16 yrs.	< 3%	normal
6 (S.C.)	18 yrs.	< 3%	normal
7 (D.H.)	8 yrs.	50%	normal

Summary

To date, we have studied 7 patients with X/XY mosaicism, one of whom showed an X/XY/XYY pattern. Four patients presented as newly born infants because of incomplete male development, ambiguity of external genitalia or Turner syndrome. The other 3 patients presented in midchildhood or early adult life.

Bilateral gonadectomy, histologic examination of the gonads for tumor or testicular tissue, and chromosome analysis from blood and gonad specimens (and usually skin) were done in these 7 patients. The Y cell line and mosaicism were always detected in the blood culture although the predominant cell line in the majority of tissues was 45,X. The Y chromosome in one of the patients failed to show the expected bright fluorescence over the long arm, and the Y chromosome of another patient previously reported[3] had a terminal nonfluorescing portion of the long arm.

Patients with masculinization showed normal height and, on laparotomy, mixed gonadal dysgenesis. Patients with Turner syndrome showed bilateral streak gonads (2) and, in one 2½-year-old girl, a bilateral gonadoblastoma. All patients with Turner syndrome were less than the third percentile in height.

All 7 patients were reared as female, 4 of them requiring surgery to diminish the size of the clitoris. All 7 patients appeared to be developing normally.

Nonrecognition or delay of the diagnosis, which still occurs in this condition, appears to be a result of the mild physical abnormalities in some patients and a clinical diagnosis of Turner syndrome supported only by a negative X-chromatin result.

Acknowledgments

We are indebted to the numerous physicians who participated in the medical and surgical management of these patients, in particular to Dr. Carole Henneman, and to Mr. Paul Brager and Mrs. Fay Kaplan for technical assistance in the preparation of the karyotypes.

References

1. Hirschhorn, K., Decker, W. H. and Cooper, H. L.: Human intersex with chromosome mosaicism of type XY/XO. *N. Engl. J. Med. 263*:1044-1048, 1960.
2. Tulinius, H., Tryggvason, K. and Hauksdottir, H.: 45,X/46,XY chromosome mosaic with features of the Russell-Silver syndrome: A case report with a review of the literature. *Dev. Med. Child Neurol. 14*:161-172, 1972.
3. Wilson, M. G., Towner, J. W., Lipshin, J. and Fleisher, A.: Identification of an unusual Y chromosome in YY mosaicism by quinacrine fluorescence. *Nature 231*:388-389, 1971.
4. Ferrier, P. E., Ferrier, S. A. and Kelley, V. C.: Sex chromosome mosaicism in disorders of sexual differentiation: Incidence in various tissues. *J. Pediatr. 76*:739-744, 1970.
5. Caspersson, T., Hulten, M., Jonasson, J. et al: Translocations causing non-fluorescent Y chromosomes in human XO/XY mosaics. *Hereditas 68*:317-324, 1971.
6. Lo Curto, F., Scappaticci, S., Zuffardi, O. et al: Non-fluorescent Y chromosome in a 45,X/46,XY mosaic. *Ann. Genet. (Paris) 15*:107-110, 1972.
7. Khudr, G., Benirschke, K., Brooks, D. and Rakoff, J. S.: XO-XY mosaicism and nonfluorescent Y chromosome. *Obstet. Gynecol. 42*:421-428, 1973.
8. Berger, R., Relier, J. P., Salmon, C. and Minkowski, A.: X/XY mosaicism with short Y. *Clin. Genet. 5*:211-217, 1974.
9. Hsu, L. Y. F., Kim, H. J., Paciuc, S. et al: Non-fluorescent and non-heterochromatic Y chromosome in 45,X/46,XY mosaicism. *Ann. Genet. (Paris) 17*:5-9, 1974.

Discussion

Dr. Puff: You had a child showing normal müllerian development, with a testis on one side and a streak on the other. How do you explain the development of a normal system on the side of the testis? Is that really normal?

Dr. Wilson: There was one patient (*Case 4, L.L.*) who had bilateral streaks grossly and bilateral gonadoblastoma which on the right side arose from apparently dysplastic testicular tissue. This was probably erroneously oversimplified on Table 3, which should read "streak grossly with dysplastic testicular tissue and gonadoblastoma" for the right gonad of this patient.

Dr. Simpson: It may be of interest that, at the time that I left the New York Blood Center one year ago, we had studied 8 patients with this mosaicism. The interesting feature, cytogenetically, was that 5 of 8 had structurally abnormal Y chromosomes. In one instance, it was an apparent nonfamilial, in-tandem duplication of the Y long arm and in the other 4 it was a dicentric. In 3 instances, as I recall, the isochromatin break in the formation of the dicentric occurred in the long arm and in the fourth instance it occurred in the short arm. This would be of interest because we know that dicentrics are unstable chromosomes, forming breakage of fusion bridge cycles. It might be that this mosaicism in many cases arises, first, from formation of a structurally abnormal chromosome and only secondarily will the monosomic line arise.

Dr. Hecht: What percentage of these patients, not the ones that you have, but all of them with XO/XY mosaicism, have gonadal tumors? How do these tumors behave?

Dr. Wilson: Gonadal tumors are found in about one fifth to one quarter. The most common tumor is gonadoblastoma, although other tumors have been found, including tumors of the reproductive system. It is very definitely a real risk. Gonadoblastoma is not a highly malignant tumor and, in fact, can be considered to be a malignancy in situ.

Dr. Bass: I have 2 questions. 1) Were any hormonal studies carried out in these patients? 2) At what age would you recommend exploration?

Dr. Wilson: I shall not answer the first question because I do not have the data here today. As for the second question, we feel that the children should be explored as soon as their general condition permits. It is not an emergency surgery, but there is no reason to wait. We actually followed the child who was 2½ years old at the time of surgery from birth and we waited to be sure that she was stable regarding her congenital heart disease, so we did temporize in her case. In several other patients, you note that we explored at 3 months of age.

Dr. Funderburk: Dr. Wilson, I am interested in the one patient you presented, I think it was the sixth one, who had the triple mosaicism. I believe you said that it was detected at age 6 due to masculinization and the child had been raised as a female, which implied that it might not have been the proper sex rearing. We recently had a newborn with this same triple mosaicism and the decision about which sex to rear the child has been very difficult and, finally, it was based more on the anatomic presence of the female genital system, rather than the cytogenetics. I wonder if you would comment about the sex rearing of this rare kind of triple mosaicism?

Dr. Wilson: The decision of the sex is really based upon the appearance of external genitalia. It is not based upon either the morphology of the gonads or the chromosome analysis. In these patients, you will note that all were raised as females, which we think was correct in these cases. Of course, if a child is raised as one sex for a time, then one needs to consider very carefully the reasons for changing the sex at a later time. A change of sex, after the neonatal period, is extremely difficult and in one sense is probably not completely possible, because of the psychologic sex identity which is normally well-established by that time. Our decision regarding the choice of sex is based on the answer to the question: In which sex will this particular child, with these external genitalia, be most functional? I think that is the right way to proceed.

Acrocephalosyndactyly and Partial Trisomy 6*

Kathleen P. Robertson, B.S., Theodore F. Thurmon, M.D.
and Margaret C. Tracy, C.T. (A.S.C.P.)

At least 2 reports have demonstrated an abnormal chromosome in Apert syndrome.[1,2] Because each case had a different chromosome aberration and this syndrome is a well-established autosomal dominant trait, such associations are probably fortuitous.

We recently encountered a patient with acrocephalosyndactyly (not Apert acrocephalosyndactyly) who had a partial trisomy for part of the long arm of chromosome 6. Other cases of malformation syndromes associated with partial C-group trisomy have had clinical pictures somewhat similar to our case, so they may represent aberrations of the same chromosome.

Case Report

The proband, a white girl born 1/31/73 to 24-year-old parents, was the product of a full-term pregnancy of a gravida 3, para 1, ab 2 mother. Birthweight, length and head circumference were 2438 gm, 4.19 cm and 34.3 cm, respectively. Her Apgar score was 0, but she responded to resuscitation. She stayed in the hospital 2 days. She had an odd appearance and slow development, choked frequently on early feedings and passed out twice after choking. There was frequent constipation. She smiled responsively at age 2 months.

Physical examination on 10/10/73 revealed a height of 67 cm (25th%) and a head circumference of 41 cm (3rd%). She had an odd facies and apprehensive demeanor. Examination of the head revealed a flat occiput, prominent vertex, hypertelorism (interpupillary distance 5.1 cm), mild micrognathia and a bow-shaped mouth (Figs. 1A and B). Examination of the hands revealed small digits held in flexion due to short

*Supported by The National Foundation-March of Dimes grant CE-39.

flexor tendons, but no actual joint contractures or stiffness (Fig. 1C). There were arches on 3 digits of each hand and simple patterns on the remainder. The total ridge count was 18. Examination of the feet revealed bilateral clubbing; on the right foot the 3rd toe overrode the 4th; on the left foot there was 2nd-3rd toe syndactyly (Fig. 1D).

G-banding and Q-banding showed that the patient had an unbalanced translocation, with a portion of the long arm of a chromosome 6 attached to the long arm of a chromosome 10; effectively, a partial trisomy 6, designated 46,XX,-10,+der(10),t(6;10)(q21;q24)mat. The portion q25-qter of the derivative chromosome 10 was deleted (Fig. 2). The patient's mother had the balanced translocation designated 46,XX,t(6;10)(q21;q24)(Fig. 3).

Discussion

The chromosome aberrations were readily apparent with banding technique but had been overlooked by another laboratory with standard Giemsa technique. In other cases,[3-7] the aberrations were seen with standard Giemsa technique. It may be assumed, therefore, that these aberrations involved more chromosomal material than our case, so they could well be clinically worse. Table 1 summarizes the findings in all the cases. As can be seen, the more severe malformations found in other cases (cleft lip, cleft palate, heart defect and kidney defect) were not found in the proband.

Findings common to most of the cases (hypertelorism, low-set ears and micrognathia) are quite common among many types of chromosome aberration. Perhaps the most striking findings in the proband were the dermatoglyphics; these departed significantly

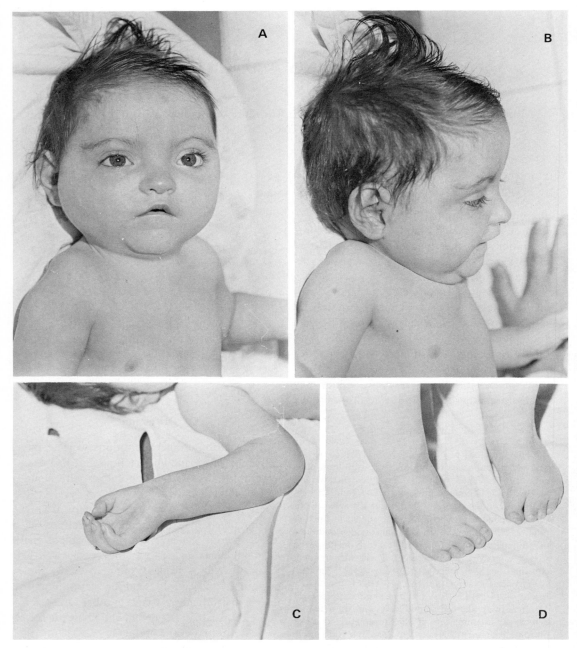

Fig. 1. Proband. A) Frontal and B) lateral views of the face. C) Hand showing flexed fingers. D) Feet showing overriding toes on right and syndactyly on left.

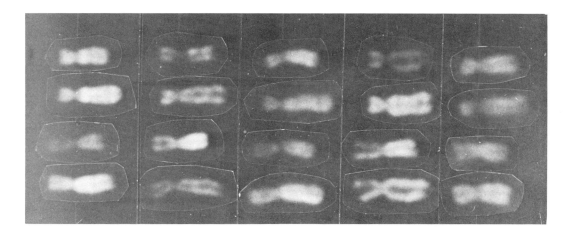

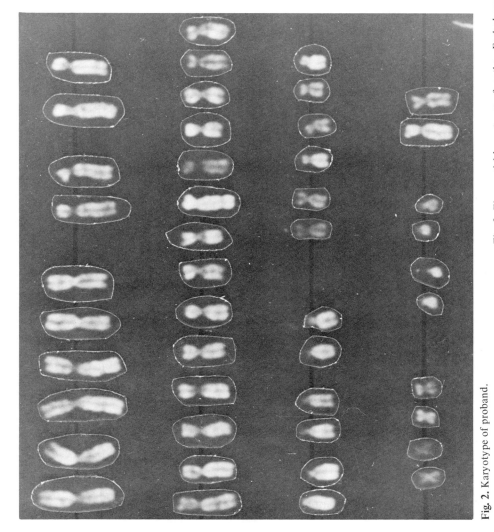

Fig. 3. Five partial karyotypes of mother. Each shows from left to right: 6, der(6)(10qter→q24::6q21→6pter), der(10)(6qter→6q21::10q24→10pter), and 10.

Fig. 2. Karyotype of proband.

**Table 1. Summary of Findings in Proband and 5 Other Cases
of Partial Trisomy C**

	Proband	Ref. 5	Ref. 7	Ref. 6	Ref. 3	Ref. 4
Hypertelorism	+	+	0	+	+	+
Acrocephaly	+	+	0	-	-	-
Flat occiput	+	-	0	+	0	0
Low-set ears	+	+	0	+	+	+
Micrognathia	+	+	+	+	-	+
Bow-shaped mouth	+	+	0	-	-	+
Cleft lip	-	-	0	+	+	-
Cleft palate	-	+	0	+	+	-
Pterygium colli	-	-	0	+	-	-
Short flexor tendons	+	0	0	0	+	0
Syndactyly	+	0	+	0	-	0
Overriding digits	+	0	0	0	+	0
Clubfoot	+	0	0	-	0	0
Faint dermal ridges	+	+	-	-	0	-
Low ridge count	+	0	-	-	0	0
Excessive arches	+	0	-	+	0	-
Heart defect	-	-	-	+	+	0
Kidney defect	-	-	-	+	-	0
Hypomentia	+	+	+	+	+	+
Chromosome aberration	+6(q21→qter)	6q+	6q+	Cq+	Cq+	Cq+

+: Present
-: Absent
0: Not mentioned in report

from those of the parents and were symmetric. These last two findings led us to perform chromosome analysis by banding technique in spite of the previous normal findings by standard Giemsa technique. Consequently, this represents an exception to previous reports[8,9] which indicated that there was little possibility of finding a chromosome aberration by banding, if the standard analysis is normal.

The reports of other partial C trisomies predated chromosome banding techniques so there is no way to be sure they represent aberrations of the same chromosome. As more C-group chromosome aberrations are reported, the clinical findings are becoming less specific. Most of the malformations seem to be a consequence of altered embryogenesis. There is a loose correlation between the amount of chromosomal material involved and the severity of the syndrome, but little specificity otherwise. The partial trisomy 10 syndrome[10] may be an exception to this statement because it had microphthalmia in addition to the nonspecific findings.

From a theoretic standpoint, the nonspecificity of malformations suggests that much of the genome is concerned with ordering of embryogenesis and that specific morphology is determined either by a higher function or by critical parts of the genome. If the latter were true, the critical parts might be mapped by exclusion, ie by excluding the parts where aberrations are associated with nonspecific findings.

From a practical standpoint, it appears necessary that banding chromosome analysis be performed in any case with these nonspecific findings. Dermatoglyphic analysis may make it possible to pick out cases more likely to have a chromosome aberration.

Summary

A partial trisomy of the long arm of chromosome 6 was found in an infant with acrocephalosyndactyly (not Apert acrocephalosyndactyly). The mother had a balanced translocation involving the long arms of chromosomes 6 and 10. Other reports of similar aberrations are reviewed.

Acknowledgments

Dr. Ernest C. Hansen of Thibodeaux, Louisiana, referred this case to us and provided an excellent data base. Ms. Ellen B. DeFraites and Ms. Jennifer Jackson assisted in the evaluation at the Louisiana Heritable Disease Center.

References

1. Dodson, W. E., Museles, M., Kennedy, J. L. and Al-Aish, M.: Acrocephalosyndactylia associated with a chromosomal translocation. *Am. J. Dis. Child. 120*:360-362, 1970.
2. Genest, P., Mortezai, M. and Tremblay, M.: Le syndrome d'Apert (Acrocephalo-syndactylie). Une observation avec un chromosome 1 anormal. *Arch. Fr. Pediatr. 23*:887-897, 1966.
3. Gray, J. E., Dartnall, J. A. and MacNamara, B. G. P.: A family showing transmission of a translocation between a 6-12 chromosome and a 21-22 chromosome. *J. Med. Genet. 3*:62-65, 1966.
4. LeJeune, J. and Berger, R.: Sur deux observations familiales de translocations complexes. *Ann. Genet. (Paris) 8*:21-30, 1965.
5. LeJeune, J., Rethore, M., Berger, R. et al: Trisomie C partielle par translocation familiale t(Cq+;Cq-). *Ann. Genet. (Paris) 11*:171-175, 1968.
6. Lindsten, J., Fraccaro, M., Klinger, H. P. and Zetterqvist, P.: Meiotic and mitotic studies of a familial reciprocal translocation between two autosomes of group 6-12. *Cytogenetics 4*:45-64, 1965.
7. Rohde, R. A. and Catz, B.: Maternal transmission of a new group C (6/9) chromosomal syndrome. *Lancet 2*:838-840, 1964.
8. del Solar, C. and Uchida, I.: Identification of chromosomal abnormalities by quinacrine staining technique in patients with normal karyotypes by conventional analysis. *J. Pediatr. 84*:534-538, 1974.
9. Kajii, T., Ohama, K., Niikawa, N. et al: Banding analysis of abnormal karyotypes in spontaneous abortion. *Am. J. Hum. Genet. 25*:539-547, 1973.
10. Yunis, J. J. and Sanchez, O.: A new syndrome resulting from partial trisomy for the distal third of the long arm of chromosome 10. *J. Pediatr. 84*:567-570, 1974.

The Cell Cycle and Chromosome Anomalies

Ian H. Porter, M.B., B.S. and Betty Paul

Since patients with Down syndrome have a decreased rate of DNA synthesis both in fibroblasts[1] and in lymphocytes[2] and since patients with trisomy 13, 18 and 21 have less than normal numbers of cells in different organs,[3] the question arises as to whether these findings may be related to delays in cell cycle times. If slowing of the mitotic cycle should prove to be characteristic of autosomal trisomies, it might help to explain the retardation of growth and development associated with these syndromes.

Patients and Methods

We determined the length of cell cycles in cultured fibroblasts from infants with trisomy 18 and 21 and other chromosomal anomalies. We compared the length of each stage and the total length of the cell cycle to diploid lines from 4 normal infants. All lines, except one obtained from a patient with trisomy 18, were in early passages and all were in a logarithmic growth phase when pulse-labeled with tritiated thymidine.

All cells were cultured in McCoy's 5A medium with 15 ml of fetal calf serum/100 ml of media, penicillin and streptomycin. Cultures were pulsed for 15 minutes at a concentration of 1 μc of tritiated thymidine (specific activity 0.36 c/mM). They were washed twice with warm Hanks balanced salt solution and the media that previously was incubated with the cells was returned to the flasks. At specific intervals, they were trypsinized, fixed in methanol-acetic acid (3−1) and the cell suspension dropped onto slides previously rinsed in cold water and dried on a 40°C hot plate. The slides were stained with 2% acetoorcein, coated with NTB-2 (Kodak film emulsion), exposed for one week at 0°C and developed in straight Dektol. The proportion of labeled mitosis was counted every 3 hours for 30 hours.

The earliest samples had no labeled mitoses. The proportion of labeled mitoses then rose to a peak as the cells which were in the S phase at the time of the pulse came through to division. Following this peak there was a trough as the cells originally in G_1 came to the end of their cycle.

The length of the S period was taken as the time between the 2 points in the first wave where 50% of the mitoses were labeled. The length of the G_2 period was taken as the time between the start of the experiment and when 50% of the mitoses were labeled. The total cycle time was the time between 2 similar points in the first and second cycle and, of course, $G_1 + M = T - S + G_2$.[4]

Results

The cell cycles in cultured fibroblasts from 3 patients with trisomy 21 showed an increase in the total length of the cell cycle accounted for particularly by an increase in the length of the G_1 phase (Table 1).

Similarly, the length of the cell cycles in cell lines from 3 patients with trisomy 18 showed an increase in the total length of the cell cycle and particularly of the G_1 phase (Table 1). One of these lines had a G_1 period which was more than 4 times that of the

Table 1. Cell Cycles of Diploid and Trisomic Cultures Determined by Pulse Labeling and Counting Labeled Metaphases

Cell Lines	$G_1 + M$	S	G_2	Total
Control:				
356	3.0	12.0	8.0	23.0
387	4.5	10.5	6.0	21.0
401	3.5	10.5	4.5	18.5
402	5.0	9.5	5.0	19.5
Trisomy 21:				
184	8.5	8.0	9.0	25.5
417	8.0	10.0	6.0	24.0
407	6.0	11.0	9.0	26.0
Trisomy 18:				
188	8.0	7.0	10.0	25.0
182	17.5	7.5	4.5	29.5
406	10.0	9.0	5.0	24.0
Trisomy 13	7.5	9.5	7.5	24.5
21/22 Translocation	7.0	6.5	7.0	20.5
46/47,+21	4.0	12.5	7.0	23.5

controls (Table 1); however this line was in culture for 16 passages before analysis. The results were similar in cells from one patient with trisomy 13 (Table 1).

The length of the cell cycle in fibroblasts from one patient with a G/G translocation Down syndrome was about the same length as our controls, although the G_1 period was longer and the period of DNA synthesis shorter (Table 1).

The length of the cell cycle in the fibroblasts from a patient with 46/47,+21 mosaicism (28% of the cells had 47 chromosomes) was increased but the G_1 phase was normal (Table 1).

Comparison of the means and standard errors between the controls and trisomy 21 and 18 shows the results to be highly significant (Table 2).

Discussion

Others have also found that the presence of an extra chromosome is associated with a prolongation of the cell cycle but particularly of the G_2 phase in the case of cells with a 47,XY,+C chromosome constitution.[5] These studies were done on cells in later passages and investigators have shown that cells in late passage may have a lengthened G_1 or G_2 phase.[6] All of our experiments were done on cell lines in early passages (<9) except one trisomy 18 line (passage 16) which did have an extremely long G_1 phase (Table 1). The pH, calf serum and temperature are factors which influence the length of the cell cycles and variations of these conditions may account for some of the observed differences among investigators.[7] Cells with less than the normal number of chromosomes, eg 45,X, appear, on the other hand, to have shorter cycles than those with a 46,XX or 47,XXX chromosome constitution and this alteration is in the G_1 phase.[8]

Although the lengthening of the cell cycle may slow the rate of cell proliferation and, therefore, retard growth, we still of course do not know how the differential rate of proliferation, which is so striking a feature of embryogenesis, is affected by anomalous chromosome constitutions. But, perhaps, the addition of a particular chromosome not only has a *general* effect on the length of the cell cycle in autosomal trisomies, but also a *specific* effect on the differential mitotic rate at certain developmental stages at times when increased activity in particular cells is required.

Table 2. Means and Standard Errors of Trisomy and Control Cultures

Cell Types	No. of Lines	Mean and S.E.			
		$G_1 + M$	S	G_2	Total
Control	4	4.0±0.46	10.6±0.52	5.9±0.77	20.5±0.98
Trisomy 21	3	7.5±0.76*	9.7±0.88	8.0±1.0	25.2±0.98†
Trisomy 18	3	11.8±2.89†	7.8±0.60	6.5±1.76	26.1±1.69†

*p < 0.01
†p < 0.05

So, in summary, lengthening of the cell cycle leads to generalized inhibition of cell proliferation which may particularly affect those stages of development that require increased cell proliferation.

References

1. Mittwoch, U.: In Wolstenholme, G. E. W. and Porter, R. (eds.): *Mongolism*. London:Churchill, 1967, p. 51.
2. Mellman, W. J., Younkin, L. H. and Baker, D.: Abnormal lymphocyte function in trisomy 21. *Ann. N. Y. Acad. Sci. 171*:537, 1970.
3. Naeye, R. L.: Prenatal organ and cellular growth with various chromosomal disorders. *Biologia Neonatorum 11*:248, 1967.
4. Sisken, J. E.: Measurement of parts of interphase. *Methods Cell Physiol. 1*:392, 1964.
5. Kuliev, A. M., Kukharenko, V. I., Grinberg, K. N. et al: Morphological, autoradiographic, immunochemical and cytochemical investigation of a cell strain with trisomy 7 from a spontaneous abortus. *Humangenetik 17*:285, 1973.
6. Macieira-Coelho, A., Ponten, J. and Philipson, L.: The division cycle and RNA-synthesis in diploid human cells at different passage levels *in vitro. Exp. Cell Res. 42*:673, 1966.
7. Mitchison, J. M.: DNA synthesis in eukaryotic cells. *The Biology of the Cell Cycle.* Cambridge: Cambridge University Press, 1972, p. 58.
8. Barlow, P. W.: Differential cell division in human X chromosome mosaics. *Humangenetik 14*:122, 1972.

Semiautomation of Chromosome Preparations*

John Melnyk, Ph.D., Garland Persinger, M.Sc. and William Porter

It has been over a decade since Arakaki and Sparkes[1] described a micromethod for culturing cells for cytogenetic analysis. Although some minor modifications have been introduced during the interim, the basic methodology has remained unchanged. Specimens are usually cultured in test tubes or vials and each is handled individually with fluids being added or removed with Pasteur pipettes. With the advent of computer technology and an increased awareness of the prevalence of chromosomal abnormalities, the need to devise new approaches in methodology to meet the expected demand is obvious. This report describes a system of processing specimens in multiple sets which is expected to increase by a factor of 8 the number of specimens that can be handled on an average day. The system is designed for high volume production of slides for analysis by a computer-controlled microscope and a karyotype system being developed by Jet Propulsion Laboratories.

The specimen preparation system consists of 12 components which were designed and constructed at this institution. This report describes 7 of the components which have been completed and tested.

Specimen Preparation System

Culture Plates

The specimen preparation system is based on a macroplate concept in which the entire process of culturing and harvesting is performed. The culture plate, which was designed after a series of experiments with various prototypes and commercially produced culture plates, is shown in Figure 1. The plate, which contains 12 wells, is 4½ inches × 3 inches × 1 1/8 inches. Each well holds 3 ml of culture fluid. The wells are spaced 1 1/8 inches from center to center and this spacing is maintained in all of the components of the system. The culture plate is manufactured† with a novel snap-off design which enables a technician to select 4, 8, 12 wells or multiples of each as required for the daily workload. The plates are made of polystyrene and are available in sterile packages with snap-on plastic caps.

Culture Medium Dispenser

The medium is pumped to a manifold‡ containing 4 needles which are spaced to coincide with the wells (Fig. 2). The pump§ is a standard unit with autoclavable tubing and syringe which is operated under a laminar flow hood.

Centrifuge Carriers

A carrier for the culture plates in centrifugation (Fig. 3) was designed. The carrier was made for the International Model UV centrifuge with a 6-place head. Each carrier can hold

*Research supported by the National Institute of Child Health and Human Development and NIH/NASA Inter-Agency Agreement 1-101-HD-30001.

†Lab-Tek Corporation, 30 W. 475 North Aurora Rd., Naperville, IL 60540.

‡Polydrop-Canalco Inc., 5635 Fishers Lane, Rockville, MD 20852.

§Filamatic Vial Filler, National Instrument Co. Inc., Baltimore, MD 21215.

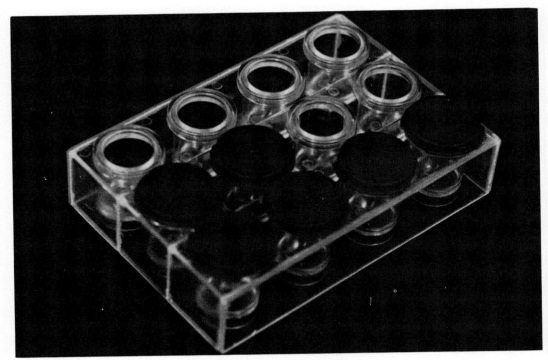

Fig. 1. Specimen culture plates.

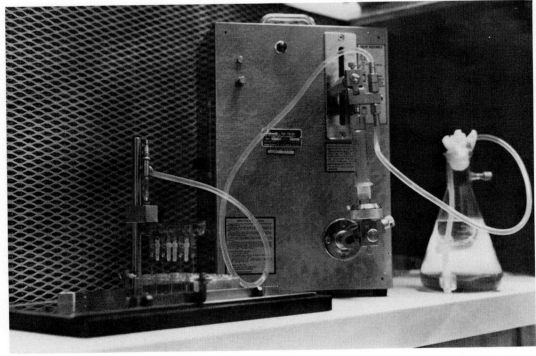

Fig. 2. Culture medium dispenser.

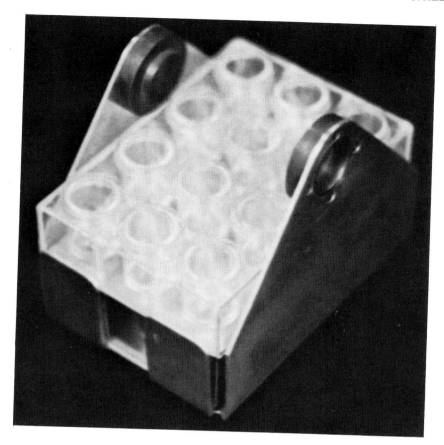

Fig. 3. Plate carrier for centrifuge.

2 stacked culture plates so that a total of 144 specimens can be centrifuged in one run.

Aspirator

Following centrifugation of the specimens, it is necessary to remove the supernatant. A 12-needle aspirator was designed and fabricated (Fig. 4A) according to the dimensions of the culture plate. The base of the unit has stops and guides which center the culture plates as they are moved manually under the unit. The suction manifold is spring-loaded and a manually operated lever lowers the needles into the wells to a depth determined by a stop which contacts the culture plate. A continuous vacuum is present in the line and the supernatant is drawn off into a flask in 1-2 seconds. After aspiration each culture tray is moved on and the lever is pulled again to lower the needles into an ultrasonic cleaner mounted beneath the aspirator (Fig. 4B). Within a few seconds any

cellular material adhering to the needles is removed and the unit is ready to aspirate the next culture plate.

Hypotonic Fluid and Fixative Dispenser

After removal of the supernatant, there are several steps involving addition of hypotonic fluid and fixatives. This is accomplished by the dispenser (Fig. 4C) which consists of 3 components: 1) a rectangular stand which supports 12 needles centered above the wells in the cuture plate, 2) a peristaltic pump (Fig. 4E) which moves the fluid from a reservoir to the needles and 3) a shaker upon which the dispensing manifold is mounted (Fig. 4D). The shaker is turned on after aspiration to re-suspend the cells and is kept in motion while the fluid is being added.

The peristaltic pump controls fluid flow to the dispenser from drop by drop to a steady flow. Since slow fixation is essential to avoid

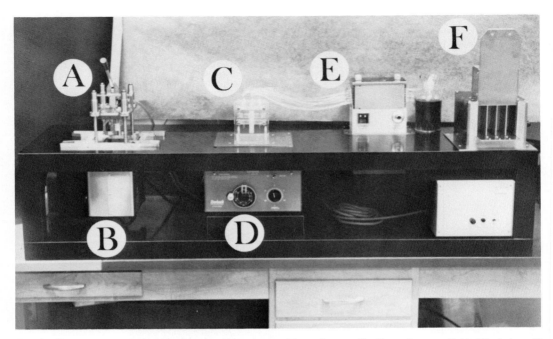

Fig. 4. Chromosome preparation bench: A) aspirator, B) sonicator, C) dispensing manifold, D) shaker, E) dispensing pump and F) slide dispenser.

excessive cell breakage, the variable flow control is of considerable importance.

Following the addition of fluid the culture plates are recycled through the centrifuge, aspirator and the fluid dispenser until the cells are adequately fixed.

Slide Dispenser

A unit was designed and made to store slides in 4 stacks and to dispense them 4 at a time. Each of the 4 stacks holds 128 premarked slides and the stacks are spaced to coincide with the wells in the cuture plates. A lever on the right hand side engages a finger-device which pushes the slides from the bottom of the stack until they are positioned under the cell dispenser.

Cell Dispenser and Needle Changer

The cell dispenser consists of a manifold with 4 removable needles (Fig. 5). Following the last fixation, aspiration and resuspension steps, the manifold is placed manually over the 4 wells of the culture plates and the needles are immersed into the suspension. A pressure plate on the manifold is depressed and released and approximately 3 drops of cell suspension are drawn into the needles. The manifold is placed over the slides and the plate is depressed again dropping the cells.

Following the dispensing of the cells the manifold is placed in a needle changer which removes the used needles. The manifold is seen in this position in Figure 5. A plate at the back of the unit activates a device which pries off the needles in one motion. The needles drop into a container and are subsequently cleaned in a sonicator and reused. The manifold is placed over a row of fresh needles on a rack (Fig. 5) and with a slight pressure 4 needles are picked up for the next preparation.

At this time plans are being prepared for additional components including a cell spreader and a slide marker. It is expected that the system will be completed and ready for clinical testing in mid-1975.

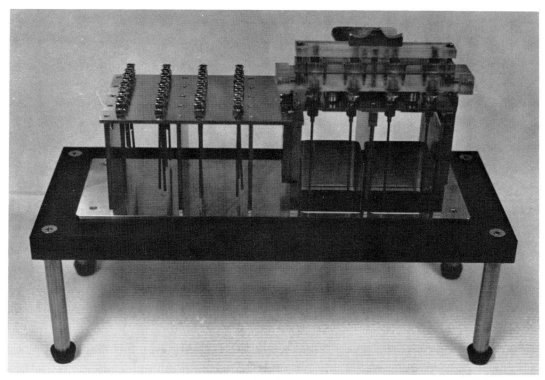

Fig. 5. Cell dispenser.

Comparison With Manual Method

Comparative Time Analysis

A comparative analysis of the time required to process 12 specimens by the tube method and the culture plate method is shown in Table 1. The figures for the tube method were based on averages of actual trials from 2 laboratories. The figures for the plate method were obtained from trials using prototype components during the first year of the project. In each step of the process, a considerable reduction in processing time is seen. The plate method provides for an overall reduction in processing time by a factor of 8.

Table 2 shows a projection for the time required to process 48, 144 and 576 additional specimens (4, 12 and 48 culture plates). It is apparent that in an 8-hour workday, the maximum number of specimens that can be processed is approximately 576. While this daily volume is beyond that of most laboratories, it would be useful for total ascertainment of transient populations (eg state hospitals for the retarded). Slides could be made in a short time and stored for subsequent analysis.

Table 1. Time of Processing 12 Specimens

| Stage | Time | |
	Tube Method	Plate Method
Centrifugation (post-culture)	10 min	5 min
Aspiration (4 times)	24 min	12 sec
Fluid dispensing (4 times)	44 min	2½ min
Slide preparation (3 slides)	9 min	3 min
	1 hr 27 min	11 min

Table 2. Time of Processing Additional Specimens

Method	Number of Specimens			
	12	48	144	576
Tube method	1 hr 27 min	5 hr 52 min	17 hr 48 min	—
Plate method	11 min	44 min	2 hr 20 min	8 hr 48 min

Comparative Cost Analysis

Table 3 shows the costs of culture vessels and materials such as culture medium, calf serum, phytohemagglutinin and antibiotics. The plastic culture tubes (16 × 125 mm) cost 10 cents each and the preliminary quotation on the cost of a 12-well culture plate is $1.75. It is quite likely that this figure will be lowered when actual production based on a permanent injection mold is realized.

Table 3. Cost Comparative

Item	Cost (per 12 specimens)	
	Plate Method	Tube Method
Culture vessel	$1.75/plate	$1.20/12 tubes
Materials	1.92	3.12
	$3.67	$4.32

Acknowledgments

The authors gratefully acknowledge the expert assistance of Douglas Alston, Bernie Munro, Grace Hirsh, Linda Revane and Ann Chapman.

Reference

1. Arakaki, D. T. and Sparkes, R. S.: Microtechnique for culturing leucocytes from whole blood. *Cytogenetics* 2:57, 1963.

Quantitative Data on Chromosome Aberrations Obtained by Computer Analysis*

Agnes N. Stroud, Ph.D. and Sayuri Harami, B.S.

Progress in human cytogenetics has advanced rapidly since the first human karyotype was published in 1956,[1] and even more so since the prenatal diagnosis of chromosomal and metabolic diseases in humans[2,3] became possible. Another major advance in the field which has made a dynamic impact in the area of genetic diseases has been the development of new chromosome staining techniques which characterize banding patterns sequentially along the chromosome. Since the first publication of fluorochrome banding of human chromosomes by Caspersson et al[4] and Giemsa banding,[5-10] the knowledge of heritable diseases associated with chromosome abnormalities has increased rapidly.

Before the new banding techniques were introduced, most of the 46 human chromosomes could only be placed in groups. When groups contained more than 2 chromosomes, the homologue of individual chromosomes usually could not be identified. In most cases, abnormal chromosomes, if present, could be recognized only if the abnormality was gross. The new chromosome banding techniques have helped to clarify some of these problems; however, there is a need for an automated system for collecting quantitative measurements on minute chromosome aberrations.

The intent of this paper is to demonstrate that, with a computer-assisted microscope and with image analysis techniques, assessment of chromosome variations can provide accurate quantitative information about chromosome structure, and do so more rapidly than manual measurements.

Materials and Methods

Abnormal chromosomes of metaphase spreads from the blood of a genetically abnormal individual (*M.G.*) and from blood irradiated in vitro with gamma rays (*A.S.*) were the source of material for analysis.

Blood cultures, banding and staining of metaphase spreads of patient *M.G.* were prepared by Dr. Jean Priest (Emory University) and sent to us for analysis. This individual had a chromosome translocated to an A-2 chromosome. The origin of the translocated material and the area of insertion along the Q segment of the chromosome were in question. The index case had multiple congenital anomalies and was presumed to be unbalanced genetically, whereas the parents were phenotypically normal.

The radiation-induced chromosome aberration was produced by irradiating whole peripheral blood from a normal person (*A.S.*) with 75

*Image Processing Laboratory, Jet Propulsion Laboratory, Pasadena, California.

This paper presents one phase of research carried out at the Jet Propulsion Laboratory, California Institute of Technology, under Research Contract NAS 7-100, sponsored by the National Aeronautics and Space Administration, and NIH Biotechnology Resource Grant RR-00443.

283

R gamma rays from a [137]Cesium source. Following irradiation, the RBCs were removed and the leukocytes placed in growth medium with the mitogen, phytohemagglutinin (PHA), to stimulate lymphocytes into division. After approximately 65 hours in culture at 37°C, the mitotic cells were blocked in metaphase for one hour with Colcemid, and then exposed for 15 minutes to 0.075 M KCl and fixed in 3 changes of methanol-acetic acid (3:1) fix. In this fixative, spreads of the chromosomes were made on cold, wet glass microscope slides. The spreads on the slides were treated with 0.05% trypsin in Hank's balanced salt solution, without Mg^{++} and Ca^{++} ions, at pH 7.0. After treatment, they were rinsed in 2 changes of the salt solution, 2 changes of 70% alcohol, and 2 changes of pure methanol. They were allowed to air dry before being dipped into a 2% Giemsa stain, buffered at pH 6.8. After the stain was washed off in buffer (pH 6.8), the spreads were briefly rinsed in tap water and air dried before being mounted in permount.

Collection of chromosome data was made with the Automatic Light Microscope System (ALMS) designed and built at the Jet Propulsion Laboratory. The ALMS is a computer-assisted microscope which has the capability of optically scanning information (chromosomes) on a microscope slide. It is equipped with objectives (100 ×, oil, planapochromat used for chromosomes), a high-resolution TV camera, a drive motor and sense switches for focusing, a motorized stage and objective-position sense switches, and an image plane scanner. The scanner digitizes a frame with maximum of 1024 × 1024 elements which covers a 100 μm square area at the specimen plane, with a 0.1 μ sample spot spacing and 256 gray levels.[11,12] The microscope is under the control of an IBM-1130 computer, which also performs elementary image analysis functions. Other complex image analyses, such as karyotyping, profile waveform analysis and generation of output pictures, were performed by the 360/44 computer.

For this study, banded metaphase chromosomes were scanned from microscope slides with ALMS and profile waveforms of the densely stained bands, and lighter interbands were obtained. The waveforms represent the average optical density at equally spaced points (0.1–0.125 μ) along the axis of the banded chromosome.[13] Information concerning the length of the chromosome, centromeric index, area, position of the bands and the distance between bands was also automatically computed. From this type of data, the amount of chromosomal material, either added or lost through deletions or translocations, was measured quantitatively.

Results

Figure 1 presents a metaphase spread of the abnormal patient (M.G.). The abnormal chromosome in question is of the A-2 group (arrow). The spread was scanned with ALMS from the microscope slide, and a printout of the computer-generated (with some manual assistance) karyotype is shown in Figure 2. Note that one A-2 chromosome is longer than its homologue due to a translocation. Measurements of the abnormal A-2 chromosome and the normal A-2 chromosome were made from the histograms (waveforms), and the data are compared in Figure 3. The normal A-2 chromosome (Fig. 3A) was divided into regions (P and Q) and band regions (1, 2 and 3) using the Paris Conference (1971) guidelines.[14] The length of the normal A-2 chromosome obtained from the measurements was 12.7 μ (corrected for banding), and the widths of P (1, 2) were 2.4 and 2.6 μ, respectively. Region Q (1, 2 and 3) measurements were 1.9, 3.7 and 2.1 μ respectively. Next to the chromosome is the profile waveform, showing the distance and location of each region along the long axis of the chromosome. The length of the abnormal A-2 chromosome was measured at 14.5 μm and is shown in Figure 3B, along with its profile waveform. The chromosome regions, band locations, and the translocation (insertion) are shown next to the histogram. The P (1) region is about 0.6 μ longer than the normal A-2 chromosome; however, differences in contraction account for this discrepancy. The translocation involves both the Q2 and Q3 regions, with a deletion of 1.3 μ

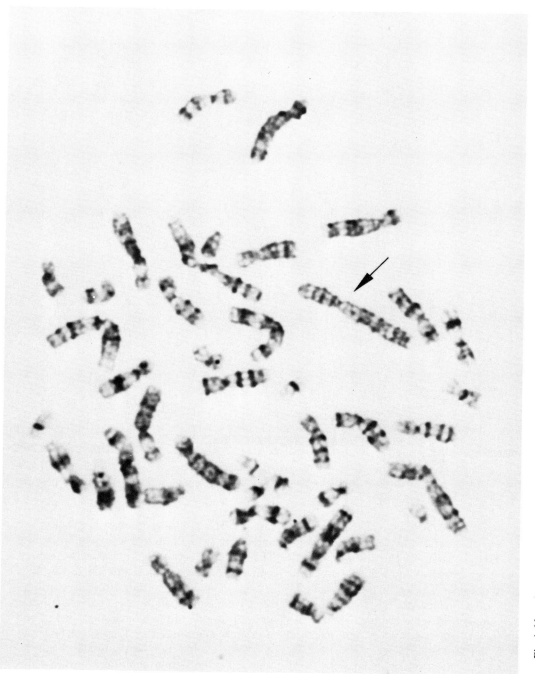

Fig. 1. Metaphase spread of a genetically abnormal lymphocyte (*M.G.*) showing the A-2 chromosome (arrow) which contains a translocation.

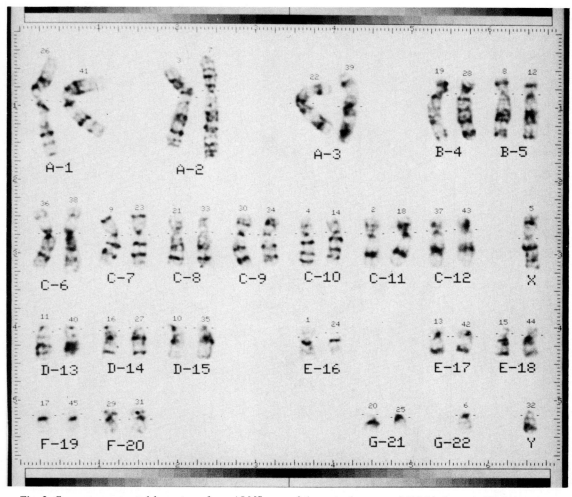

Fig. 2. Computer-generated karyotype from ALMS scan of the metaphase spread (*M.G.*) shown in Figure 1. The abnormal chromosome is A-2, No. 7, and its normal homologue is A-2, No. 3. Some manual assistance was necessary to complete the karyotype.

of chromosome material at the 2q5 and 3q1 bands, and an insertion of 3.2 μ in this same region. The histogram of the inserted material does not correspond to any band region of the A-2 chromosome. The origin of this material was not known, since the other chromosomes in the complement were normal. The father's chromosomes were examined and were all found to be normal; however, there was the possibility that the extra material was derived from the mother, whose chromosomes were not examined.

Figure 4 is a partial metaphase spread with the radiation-induced chromosome·aberration (arrow). The abnormal chromosome is dicentric and belongs to the B group of chromosomes. The computer-generated, manually assisted printout of the complete metaphase spread is shown in Figure 5. Data from the profile waveform show that the dicentric was a translocation to one of the B-5 chromosomes of one of the X chromosomes, after a deletion had occurred in the B-5 chromosome. Figure 6 represents the chromosome and profile waveforms of A) the X chromosome, B) the normal B-5 chromosome and C) the dicentric formed from the break and rejoining of the B-5 with the X. In the waveform data, a break occurred

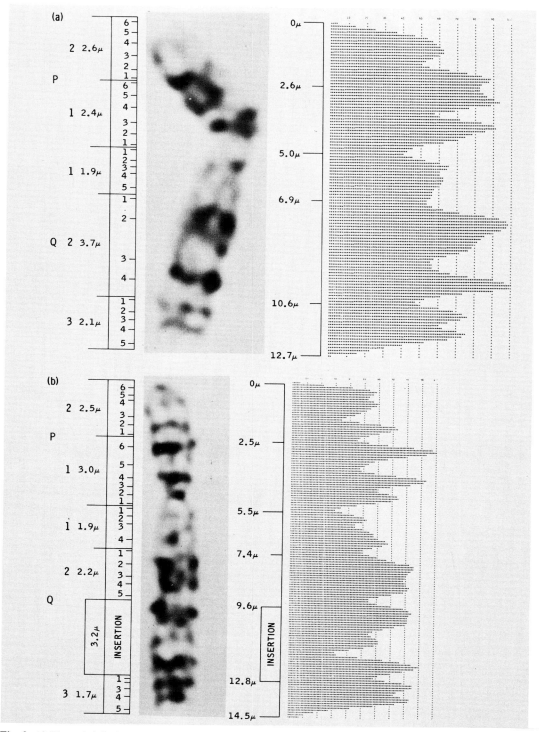

Fig. 3. A) Normal A-2 chromosome and B) the abnormal A-2 chromosome. The chromosomes are divided into regions. The short arm represents the P region, and the long arm the Q region, and the regions are further subdivided (1, 2 and 3). The histogram of the chromosomes, which represents the profile waveform, is shown to the right of the chromosomes. The translocation of chromosome B-5 (3B) is represented by a block diagram (insertion) to indicate that 3.2 μ of foreign chromosomal material was inserted.

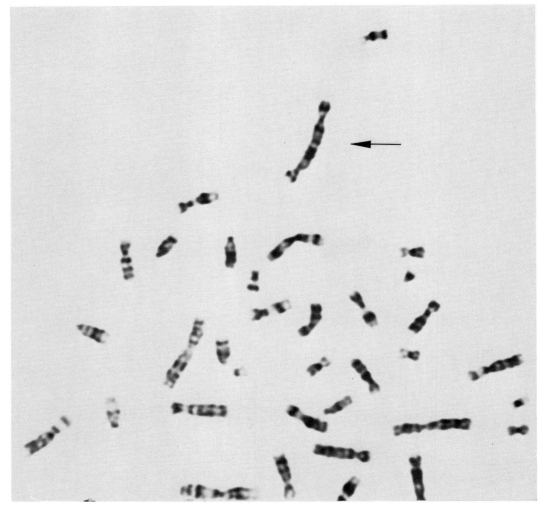

Fig. 4. Partial metaphase spread (*A.S.*) of a lymphocyte which received 75 R of [137]Cesium gamma rays. A dicentric chromosome (shown by the arrow) was radiation-induced.

at the end of the B-5 chromosome at 3q3, where 1.0 μ of material was lost and 0.3 μ of the X chromosome at 2q7 and 2q8 was masked but not lost in the rejoining. Figure 7 shows the dicentric chromosome, its profile waveform (right) and a diagrammatic scheme of the P and Q regions to demonstrate the area of rejoining of one of the X chromosomes (top) to one of the B chromosomes (bottom) after a terminal deletion of the B chromosome. The diagram shows 0.3 μ of the X chromosome (terminal end) masked in the rejoining with the terminal end of the B chromosome of which 0.5 μ was

deleted and 0.5 μ masked in forming the dicentric.

Discussion

The recently developed chromosome staining techniques which produce characteristic banding patterns provide challenging and new problems for computer-assisted chromosome identification. The development of a feature-ordering algorithm[13] for producing profile waveforms of banded chromosomes has enabled us to quantitatively assess a chromosome translocation from the blood of a genetically abnor-

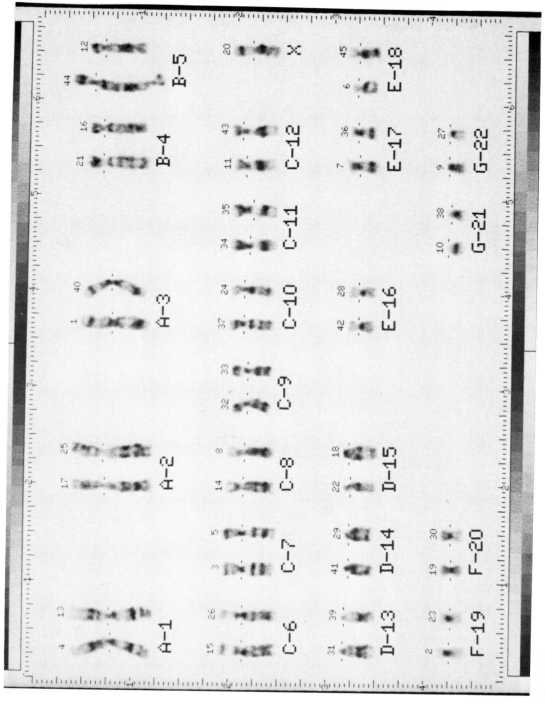

Fig. 5. Computer-generated karyotype from ALMS scan of the metaphase spread (Fig. 4) containing the dicentric. The dicentric is one of the B-5 chromosomes and is shown with its homologue. Some manual assistance was necessary to complete the karyotype.

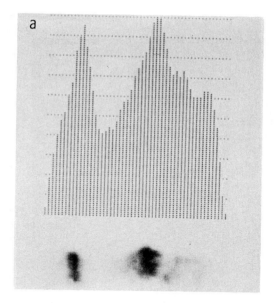

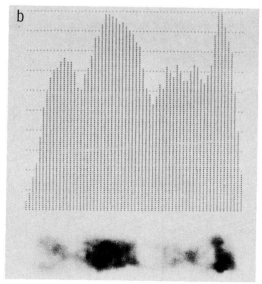

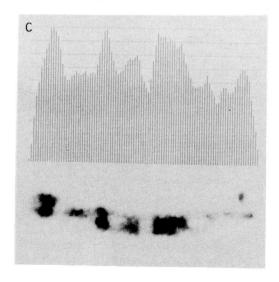

Fig. 6. Chromosomes and profile waveforms of A) the X chromosome, B) normal B-5 chromosome and C) dicentric.

mal child and a radiation-induced chromosome aberration (dicentric) produced in vitro. The data show that the translocation involved 3.2 μ of chromosomal material and the dicentric 0.5 μ which was deleted from one of the B chromosomes; 0.3 μ of material from the X chromosome was masked when the rejoining of the B and X chromosomes occurred.

It is possible from this type of profile waveform analysis to characterize anomalies within 0.1 μ so that insertions or deletions can be measured accurately. Although these results are preliminary, it appears that computer analysis of chromosomes can provide quantitative data on chromosome structure heretofore unavailable.[15,16] The ALMS speeds up collec-

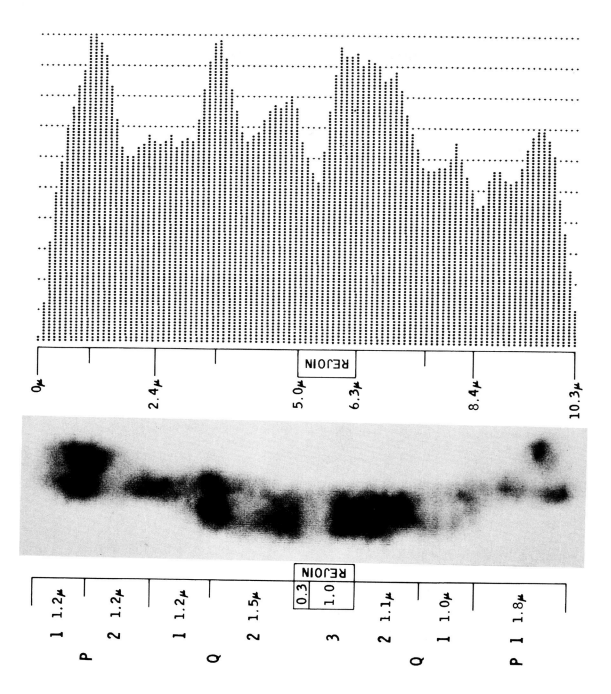

Fig. 7. Profile waveform (right) and dicentric chromosome (left) representing the fusion of one of the X chromosomes (above) with one of the B-5 chromosomes (below) after a terminal deletion of the B chromosome. The P region represents the short arm of the chromosome and the Q region, the long arm. Note rejoining occurred at the terminal ends of both chromosomes (Q) where 0.3 μ of chromosomal material of the X chromosome was masked in the fusion and 1.0 μ of the B chromosome was involved but 0.5 μ was deleted prior to fusion.

tion of information, making such studies applicable to large-scale biologic monitoring. It could lead to the application of automated systems in studies of basic mechanisms of genetic and radiation-induced chromosome damage.

References

1. Tjio, J. H. and Levan, A.: The chromosome number of man. *Hereditas 42*:1, 1956.
2. Milunsky, A., Littlefield, J. W., Kanfer, J. N. et al: Prenatal genetic diagnosis. *N. Engl. J. Med. 283*:1370, 1970.
3. Warkany, J.: *Congenital Malformations*. Chicago: Year Book Publishers, Inc., 1971, p. 1309.
4. Caspersson, T., Zech, L., Johansson, C. and Modest, E. J.: Identification of human chromosomes by DNA-binding fluorescent agents. *Chromosoma (Berl.) 30*:215, 1970.
5. Arrighi, F. E. and Hsu, T. C.: Localization of heterochromatin in human chromosomes. *Cytogenetics 10*:81, 1971.
6. Sumner, A. T., Evans, H. J. and Buckland, R. A.: A new technique for distinguishing between human chromosomes. *Nature (New Biol.) 232*:31, 1971.
7. Yunis, J. J., Roldan, L., Yasmineh, W. G. and Lee, J. C.: Staining of satellite DNA in metaphase chromosomes. *Nature 231*:532, 1971.
8. Seabright, M.: A rapid banding technique for human chromosomes, *Lancet 1*:971, 1971.
9. Patil, S. R., Merrick, S. and Lubs, H. A.: Identification of each human chromosome with a modified giemsa stain. *Science 173*:821, 1971.
10. Borgaonkar, D. S. and McKusick, V. A.: Human chromosome fluorescence, *Johns Hopkins Med. J. 128*:75, 1971.
11. Castleman, K.: Pictorial output for computerized karyotyping. In Wright, S. W., Crandall, B. F. and Boyer, L. (eds.): *Perspectives in Cytogenetics*. Springfield:Charles C Thomas, 1972, p. 316.
12. Caspersson, T., Castleman, K. R., Tomakka, G. et al: Automatic karyotyping of quinacrine mustard stained human chromosomes. *Exp. Cell Res. 67*:233, 1972.
13. Wall, R. J.: *The Gray Level Histogram for Threshold Boundary Determination in Image Processing with Applications to the Scene Segmentation Problem in Human Chromosome Analysis*. (Thesis for degree of Doctor of Philosophy in Engineering, University of California, Los Angeles, 1974.)
14. Bergsma, D. (ed.): *Paris Conference (1971): Standardization in Human Cytogenetics*. Birth Defects: Orig. Art. Ser., vol. VIII, no. 7. White Plains:The National Foundation—March of Dimes, 1972.
15. Stroud, A. N. and Ingram, M.: Radiation-induced chromosome aberration: Computer analysis with the ALMS system. (Abstract) *J. Cell Biol. 54*:254a, 1971.
16. Stroud, A. N., Harami, S. and Nathan, R.: Profile waveform analysis of interphase nuclei showing premature chromosome condensation. (Abstract) *Am. J. Hum. Genet. 25*:76a, 1973.

Discussion

Dr. Gordon: At the last Birth Defects Conference, in Boston, I presented, on behalf of my colleagues, a preliminary report on our experience at the Mayo Clinic with this kind of system for analyzing chromosomes. I am happy to say that we have made progress and it is now a routine clinical tool in our laboratory. The important point to make is one which I think deals with the question which was raised by a speaker from the floor a little earlier, in which Dr. Richard Warren of Miami pointed out that we were overinterpreting some of our opinions on G and other bands. I think he is correct. Our experience has been that we have made a particular diagnosis by the ordinary method of examining a G-banded preparation, and after we have done videodensimetric analysis, with this automated type of technique very similar to the one just described, we have had to change our mind. I think that we are going to find in the future that not only will this become a more accurate way of looking at what we now know about banded chromosomes, but I think that we are also going to see a lot more in the chromosome with this technique. Dr. Stroud pointed out the fact that she was having some difficulties with comparison nomenclature. I do think that once this kind of method of examining chromosomes becomes more advanced, both in depth and in width, so to speak, when more people have experience with it, we will have to change the comparison nomenclature. We now have to sort of twist our data to make it fit the pattern comparison nomenclature, which I think is not correct. I recall the old days of electrocardiography when one had to damp down the electrocardiogram so that he only got P, Q, R, S, T and U waves. It is quite easy to get about 40 waves on the electrocardiogram, and by using an instrument such as the Ram Tech for displaying and analyzing a banded chromosome, one could produce far more detail than the Paris people ever dreamt of. So, somewhere along the line, I think that we are going to have to review our concepts of the normal band pattern for normal chromosomes. I would like to confirm what Dr. Stroud has said, of how valuable a tool it is already in our hands for helping to sort out some clinical cytogenetic problems.

Dr. Warren: I would like to inquire as to the cost of these set-ups?

Dr. Stroud: That unit probably costs about $100,000. But we are in the process of building a second unit, with a small computer, which will probably cost about $75,000.

Dr. Warren: That would be a real bargain!

Moderator: Dr. Gordon, have you given any thought about what your unit will cost?

Dr. Gordon: It will cost about $8,000. I rather upset some people at the Boston Birth Defects Conference by saying that our entire set-up has cost us to date $520. As a matter of fact, our cost has now gone almost over $1,000. This is mainly owing to the fact that we are very good scroungers of equipment. We also get our computer time for nothing. We did not buy a computer. We have now run into a huge expense because we have had to hire a programmer, and that is costing us about $10,000 annually. But, in fact, given a computer, the kind of equipment which we are using, the television camera which we adapt to an ordinary microscope and then feed into the digitizing equipment, our expectation is that the overall cost, eventually, will be on the order of $30,000, provided that the market does not go up too quickly. But, given the computer, which most major institutions seem to have on-line, I think that this will not be that expensive, because we simply adapt the television camera to an ordinary microscope and the overall cost, then, for the microscope is $12,000, and the cost for the television camera is $9,000, then the transforming unit, the digitizing unit, is the most expensive part of the apparatus, which is about $25,000.

Dr. Stroud: They can be built for less. The microscope we are using is a spin-off from the space sciences. It was originally built to go to Mars, and money ran out for completion of this prototype so we obtained it and use it for this purpose. We are also using the image processing facility laboratory, where all the photographs that come back from the moon and Mars and Jupiter and from outer space are enhanced. So, in a sense, it does not cost us that much money. We are just using the facilities which have already been paid for.

A New Approach to Prenatal Diagnosis Using Trophoblast Cells in Maternal Blood*

Mostafa Raafat, M.D., Sc.D., James B. Brayton, D.V.M., M.P.H., M.D.,
Virginia Apgar, M.D.† and Digamber S. Borgaonkar, Ph.D.

Amniocentesis has been extensively used for prenatal diagnosis of certain genetic disorders.[1-4] In spite of its considerable value, this procedure carries definite, though infrequent, fetal and maternal risks. These complications include bleeding, infection, abortion, fetal injuries, fetomaternal sensitization, etc.[5-9] Moreover, therapeutic abortions following amniocentesis are usually induced late in the second trimester and are more risky than those induced earlier in pregnancy.[8]

The aim of the present work is to explore the possibility of using trophoblast cells recovered from the maternal circulation, instead of amniotic cells, for prenatal diagnosis. If this could be done, the complications arising from amniocentesis could be avoided. It would also be possible to induce earlier and less risky abortions, since human trophoblast cells start to deport into the maternal circulation early in the first trimester of pregnancy.[10-12]

The following is a short report on the studies performed to evaluate this approach in experimental models. The details of this work will be published separately.[13-15]

Experiment I

This experiment was designed to test the efficiency of our method for detection and recovery of trophoblast cells suspended in the maternal blood.

Healthy human placental tissue was obtained from early abortions and cut into tiny pieces in petri dishes containing a few milliliters of TC 199 medium. The trophoblast-199 suspension was then mixed with a 20 ml sample of heparinized peripheral blood taken from the same patient. The resulting trophoblast-blood suspension, containing known amounts of trophoblast cells (Fig. 1A), was then divided into 2 tubes which were allowed to stand in the refrigerator for 4 hours and 24 hours, respectively. Smears were then made from the supernates, buffy coats, and red cell sediments of both tubes (Figs. 1B and C). The remaining buffy coat was kept for the tissue culture studies (**Experiment II**). The smears were stained with Giemsa stain and examined for the number and condition of the trophoblast cells and leukocytes, and for the amount of RBCs in the background.

Sixty-one percent of the suspended trophoblast cells were recovered from the buffy coat after 4-hour sedimentation and 82% after 24 hours. The recovered trophoblasts were seen as well-preserved single cells (Fig. 2A) and as small groups of cells (Fig. 2B), which were easily identified by their large size and tendency towards multinucleation. In addition, syncytial

*Supported in part by a grant from The National Foundation-March of Dimes, Genetics Center grant GM 19489 and by a Genetics Training grant No. GM 00795 from the USPHS.
†Deceased August 7, 1974.

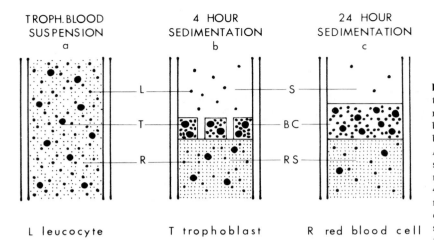

TROPH. BLOOD SUSPENSION
a

4 HOUR SEDIMENTATION
b

24 HOUR SEDIMENTATION
c

L leucocyte   T trophoblast   R red blood cell

S supernate   BC buffy coat   RS red sediment

Fig. 1. Diagram showing the methods used for recovery of the trophoblast cells from trophoblast-blood suspension. A) Trophoblast-blood suspension before sedimentation. B) After 4-hour sedimentation, notice the patchy buffy coat. C) After 24-hour sedimentation, notice the complete buffy coat.

masses (Fig. 2C) and even big portions of chorionic villi (Fig. 2D) were also seen. The 24-hour sedimentation method was preferred to the 4-hour method since it yielded more trophoblast cells and leukocytes, and showed fewer RBCs in the background.

Experiment II

This experiment was designed to compare the growth potentials in vitro of the trophoblast cells recovered from the maternal blood suspension (**Experiment I**), with those directly explanted from the placenta of the same patient.

Trophoblast cells, obtained from both sources, were cultured in T30 plastic flasks. Half the flasks were lined with thin layers of reconstituted rat-tail collagen, which was prepared following a modification of the technique of Ehrmann and Gey.[16] Three culture media were used: TC 199 with 33% fetal bovine serum (FBS), Eagle's MEM with 15% FBS, and Gibco diploid growth medium with 10% FBS. The cultures were incubated at 37°C in a gas phase of 5% CO_2 in air. They were periodically examined for cell morphology, growth rate and the sequence of events in culture.

In all the systems used, trophoblast cells grew actively while leukocytes did not grow and gradually degenerated. Apart from a slight delay in the initial migration, the blood-recovered trophoblast cells behaved in a similar manner to those directly explanted from the placenta. The cells grew better on the collagen substrate than on the plastic surface. The 3 media supported the growth of trophoblast cells equally well. The third medium, however, was preferred because of its lower serum content.

About 80% of the explants produced pure epithelial monolayers of trophoblast cells which grew actively for about 4 weeks (Fig. 3A). During this phase of active growth, many mitotic figures were seen (Fig. 3B). Numerous microvilli were also noticed projecting from the free borders of the cells (Fig. 3C). After 4-6 weeks small gaps started to appear in the monolayers (Fig. 3D) and gradually expanded. This was accompanied by progressive degeneration of the trophoblast cells.

About 20% of the explants produced a mixed population of trophoblast and fibro-spindle cells. Sometimes a few histiocytes were also seen. These mixed cell cultures were kept growing for about 20 weeks before they started to degenerate. They were transferred several times with gradual disappearance of the trophoblast cells and overgrowth of the fibroblasts.

Collagen lysis was frequently observed, particularly in the mixed cell cultures. Cytogenetic studies revealed a high incidence of polyploidy (20%) mainly in the 4n range. Satisfactory karyotypes were made from both types of cultures (Fig. 4).

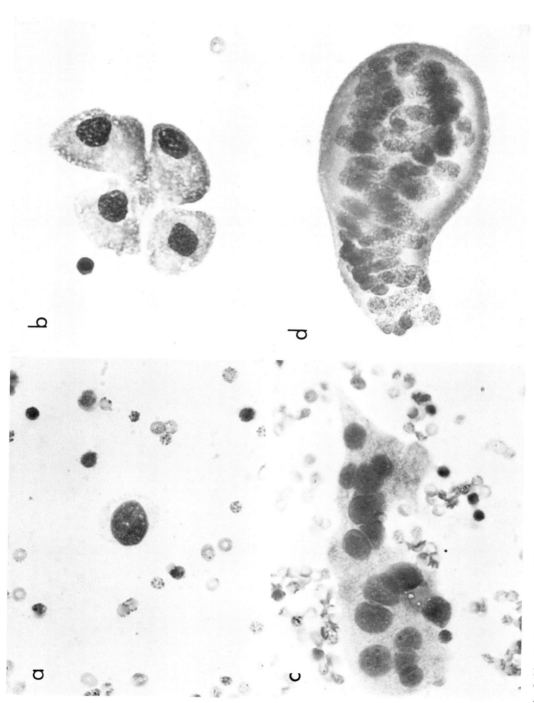

Fig. 2. Morphologic patterns of the recovered trophoblast. Smear stained with Giemsa. Notice the well-preserved condition of the trophoblast cells and their large size as compared to the leukocytes and RBCs in the background. A) A single cytotrophoblast cell (×320). B) A group of cytotrophoblast cells (×320). C) A mass of syncytotrophoblast (×320). D) A big portion of a primary chorionic villus (×160).

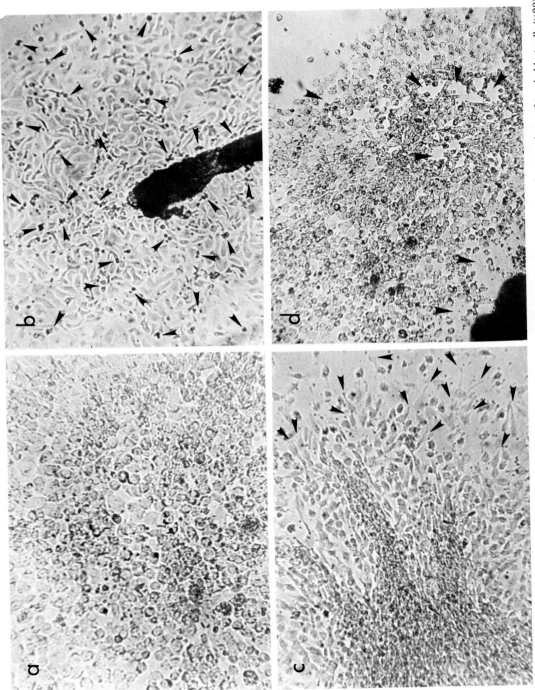

Fig. 3. Growth morphology of the *in vitro* recovered trophoblasts. A) Three-week-old culture showing an extensive monolayer of trophoblast cells (×90). B) Two-week-old culture showing a large number of dividing cells (×60). C) Three-week-old culture showing microvilli projecting from the free borders of trophoblast cells (×60). D) Five-week-old culture, showing small gaps in the trophoblast monolayer (×60).

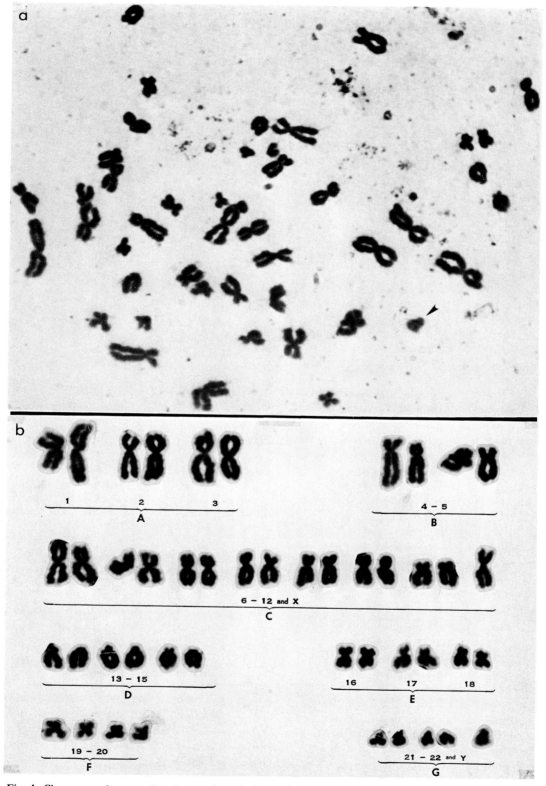

Fig. 4. Chromosomal preparation from a 2-week-old trophoblast culture. Giemsa stain. A) Metaphase spread showing 46,XY. The arrow points to the Y chromosome. B) Karyotype of the same spread.

Experiment III

This experiment was designed to recover the trophoblast cells from the blood circulation of pregnant rhesus monkeys (*Macaca mulatta*). Due to the large size of these cells, they are filtered in the pulmonary capillaries and do not reach the peripheral circulation.[11,17,18] Therefore, for successful recovery, blood samples should be obtained along the venous drainage of the placenta, somewhere between the uterus and the lungs. The higher we go into the inferior vena cava, the more complete will be the sampling, since the drainage of the ovarian veins will be included.[17-19]

The monkeys were given a mild sedative 15 minutes before catheterization. Then by simple venipuncture, a thin radiopaque catheter was introduced into the femoral vein, along the inferior vena cava until its tip reached above the left renal vein (Fig. 5). There was no need for general anesthesia, x-ray confirmation of the catheter level, or for an open incision on the femoral vein. A 10 ml blood sample was then drawn using a heparinized syringe. Attempts were made to recover and grow the trophoblast cells which might be present in the sample, following the methods mentioned in **Experiments I** and **II**. Control samples were taken from the peripheral blood of the pregnant monkey and the male partner.

So far 10 pregnant monkeys have been catheterized: 4 in the second month of gestation and 6 in the third and fourth months. The total gestation period in the rhesus monkey is 5½ months. No trophoblast cells could be detected in either the smears or the cultures examined. The negative results may be due to the lack of deportation of trophoblast cells into the maternal circulation at the time of sampling, thus confirming the observations of previous investigators who were also unable to find trophoblast cells in the lungs of pregnant experimental animals including the monkey.[20,21] Therefore it seems that the trophoblast deportation phenomenon, which is generally observed in pregnant women, is rather specific to the human and does not occur in the monkey. This is possibly related to the struc-

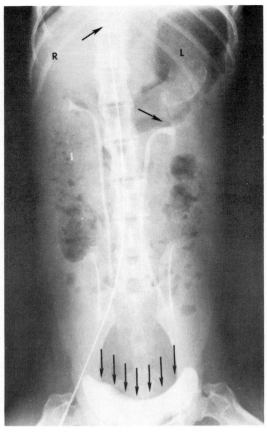

Fig. 5. An IVP of a 46-day pregnant rhesus monkey with the catheter in the inferior vena cava. The upper arrow points to the tip of the catheter. The middle arrow points to the level of left renal vein. The lower arrows point to the indentation in the bladder caused by the pregnant uterus.

tural differences, which are known to exist between the placentas of the 2 taxa.[23] However, more monkeys will need to be catheterized early in pregnancy before reaching definite conclusions.

Summary and Conclusions

A new approach to prenatal diagnosis, using the trophoblast cells in maternal blood, has been proposed. This approach would hopefully avoid the risks of amniocentesis and help induce earlier abortions.

Three experiments were performed for the evaluation of this approach. In the first experiment human trophoblast cells were successfully recovered from a trophoblast-blood suspension by slow cold sedimentation. In the second experiment, the recovered human trophoblast cells were successfully grown in culture for several weeks and satisfactory karyotypes were prepared from them. In the third experiment attempts were made to recover the trophoblast cells from the inferior vena caval blood of pregnant monkeys, but were not successful. The absence of trophoblast cells in catheter specimens is probably due to the lack of their shedding into the maternal circulation of the monkey.

We recommend trying this new approach in pregnant women since it proved to be simple, safe and efficient in experimental models. Moreover, the trophoblast deportation phenomenon seems to be specific to the human placenta.

* * *

This chapter is dedicated to the memory of Dr. Virginia Apgar, who died during the preparation of the manuscript. Without her inspiration and continuous support, this work would not have been possible.

References

1. Valenti, C., Schutta, E. F. and Kehaty, T.: Cytogenetic diagnosis of Down's syndrome in-utero. *JAMA 207*:1513-1515, 1969.

2. Nadler, H. L. and Gerbie, A. B.: Role of amniocentesis in the intrauterine detection of genetic disorders. *N. Engl. J. Med. 282*:596-599, 1970.

3. Shih, V. E. and Littlefield, J. W.: Argininosuccinase activity in amniotic fluid cells. *Lancet 2*:45, 1970.

4. Shneck, L., Valenti, C., Amsterdam, D. et al: Prenatal diagnosis of Tay-Sachs disease. *Lancet 1*:582-584, 1970.

5. Liley, A. W.: The technique and complications of amniocentesis. *N. Z. Med. J. 59*:581-586, 1960.

6. Burnett, R. G. and Anderson, W. R.: The hazards of amniocentesis. *J. Iowa Med. Soc. 58*:130-137, 1968.

7. Creasman, W. T., Lawrence, R. A. and Thiede, H. A.: Fetal complications of amniocentesis. *JAMA 204*:949-952, 1968.

8. Fuchs, F.: Amniocentesis and abortion. Methods and risks. In Bergsma, D. (ed.): *Intrauterine*

Diagnosis, Birth Defects: Orig. Art. Ser., vol. VII, no. 5. Baltimore:Williams & Wilkins Co. for The National Foundation-March of Dimes, 1971, pp. 18-19.

9. Cook, L. N., Shott, R. J. and Andrews, B. F.: Fetal complications of diagnostic amniocentesis. A review and report of a case with pneumothorax. *Pediatrics 53*:421-424, 1974.

10. Bardawil, W. A. and Benjamin, L. T.: The natural history of choriocarcinoma: Problems of immunity and spontaneous regression. *Ann. N. Y. Acad. Sci. 80*:197-261, 1959.

11. Salvaggio, A. T.: Deportation and destruction of the trophoblast. In Thiede, H. A. (ed.): *Transcript of the First Rochester Trophoblast Conference,* 1961, pp. 89-97.

12. Hertig, A. T.: Implantation and early development. In Thiede, H. A. (ed.): *Transcript of the First Rochester Trophoblast Conference,* 1961, pp. 2-27.

13. Raafat, M., Apgar, V., Borgaonkar, D. S. and Brayton, J. B.: The use of circulating trophoblast cells for prenatal diagnosis: I. Testing the efficiency of our method for detection and recovery of human trophoblast cells from maternal blood suspension. (In preparation.)

14. Raafat, M., Borgaonkar, D. S., Apgar, V. and Brayton, J. B.: The use of circulating trophoblast cells for prenatal diagnosis: II. In vitro behavior of human trophoblast cells recovered from maternal blood suspension. (In preparation.)

15. Raafat, M., Brayton, J. B., Apgar, V. and Borgaonkar, D. S.: The use of circulating trophoblast cells for prenatal diagnosis: III. An attempt to recover and grow trophoblast cells from the blood circulation of pregnant rhesus monkeys. (In preparation.)

16. Ehrmann, R. L. and Gey, G. O.: The growth of cells on a transparent gel of reconstituted rat-tail collagen. *J. Natl. Cancer Inst. 16*:1375-1403, 1956.

17. Thomas, L., Douglas, G. W. and Carr, M. C.: The continual migration of syncytial trophoblasts from the fetal placenta into the maternal circulation. *Trans. Assoc. Am. Physicians 72*:140-148, 1959.

18. Douglas, G. W., Thomas, L., Carr, M. et al: Trophoblast in the circulating blood during pregnancy. *Am. J. Obstet. Gynecol. 78*:960-973, 1959.

19. Ramsey, E. M.: Circulation in the uterus and the intervillous space in the primate placenta. In Thiede, H. A. (ed.): *Transcript of the Third Rochester Trophoblast Conference,* 1965, pp. 6-27.

20. McKay, D. G.: Comment on paper by Douglas, G. W. (ref. 22). In Thiede, H. A. (ed.): *Transcript of the First Rochester Trophoblast Conference,* 1961, p. 78.

21. Hertz, R.: Comment on paper by Douglas, G. W. (ref. 22). In Thiede, H. A. (ed.): *Transcript of the First Rochester Trophoblast Conference,* 1961, p. 78.

22. Douglas, G. W.: Deportation and destruction of the trophoblast. In Thiede, H. A. (ed.): *Transcript of the First Rochester Trophoblast Conference,* 1961, pp. 70-80.

23. Ramsey, E. M. and Harris, J. W. S.: Comparison of uteroplacental vasculature and circulation in the rhesus monkey and man. In *Contributions to Embryology,* Carnegie Institution of Washington Publication 625. Baltimore:Garamond/Pridemark Press, 1966, vol. 38, no. 261, pp. 59-70.

Case Reports

A — The Floating-Harbor Syndrome

Jaako Leisti, M.D., David W. Hollister, M.D. and David L. Rimoin, M.D., Ph.D.

M.M. (HH 308280) was born in 1964 and has been followed at HGH since age 3 months because of failure to thrive, growth retardation, unusual facial appearance and delayed development of speech.

The patient was the product of a 9-month gestation. The mother was 23 years old (gravida 3, para 3, ab 0) and the father 30 years old. They were not consanguineous. Two healthy sibs were of average height, and the family history was negative for short stature. The birthweight was 3300 gm, length 43 cm and head circumference 32.5 cm. The peculiar facies with large nose and deep-set eyes, was noticed soon after birth.

The patient had grown very slowly and this had been further characterized by a greatly retarded bone age (at age 4½ years, BA was 9 months; at age 9 9/12 years, BA was 4 2/12 years). Motor development had also been slightly retarded. Language development had been definitely retarded because of expressive aphasia, while intellectual development according to testing had progressed at average level. General health of the patient had been quite satisfactory, but he had had recurrent otitis media and had also suffered from allergic rhinitis and eczema. The pseudoathrosis-type anomaly of the right clavicle was first noticed at age 2. Dilatation of the urethra had been performed because of meatal stenosis and stricture of the fossa navicularis.

Physical examination at age 9 9/12 years showed a white male with proportionate short stature and unusual facial appearance (Fig. 1). His height was 103 cm, U/L ratio 0.95, and weight 15 kg. The skull appeared dolichocephalic with a prominent occiput. The facies appeared triangular with wide forehead, hypoplastic maxilla and small mandible with slight mandibular overbite. The nose appeared large and had a broad base. The eyes appeared normal but deep-set and the eyelashes were long. The palate was narrow due to hypertrophy of the maxillary alveolar ridge. The ears were low-set and posteriorly rotated. The neck appeared short with normal posterior hairline and the chest was wide. No abdominal organomegaly was palpated; the penis was small and both testes were descended. The hands were small with short stubby fingers, the 5th fingers showing slight clinodactyly with hypoplastic middle phalanges. The fingers were also slightly hyperextensible. The flexion creases and dermatoglyphics of the palms were considered normal. The 4th and 5th toes were slightly incurved. There was also mild limitation of extension at the elbows.

X-ray studies and laboratory data showed no significant abnormal findings. Among others, the karyotype was normal 46,XY (with ASG-banding), and growth hormone and cortisol responses to insulin-induced hypoglycemia were normal.

This patient's appearance is identical to that of a patient described by Pelletier and Feingold as their *Case 1* in *Syndrome Identification* (I(1):8, 1973). Indeed, each mother identified the other child's photograph as her own son. Because these 2 patients were studied at the Boston Floating and Harbor General Hospitals, we tentatively propose the name "Floating-Harbor syndrome" for this disorder.

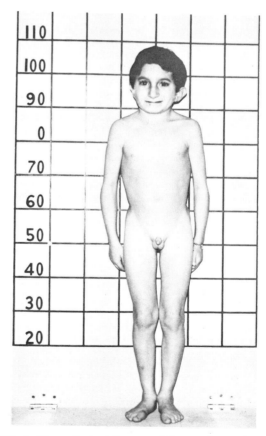

Fig. 1. The patient at the age of 9 years 9 months. Note the low-set ears, long nose and the shallow maxillary region.

B — Humeroradial Ankylosis Associated with Other Congenital Defects (The "Boomerang Arm" Sign)

Jaakko Leisti, M.D., Ralph S. Lachman, M.D. and David L. Rimoin, M.D., Ph.D.

B.S. (HH 630955), a product of a normal pregnancy and delivery, was born in 1960 to a 33-year-old mother and a 27-year-old father. Several congenital defects were noted after birth, including flexion contractures of elbows, hips and knees; bilateral dislocation of the hips; bilateral clubfoot (right side more severely affected); micrognathia; and cleft of the soft palate. The birthweight was 2270 gm and length 40 cm. The family history was negative as to congenital anomalies and the patient's 2 brothers were healthy. The motor milestones were achieved late but mental development had been normal. The patient had undergone several operations: right Achilles tenotomy at age 7 months; correction of cleft palate at 15 months; surgery of the left hip at age 4; dextrorotation osteotomy of the proximal right tibia at age 9; and repair of a strangulated right inguinal hernia at age 7.

Physical examination at age 13 showed a short young man with severe changes in his limbs (Fig. 1). Height was 117 cm (< 3rd%), span was 100 cm and U/L ratio, 1.2. The facies appeared peculiar with small nose, long philtrum and small chin. The chest appeared asymmetric, with left side and left shoulder somewhat depressed, and there was slight scoliosis and accentuated lumbar lordosis. No abdominal organomegaly was present. The right testis was not descended.

Both shoulders presented with slight limitation of movements, the elbows were ankylotic with a 90° angle between the arms and forearms, while the wrists showed normal flexion. The fingers were somewhat loose-jointed but were otherwise normal. Both hips, especially the left one, showed severe flexion contractures. Slight flexion contracture was also noticed in both knees and limitation of movements was present in both ankles. The right lower limb was shorter than the left.

X-ray studies revealed a complete ankylosis of both humeri and radii (Fig. 2). There was dislocation of the left hip with no formation of the acetabulum (Fig. 3). On the right, the acetabulum was present

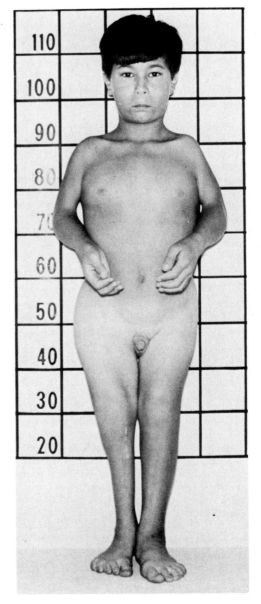

Fig. 1. The patient at the age of 13. Note the asymmetry of the lower limbs and the peculiar facies. The elbows are fixed at a 90° angle.

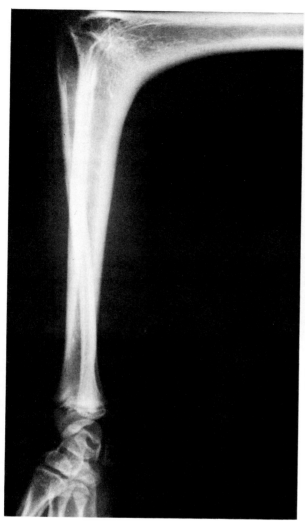

Fig. 3. AP view of pelvis. Note the absence of left acetabulum, deformed right acetabulum and marked right coxa vara producing a curved femur.

Fig. 2. Lateral view of right arm. Note the complete anklyosis of the humeroradial joint.

with deformity of the roof and dislocation of the hip and marked coxa vara. The femurs showed lateral bowing.

The presence of complete humeroradial ankylosis, resembling an Australian boomerang radiographically, is quite unusual, but has been described with a variety of different developmental defects.

Addendum

A similar constellation of anomalies has been described by Daentl et al in *J. Pediatr.* 86:107, 1975 under the name "Femoral hypoplasia — unusual facies syndrome."

C — Progeroid Syndrome

Marshall D. Levine, M.D., Elaine Alexander, M.D. and David L. Rimoin, M.D., Ph.D.

J.M. (HH 561150) was a 7-year-old female with many progeroid features, normal mentation and improving motor development. She was the 2.88 kg, 53.34 cm product of a normal, full-term, uncomplicated pregnancy. At birth it was noted that the right wrist was abnormally flexed with abduction of the thumb and hyperextension of the other joints of the hand. Radiographs were normal.

As an infant the patient apparently had intolerance to milk and other foods, with failure to thrive. In February 1968, she began on a meat-based diet with some improvement in temperament and a slight weight gain. Evaluation for failure to thrive at that time revealed epicanthal folds, asymmetry of the skull, slight pectus, diffuse hypotonicity with marked decrease in muscle mass, generalized hyporeflexia with sustained clonus in the lower limbs, hypertrichosis, synophyrs and marked diaphoresis. No definite diagnosis was made.

Reevaluation approximately one year later revealed, in addition to the above-mentioned findings, marked diaphoresis, asymmetry of the head with hyperplasia of the right side and right microdontia, gingival hypertrophy and a high-arched palate. A pneumoencephalogram revealed asymmetry of the lateral ventricles with the left slightly larger than the right, mild paraventricular atrophy, and gas accumulation over the left parietal-temporal areas with the sulci appearing larger than normal. Brain scan, EEG and echoencephalogram were normal.

Skull x-ray films revealed arrested hydrocephalus with elevation of the petrous ridges and prominent parietal regions. The right side of the skull was larger than the left. Karyotype and IVP were normal.

Patient's developmental milestones were all markedly delayed with the exception of language which was normal. At age 5 months weight was at the 3rd percentile while height was less than the 50th. At 17 months weight (6.36 kg) and height (71.12 cm) were both less than the 3rd percentile.

Family history revealed that the patient has 3 older sibs (2 females and 1 male), each of whom probably had bilateral congenital dislocation of the hip and anterior tibial torsion. One other normal sib died of flu and the patient's mother had one spontaneous abortion. Her father and one of his male sibs probably had congenital dislocation of the hip. Her parents were unrelated and from large families.

The patient was first admitted for evaluation at the age of 4½ years (Fig. 1). At that time her weight (8.17 kg) and height (81.28 cm) were both below the

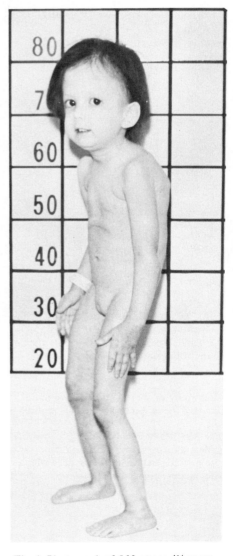

Fig. 1. Photograph of *J.M.* at age 4½ years.

3rd percentile. She appeared emaciated and much older than her stated age of 4. Pertinent findings included transiently elevated blood pressure; moderate diaphoresis; thin, transparent, diffusely red-purple skin; a prominent venous pattern over the head and chest; hypotrichosis with very fine graying hair, scanty eyebrows and short eyelashes; asymmetric prominence of the right parietal-temporal region; frontal and parietal bossing; triangular-shaped face with striking micrognathia and maxillary hypoplasia; small orbits; epicanthal folds; antimongoloid slant to the palpebral fissures; beak-like small nose; low-set posteriorly rotated small ears; high-arched palate, gingival hypertrophy; dental dysplasia; bilateral Harrison grooves; kyphoscoliosis; 15% limitation of extension of the knees bilaterally with hyperextensibility of other joints; bilateral coxa valga; bilateral cubitus varus; markedly decreased muscle mass; a broad-based unsteady gait with bent knees (horse rider's stance); and a coarse tremor of the tongue.

The following normal data were obtained: CBC, SMA 12, lytes, creatinine, creatinine clearance, total lipids, cholesterol, triglycerides, ECG, chest radiograph, EMG, nerve conduction studies and skin biopsy for light and electron microscopy. CPK was slightly elevated. Immunoglobulins revealed a slight decrease in IgG and serum protein electrophoresis revealed a slight decrease in the gamma globulin content. Growth hormone, insulin, cortisol, blood sugar, VMA and HVA measurements were all normal.

Psychologic testing revealed a bright normal child.

In the following 2 years the patient's motor development and skeletal deformities had markedly improved. Her muscle mass was still markedly deficient but her hypotonia had significantly improved. Her hair growth also appeared better. She thus had many of the physical features of progeria, but the definite improvement in muscle tone, motor abilities and hair growth over the past 2 years make this diagnosis somewhat unlikely.

D — An Unusual Short Stature Syndrome

Jaakko Leisti, M.D., Gerald Sugarman, M.D. and David L. Rimoin, M.D., Ph.D.

This child had an unusual constellation of anomalies consisting of short stature, failure to thrive, mental retardation, microcephaly, deafness and peculiar facies. She was born in 1967 with a birthweight of 1.90 kg. Family history and data on pregnancy were not known, but the child was apparently born at term to a mother who was a heroin addict. Since the age of 7 months, the child has been raised in foster homes.

The patient (HH 532979) was first seen at HGH in May 1971 at the age of 4 4/12 years because of short stature, developmental retardation and deafness. The motor milestones were reached late; the patient sat at 24 months, stood and walked at about 4 years. Intelligible words appeared also at 4 years; impaired hearing was detected at age 2 when a hearing aid was also prescribed. Physical growth has been very slow with the height remaining 7-8 SDs below the mean for sex and age, while the bone age has closely followed the chronologic age. First teeth erupted at 23 months. Her mental and motor development greatly improved when she was placed with her current foster mother at age 3.

Physical examination at age 6 10/12 years showed a very small gracile female with peculiar facial appearance (Fig. 1). Height was 98.43 cm and weight 10.90 kg. Body proportions were normal. The head was microcephalic with a circumference of 43 cm and with a flat occiput. The face appeared elongated and slightly pinched, with slight malar hypoplasia, downward slanting palpebral fissures and a beaked nose. The palate was highly arched and the chin small. There were both frontal and muchal hemangiomata; the posterior hairline was low-set and the neck was long with slight bilateral pterygium. The chest, abdomen and external genitalia appeared normal. A grade 2/6 cardiac systolic murmur was audible. The limbs were well-proportioned but thin. The fingers were short with hyperextensible joints. There were bilateral simian creases: the axial triradii were distally located and 5 fingers showed arches.

The patient was alert, easily irritated and obviously retarded. The gait was wide-based and there was a slight intention tremor in the hands. Hearing was significantly reduced bilaterally.

Skeletal x-ray findings and pneumoencephalograms were normal, as was an upper GI series. Karyotype with ASG-banding was normal 46,XX. EEG was normal and laboratory results have been essentially normal with decreased absorption of D-xylose on repeated occasions but with normal fecal fat content.

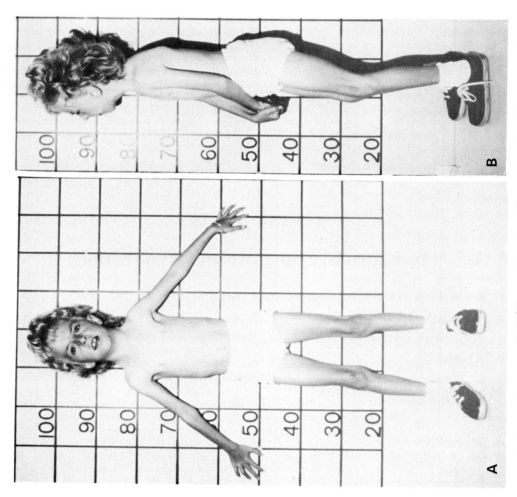

Fig. 1. A and B) the patient at age of 6 10/12 years. Note the gracile appearance, broad neck with pterygium and unusual facial features.

E — Unusual Congenital Anomalies

Marshall D. Levine, M.D., Jerome Rotter, M.D. and David L. Rimoin, M.D., Ph.D.

V.R. (HH 630728) is a 14-year-old female who has an unusual constellation of anomalies consisting of short stature, microcephaly, hypotelorism, congenital cardiac and congenital skeletal disease. She was the 1417.5 gm, 7-month product of a 34-year-old white female and a 39-year-old white male. Apparently no obvious abnormalities were noted at birth. In the neonatal period she had a very severe problem with diarrhea and it was 3 months before she gained the weight necessary to be discharged from the hospital. At 3 months of age she was noted to have a heart murmur. Catheterization subsequently revealed an atrial septal defect (ASD), a small patent ductus arteriosus (PDA) and a persistent left superior vena cava. The ASD (ostium secundum) and the PDA were corrected at age 4 without sequelae.

At approximately age one she developed a urinary tract infection. IVP was negative. Urethral stenosis was diagnosed and she was treated with urethral dilatation. No further GU problems were noted until 1972, when she developed cystitis. She responded well to antibiotics and urethral dilatation without subsequent problems.

Since age 4 she has had multiple episodes of bilateral serous otitis media with recurrent sinusitis. Adenoidectomy and bilateral polyethylene tube placement on 2 occasions have not helped. Sinus x-ray films are unrevealing except for demonstrating maxillary and ethmoid sinusitis. She is almost totally deaf but she reads lips well.

For many years the patient has been troubled with a chronically dislocating right elbow. No history of trauma was associated with the initial episode. She has not been bothered by this problem in the last 2½ years, even though she is a very active roller skater.

Her mental and motor landmarks have been normal with exception of the limitations engendered by her deafness. However, she has always been very small in height and weight.

Her father, mother and an 8-year-old male sib are all healthy. There is no consanguinity in the family. There is no similar constellation of abnormalities in any other family member.

On physical examination, the patient was a short (142.5 cm), thin (31.326 kg), microcephalic (48 cm), hypoteloric (interpupillary distance 3.9 cm; outer canthal distance 6.8 cm), postpubertal white female (Fig. 1). Pertinent findings included a mild peripheral facial palsy on the right; a high-arched palate; a persistent epicanthus on the right; bilateral scarring of the tympanic membranes; acne, especially on the face; a healed vertical scar on the chest from previous cardiac surgery; radial deviation of the right 2nd finger distal to the PIP joint; camptodactyly at the PIP joint and clinodactyly of both 5th fingers; poorly developed digital creases, especially in the 2nd finger at the PIP joints; and distal axial triradii bilaterally. Karyotypic analysis revealed 46,XX with normal ASG bands.

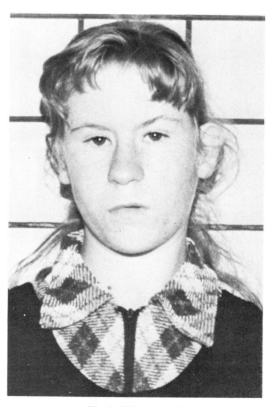

Fig. 1. *V.R.* at age 14.

F — Unusual Skeletal Anomalies

Marshall D. Levine, M.D., Ralph Lachman, M.D. and David L. Rimoin, M.D., Ph.D.

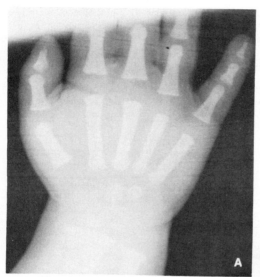

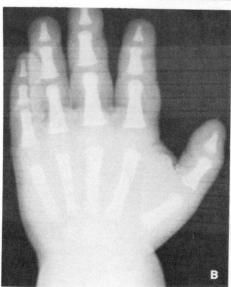

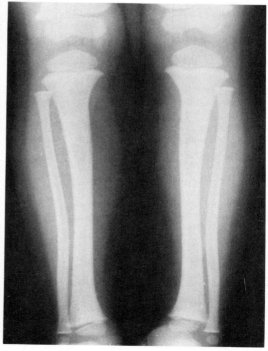

T.L. (HH 516297) is presented because of unusual skeletal x-ray findings of unknown etiology. X-ray examination at age 20 months revealed thin trabeculated metacarpals (2 to 5) with bulbous proximal ends (Fig. 1). A subsequent skeletal survey 7 months later revealed, in addition, bilateral hypoplasia of the radial head, bilateral anterior and medial bowing of the tibia, and medial bowing of the fibulas (Fig. 2). Follow-up x-ray examination when the patient was age 3 revealed the same findings in the hands and long bones as well as similar changes in the feet. Bone age has been consistent with chronologic age. The patient's growth and development have been normal except for transient inappropriate ADH hypersecretion.

Fig. 1. A and B) Radiographs at 20 months reveal thin trabeculated metacarpals (2-5) with bulbous proximal ends bilaterally.

Fig. 2. Radiograph at 27 months reveals bilateral medial bowing of the tibia and the fibula.

G — Familial Frontal Dysplasia

Marshall D. Levine, M.D., David L. Rimoin, M.D., Ph.D. and Ralph Lachman, M.D.

J.E. (HH 266800) (Fig. 1) and *K.E.* (HH 379620) (Fig. 2) are brothers whose facies resembled those seen in frontal metaphyseal dysplasia but who have no metaphyseal abnormalities or other malformations. Their facies were characterized by a flat sloping forehead with an extremely prominent supraorbital ridge, malar hypoplasia, a prominent mandible, maxillary midline diastema, and a decrease in the size of the pulp chambers. X-ray films revealed that the ridge in the younger brother (*K.E.*) was bony (Fig. 3A), but the older brother's prominence represented a markedly enlarged frontal sinus covered by a thin layer of bone (Figs. 3B and 4).

The family history revealed that their father and paternal grandfather each had a similar facial appearance, but the brothers refused to have any of their relatives examined. Their only sib, an older sister, was said to have a slight supraorbital prominence. She has 3 healthy female children and one questionably affected male child. The older brother has 3 daughters, the oldest of whom was said to have a small supraorbital prominence. The younger brother has a boy with a marked supraorbital ridge and an unaffected girl.

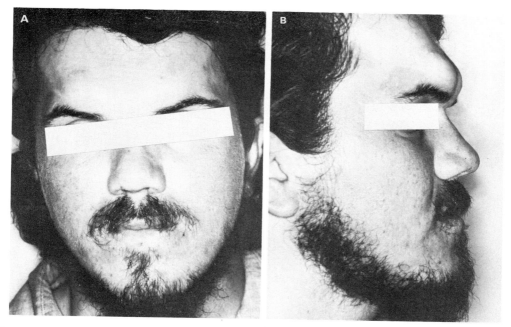

Fig. 1. *J.E.* A) Note the malar hypoplasia and prominent supraorbital ridge and B) the flat sloping forehead with an extremely prominent supraorbital ridge and prominent mandible.

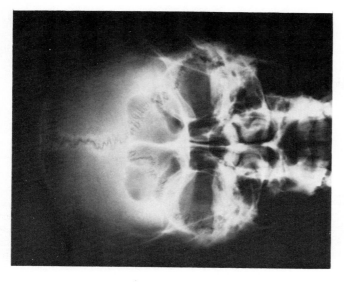

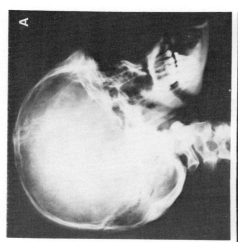

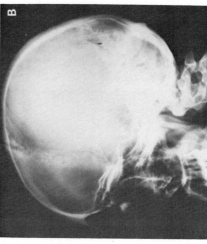

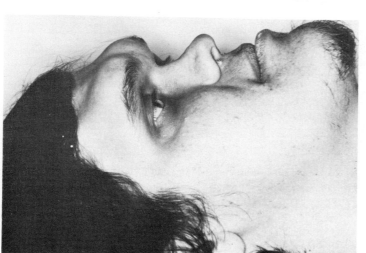

Fig. 4. *J.E.*, note the prominent sinuses.

Fig. 3. Note the difference in the composition of the supraorbital ridges in the 2 brothers. A) In *K.E.* the supraorbital ridge is composed entirely of bone. B) In *J.E.* the supraorbital ridge is composed of a prominent frontal sinus covered by thin layer of bone.

Fig. 2. *K.E.*, note the similarity to *J.E.* with the flat sloping forehead, extremely prominent supraorbital ridge and prominent mandible.

H — The Turner Phenotype Associated with Unbalanced X/Autosome Translocation

Jaakko Leisti, M.D., Michael M. Kaback, M.D. and David L. Rimoin, M.D., Ph.D.

S. McC. (HH 620082) was a 29-year-old black female who was referred because of short stature, primary amenorrhea and multiple minor anomalies.

The patient was a term product of a 27-year-old mother (gravida 6, para 4, ab 2) and a 32-year-old father. The family history was negative as to short stature, primary amenorrhea or somatic anomalies, and the 3 healthy sibs are of average height. The mother's 2 miscarriages occurred during the first and second trimester of pregnancy.

The pregnancy was uneventful except for threatened abortion during the seventh month. Birthweight was 2438 gm and no malformations were noted at birth. Both physical and mental development have been slow and she reached her motor milestones late. At age 17 years she was diagnosed as having a goiter and hypothyroidism and was started on thyroid. Because of the primary amenorrhea and lack of secondary sexual development, progesterone and estrogen therapy was started as well, which resulted in regular periods and development of breasts and pubic hair. At age 27, elevated blood pressure (140-150/100-110) and hyperglycemia with glucosuria were found.

Physical examination at the age of 28 years revealed a black female with short stature and somewhat unusual facial features (Fig. 1). Her height was 136 cm, U/L ratio 1.1 and weight 50 kg. The patient was obese and showed secondary sexual characteristics secondary to the substitution therapy. Her head was small and brachycephalic with a circumference of 50 cm. The posterior hairline was normally located. The face showed abundant lanugo-like hair and deep-set eyes with exotropia of the right eye. The palate was normal and the chin was small with malocclusion of teeth. Auricles were normal and no pterygium was found. The chest appeared wide; there was slight bilateral cubitus valgus and both hands and feet appeared small. Both 4th metacarpals were short and the 5th fingers were short and clinodactylic. The nails were hyperconvex and deep-set. Simian creases, proximal axial triradii and interdigital loops in both the 3rd and 5th interspaces were found bilaterally. The 1st and 2nd toes were widely spaced and the 4th and 5th toes were very short.

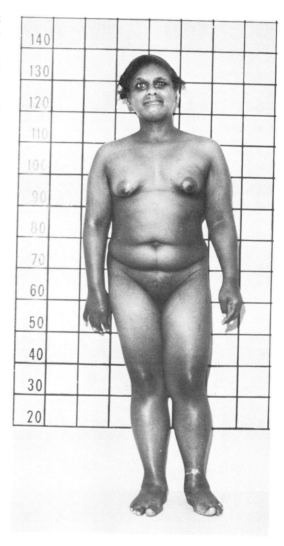

Fig. 1. The patient at age 27 years, following cyclical estrogen therapy.

Chromosome analysis of peripheral lymphocytes showed the mother of the patient to be a carrier of a balanced translocation between an X chromosome and chromosome 9, with the majority of the long arm of X being translocated to the very distal portion of the long arm of chromosome 9 [karyotype: 46,X,t(X;9)(q11;q32)] (Fig. 2). The patient had 46 chromosomes also, but her karyotype was unbalanced with only one X, 2 normal chromosomes 9, and the long translocation chromosome [karyotype: 46,X,-X,+der(9),t(X;9)(q11;q32)mat] (Fig. 3). Both mother and daughter were sex-chromatin positive, but in the mother's cells the normal X was late-labeling while in the patient's cells the translocation chromo-some (der 9) was late-labeling, with the label spread along the adjacent autosome 9.

Thus, this family represents differential inactivation of the X chromosome in the mother and daughter. In the translocation chromosome of the patient, the inactivation has spread to the adjacent autosome, explaining why she does not have the full clinical features of trisomy 9. This case is also an example of the rare adjacent-2 type of segregation.

This patient was previously described as a 6/9 translocation (Rohde, R. A. and Catz, B.: Maternal transmission of a new group-C (6/9) chromosomal syndrome. *Lancet* 2:838-840, 1964).

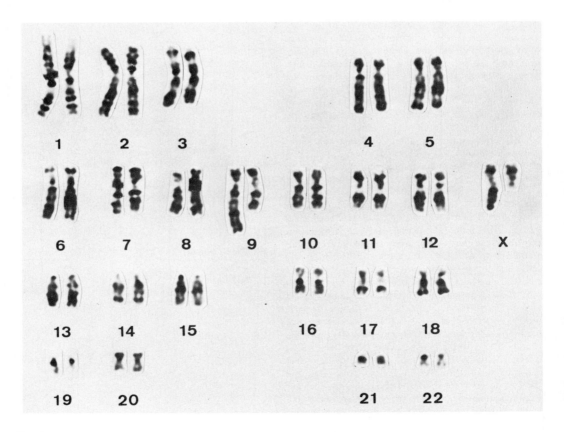

Fig. 2. Karyotype of the mother showing a reciprocal translocation between an X chromosome and a chromosome 9. [46,X,t(X;9)(q11;q32)] (ASG-Giemsa).

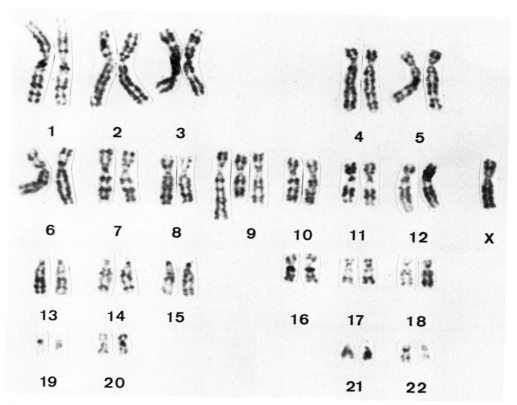

Fig. 3. Karyotype of the proposita [46,X,-X,+der(9),t(X;9)(q11;q32)mat]. Note the presence of 2 normal chromosomes 9 and one X chromosome, in addition to the translocation chromosome (ASG-Giemsa).

I — Cri-Du-Chat and Trisomy 13 Syndromes in an Infant with an Unbalanced Chromosomal Translocation

Jaakko Leisti, M.D., Michael M. Kaback, M.D. and David L. Rimoin, M.D., Ph.D.

G.T. (HH 613318) was hospitalized at HGH because of multiple anomalies at the age of 2 days and died at the hospital at the age of 2 months.

The patient was the product of a 39-week pregnancy to a 38-year-old mother (gravida 9, para 4, ab 5) and a 40-year-old father. Birthweight was 2040 gm, length 44 cm. The family history was negative as to congenital anomalies, and the mother's 5 abortions had all occurred during the first trimester. There were no complications during labor or delivery, and the child did well during the first days of life. Her cry, however, was peculiar with a high-pitched quality resembling a cat's meowing. Gradually signs of cardiac insufficiency developed which required digitalization. Later apneic spells appeared and the patient died in apnea at the age of 2 months.

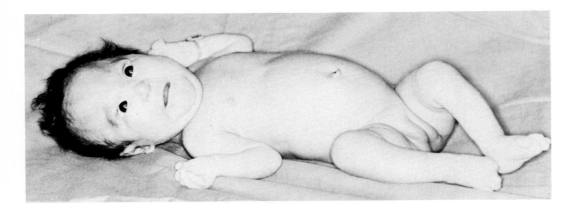

Fig. 1. The patient at the age of one month. Note the round face with widely spaced eyes, slightly protuberant nasal bridge, the small nose, the abnormal positioning of the fingers and remnants of the supernumerary digits after ligation.

Physical examination revealed a markedly abnormal child with multiple anomalies and muscular hypertonia (Fig. 1). The head appeared microcephalic with a circumference of 30 cm and had widely open anterior and posterior fontanels. The forehead was sloping and had a wide hemangioma. The face had a round appearance; the eyes were wide-set and the nasal bridge was slightly protuberant. There were bilateral epicanthic folds. The nose was small and stubby; the chin was small and retracted and the palate was highly arched (Fig. 2). The ears appeared small, dysmorphic and low-set. The neck was short with abundant loose skin posteriorly but the posterior hairline appeared normal. Chest and abdomen were normal to inspection and palpation; a grade 3/6 systolic murmur was audible. The genitalia were normal female. The skin presented with marked cutis marmorata discoloration.

Postaxial polydactyly was present in all 4 limbs. Bilateral simian creases were present on both palms and the fingers showed abnormal positioning with overriding.

The autopsy revealed a patent ductus arteriosus, bicornuate uterus and slightly diffusely dilated cerebral ventricles.

Chromosome analyses of peripheral lymphocytes showed that the mother was a carrier of a balanced reciprocal translocation between chromosome 5 and 13 (as verified by G-banding techniques), with practically all of the long arm of chromosome 5 being translocated to the short arm of chromosome 13 (Fig. 3). Her karyotype was interpreted as probably being 46,XX,t(5;13)(?q11;p11). The patient's karyotype was unbalanced with only one normal chromosome 5, 2 normal chromosomes 13, and the long translocation chromosome (der 13) (Fig. 4). Thus she had an additional long arm of chromosome 13 and deficient short arm of chromosome 5. She thus represented a duplication-deficiency syndrome with the clinical signs of both the cri-du-chat and trisomy 13 syndromes.

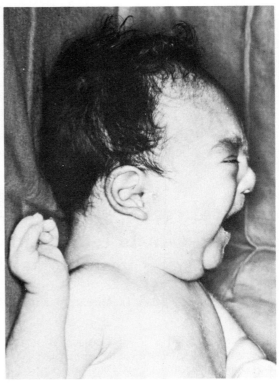

Fig. 2. The forehead is sloping; the ears are low-set, small and dysmorphic. The chin is small.

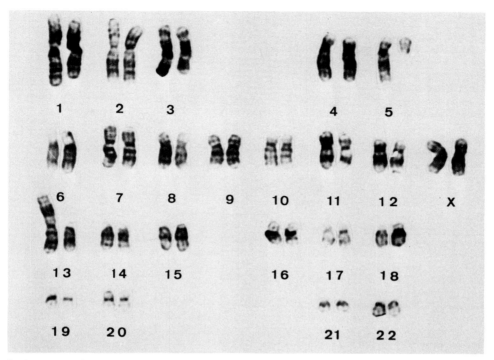

Fig. 3. Karyotype of the mother shows a reciprocal translocation between a chromosome 5 and a chromosome 13 (Trypsin-Giemsa).

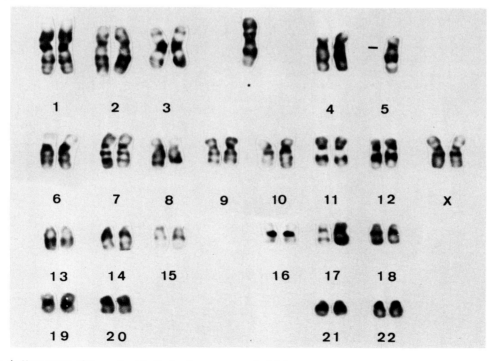

Fig. 4. Karyotype of the patient indicates the presence of additional long arm of chromosome 13 translocated to chromosome 5, which has lost its short arm (Trypsin-Giemsa).

Selected Abstracts

Selected Abstracts

WILMS TUMOR: A BIRTH DEFECT? *S. E. Allerton, J. W. Beierle* and *D. R. Powars*, Dept. of Biochemistry, Microbiology, School of Dentistry and Dept. of Pediatrics, School of Medicine, University of Southern California, Los Angeles, CA.

Wilms tumor (nephroblastoma) is a leading form of cancer in infants and young children. This tumor is believed to originate during embryonic or fetal development and is only rarely found in adults. In some cases the tumor is associated with aniridia, GU defects, hemihypertrophy or the numerous abnormalities characteristic of Beckwith-Wiedemann syndrome. Also, the tumor has been reported to occur in twins, sibs and 2-3 successive generations of families. These considerations suggest that Wilms tumor may be a birth defect arising from some oncogenic/teratogenic agent in prenatal development or via genetic penetrance in some families. We have been developing a combined biochemical/immunologic approach aimed at early diagnosis and follow-up monitoring of Wilms patients. We find that large amounts of a proteoglycan (3-5S) can be extracted from the tumor with isotonic EDTA and other chelating agents. A related hyaluronic acid-like mucopolysaccharide can often be detected in the serum and ultrafiltered urine concentrate. The tumor mucin precipitates from solution at pH 4 and gives a single precipitin line vs rabbit antibody in the double immunodiffusion technique. Another antigen (fetuin-like) is also present in the tumor extract. These findings provide a basis for developing more sensitive assays for detecting the antigens and mucopolysaccharide in sera from Wilms patients, their sibs and their parents. The results, combined with information on prenatal care and family medical histories, could provide new insights concerning factors associated with the development of this tumor.

ABSENCE OF PECTORALIS MAJOR MUSCLE IN 2 SISTERS ASSOCIATED WITH LEUKEMIA IN ONE OF THEM. *S. Armendares* and *I. Rostenberg*, Sección de Genética, Departamento de Investigación Científica, I.M.S.S., México, D.F., México

We have observed a family with 2 female sibs affected with absence of pectoralis major muscle without ipsilateral upper limb defects, in which the older sib (*Patient 1*) developed acute lymphocytic leukemia at 4 years of age. On physical examination, *Patient 2* (the younger sister of *Patient 1*) revealed, in addition to absence of the left pectoralis major muscle, an angioma on the right side of the neck. At 9 months of age she developed a right hemiparesis. Cerebral angiography disclosed the presence of abnormal vessels in the parietal operculum in the capillary phase compatible with capillary angioma or telangiectasia. A niece of the father of the propositi died at 3 years of age of acute leukemia. The peculiarities of the cases reported here are discussed with reference to the possible association between muscle anomalies and acute leukemia, as suggested by the fact that at least 3 cases have been described as having both Poland anomaly and acute leukemia. The abnormal vessels observed in the parietal operculum of *Patient 2* and their relationship to absence of pectoralis major muscle and to acute leukemia in her sib and first cousin is discussed, since in another angiomatous syndrome, ataxia-telangiectasia, the association with acute lymphocytic leukemia is well-established. In our cases ataxia-telangiectasia was ruled out on clinical grounds, as well as the normal serum levels of immunoglobulins, adequate responsiveness of lymphocytes to phytohemagglutinin stimulation and normal chromosomal studies in *Patient 2*.

TOWARD A PHYSICAL COMPOSITE OF XYY MAN. *F. A. Baughman, Jr., J. V. Higgins* and *J. D. Pool*, Blodgett Memorial Hospital, Grand Rapids and Michigan State University, East Lansing, MI.

In 1972, Baughman and Mann reported the ascertainment of 6 XYY males in a neurologic practice. To date we have ascertained 9 such patients. This report deals with the frequency of certain of their physical abnormalities. The endocrine and behavioral aspects will be the subjects of separate reports.

Cowling et al (1969) described a 20-year-old XYY male with varicose veins, deep-vein thrombosis and pulmonary emboli. Rohde (1963) and Borgaonkar et al (1970) have indicated an increased frequency of varicose veins in Klinefelter syndrome and in the XXYY syndrome, respectively. Four out of 5 patients examined for varicose veins were affected. Two have had recurrent thrombophlebitis and pulmonary emboli.

Baughman et al (in press) determined that a spectrum of elbow abnormalities exists in sex chromosome aneuploidy; maximal cubitus valgus is seen in XO, decreasing degrees of valgus in XX and XY, respectively, approaching cubitus rectus in cases with one supernumerary X or Y, with cubitus varus and radioulnar synostosis and radial head dislocation where there are multiple supernumerary sex chromosomes. Frank cubitus rectus and cubitus varus — obvious deviations from the normal range (XY:2-24° valgus) — were found in 7 of 10 elbows of 5 XYY males.

Daly (1969) reported essential tremor in 10 of 12 institutionalized XYY males while Baughman et al (1973) reported essential tremor as a frequent component of the male supernumerary X chromosome syndromes. Essential tremor was present in 2 of the 9 XYY patients presently reported.

Nodulocystic acne (held by Voorhees (1970) to be a feature of the XYY phenotype) was encountered in 5 of our 9 patients.

Four of our 5 XYY patients are disproportionally taller than their parents and sibs. By comparison, tall XYY suspects whose chromosomes proved to be normal usually had parents of comparable tallness.

There have been numerous reports of epilepsy and abnormal EEGs. Two of our patients had convulsions in infancy. A third had petit mal at 7 years of age and now, at 33 years of age, has had 2 idiopathic generalized seizures. In a fourth patient the diagnosis of psychomotor epilepsy remains questionable. These 4, ranging in age from 15-33 years, all have moderate-to-marked diffuse EEG abnormality. In 4 of the remaining 5 patients, the EEG was normal or just mildly abnormal.

MANDIBULOFACIAL DYSOSTOSIS (TREACHER COLLINS SYNDROME): CORRELATION OF SOFT TISSUE AND SKELETAL ABNORMALITIES. *S. M. Blain, R. E. Stewart, J. F. Mulick* and *J. Snyder*, UCLA Center for Craniofacial Anomalies, Harbor General Hospital, Division of Medical Genetics, Kaiser Permanent Cleft Palate Team in Los Angeles, CA.

Since the original reports by G. A. Berry and E. Treacher Collins, there have been more than 250 similar cases of the Treacher Collins syndrome reported in the world's medical and dental literature. Franceschetti, Zwahlen and Klein made extensive reports on this condition and called it mandibulofacial dysostosis.

The clinical findings as originally described by Franceschetti and Klein consisted of essentially antimongoloid palpebral fissures, lower eyelid colobomas, hypoplasia of the facial bones, malformation of the external and perhaps middle ear, macrostomia, blind fistulas between the angle of the ear and the mouth, atypical hair growth extending towards the cheeks and occasionally additional anomalies, ie facial clefts and skeletal deformities.

To date, reports concerning the radiographic and cephalometric findings in mandibulofacial dysostosis have lacked a detailed description of the dysmorphic changes in the craniofacial complex.

Eleven previously unreported cases of Treacher Collins syndrome demonstrate the variability which exists within this syndrome and indicate that such clinical variability is determined by underlying bony abnormalities of the facial skeleton.

The relationships of the various segments of the facial skeleton and the cranial base, as determined by cephalometric radiographs, deviate significantly from normal and account for the soft tissue malformations giving rise to the typical facies of this syndrome. The occurrence and severity of lower lid colobomas are related to discrepancies in the infraorbital margin. These discrepancies range from minor notching to frank clefts and agenesis of the infraorbital rim.

In addition, the severity of malar hypoplasia is directly related to the extent of zygomatic arch dysgenesis ranging from hypoplasia to complete aplasia of the maxillary, frontal, temporal and malar bones which constitute the zygomatic arch complex.

Our data substantiate the wide variability reported in the dysmorphic changes of the mandible. These consist of antigonial notching and hypoplastic changes of the ascending portion of the mandible ranging from minor hypoplastic changes of the condyles and coronoid processes to complete absence of these structures.

Our findings support Pruzansky's observation that dysmorphic changes in the mandible can be correlated with the overall severity of facial abnormalities. We have shown that this reasoning is applicable to other skeletal features of the Treacher Collins syndrome as well.

A DISTINCT AND UNUSUAL SYNDROME WITH CHARACTERISTIC FACIES, SHORT STATURE, BONY DEFECTS, AORTIC CALCIFICATION WITH AORTIC VALVULAR STENOSIS, ABNORMAL DENTITION, HYPOTONIA, LENTIGINOSIS AND PSORIASIS. *A. C. Brown, W. H. Plauth, B. B. Gay, Jr., D. R. Blackston, J. S. Giansanti and P. J. Mattina, Jr.,* Division of Dermatology, Dept. of Medicine, Dept. of Pediatrics, Henrietta Egleston Hospital for Children, School of Dentistry, Emory University School of Medicine, Atlanta, GA.

Singleton and Merten recently reported an unusual syndrome in 2 children with widened medullary cavities of the metacarpals and phalanges, aortic calcification and abnormal dentition (*Pediatrics Radiology 1*:2, 1973). In 1972, Polani and Moynahan (*Q. L. Med. XLI*: 205-225, 1972) reported a new syndrome of progressive cardiomyopathic lentiginosis in 8 patients, consisting of multiple symmetric lentigines, left-sided obstructive cardiomyopathy, associated growth retardation and, at times, slight intellectual impairment. Our case adds characteristic facies, normal intelligence, short stature, hypotonia, psoriasis and includes the previously described unusual calcification of the ascending aorta. This 14-year-old white male patient, therefore, has features of both

syndromes; however, echocardiogram did not show asymmetric hypertrophy of the ventricular septum or abnormal anterior movement of the anterior mitral valve leaflet. Cardiac catheterization revealed the presence of critical valvular aortic stenosis. The patient is currently asymptomatic with some exercise restriction and aortic valve surgery may be required in the future. The authors present a further case of widened medullary cavities of the metacarpals and phalanges, aortic calcification, abnormal dentition and stress the previously undescribed psoriasis, characteristic facies, hypotonia, short stature and normal intelligence of this unusual syndrome.

STRUCTURAL X ABNORMALITIES IN TURNER SYNDROME. *M. Buyse, J. W. Towner and M. G. Wilson,* Dept. of Pediatrics, Los Angeles County-University of Southern California Medical Center and University of Southern California School of Medicine.

Monosomy of the X chromosome was the original karyotype identified in patients with Turner syndrome. Subsequently, a variety of types of X chromosome mosaicism and structural X abnormalities were described in patients with Turner syndrome. Approximately 50% of patients with Turner syndrome are reported to have monosomy of the X chromosome. The most frequently found mosaic karyotype has been reported to be 45,X/46,XX. The remainder of reported karyotypes usually have a structural abnormality of one X chromosome such as a simple deletion, a ring or an isochromosome, and are often accompanied by a 45,X line.

We reviewed the karyotypes of 27 patients with Turner syndrome and an X-chromosome abnormality referred to our medical center from 1966 to the present. One half (14) were 45,X, as expected; one was 45,X/47,XXX mosaic and the remaining patients had a structural X abnormality. An isochromosome for the long arm of X was the most frequent structural aberration and was present in 8 patients, 5 of whom had an additional 45,X cell line. The remaining patients had a variety of structural abnormalities: a deletion of the short arm of X, a ring X chromosome mosaic with 45,X and an isochromosome of the short arm of X mosaic with 45,X. Notable is the absence of 45,X/46,XX mosaicism. We suggest that the karyotypes of patients with 45,X/46,XX be reexamined with the newer staining techniques to determine whether some of these represent an undetected structural X abnormality.

THE RUSSELL-SILVER SYNDROME IN DISCORDANT MONOZYGOTIC TWINS. *J. A. Campbell, E. H. Harley* and *W. K. McCord*, Dept. of Pediatrics, Naval Regional Medical Center, San Diego, CA.

The clinical findings of short stature, asymmetry, craniofacial dysostosis and hypergonadotropism have been described and reported by different authors as a single clinical entity under the name of Russell-Silver syndrome. Although most reported cases have been sporadic, it has been postulated that there is a genetic etiology, since it is concordant in monozygotic twins, nonconcordant in fraternal twins and occurs in sibs from parents with a common ancestor. Its sporadic occurrence when there is no history of consanguinity has been attributed to probable fresh dominant mutations.

We present a case of the Russell-Silver syndrome which occurred discordantly in apparently monozygotic twin sisters. Characteristic findings in the affected twin included low birthweight, short stature, craniofacial dysostosis with triangular facies, broad forehead, downturned corners of the mouth, mild asymmetry, clinodactyly of the 5th fingers, partial syndactyly of the 2nd and 3rd toes, hyperextensible joints, excessive sweating and retarded bone age. Both twins had normal female karyotypes. Supporting evidence of monozygosity included HL-A typing and blood group antigens for 22 systems being identical in the twins, yet inconsistent when such typing was compared to that of the parents.

MENTAL RETARDATION, PECULIAR FACIES AND DOLICHOMORPHISM IN 2 FEMALE COUSINS. *J. Cantú, A. Hernández* and *C. Pacheco*, Departamento de Investigación Científica, I.M.S.S. and Hospital Psiquiátrico Infantil "Dr. Juan N. Navarro," S.S.A., México, D.F., México.

Two female first cousins were found to be concordant for the following abnormal features: mental retardation, peculiar flat facies with low nasal bridge, wide nose, ocular hypertelorism, epicanthal folds, dental abnormalities

and a generalized dolichomorphism. Their 2 fathers were brothers, but their mothers were not related, either to each other or to their husbands; however, all 4 of them came from an isolated village in Michoacan, Mexico, where inbreeding is common. Extensive bibliographic inquiry leads to the belief that this is a new syndrome with a probable autosomal recessive inheritance.

CONGENITAL ABSENCE OF GLUTEAL MUSCLES: REPORT OF 2 SIBS. *A. Carnevale* and *V. del Castillo*, Dept. of Genetics, Hospital del Nino IMAN, Mexico City.

Congenital absence of hypoplasia of muscles has been estimated to occur with a variable frequency between 1 in 4000 and 1 in 10,000. Among individual muscle aplasias, that of the pectoralis has been observed most frequently. Congenital absence of abdominal muscles, palmaris longus and peroneus tertius have also been reported.

The purpose of this presentation is to describe a family in which 2 sibs, a male and a female, have bilateral aplasia of gluteal muscles that has not yet been reported. No other malformations were present except for a spina bifida at the sacral level.

There was inability for flexion of the hip but abduction was complete; walking with outward rotation and abduction deformation of the hip was possible between 3 and 4 years of age.

X-ray studies failed to show any skeletal abnormality. Electromyography and biopsy of the gluteal region confirmed the aplasia of gluteus maximus and probably of gluteus medius.

Mild mental retardation occurred in both children. Whether this finding is part of the syndrome or an independent alteration is discussed.

The presence of 2 sibs with the same congenital malformation, with normal parents, is suggestive of an autosomal recessive mode of inheritance.

RETHORE SYNDROME: TRISOMY OF THE SHORT ARM OF CHROMOSOME 9. *W. R. Centerwall* and *J. F. Wyatt*, Dept. of Pediatrics, Loma Linda University Medical Center, Loma Linda, CA and *J. W. Beatty-DeSana* and *M. J.*

Hoggard, Georgia Retardation Center, Georgia Department of Human Resources, Atlanta, GA.

Rethore and her collaborators in 1970 reported on 5 children with a newly recognized chromosomal-clinical syndrome. As of 1973, the list had increased to 13; and we are now presenting the 14th case, making in all, 7 boys and 7 girls. All these children have extra chromosome material identified as the short arm of a No. 9 chromosome. This tripling of the usual diploid dose is called trisomy 9p. Eleven of the 14 cases, including ours, have been translocations; but this is the first which is known to have involved chromosome D14. Our 3-year-old boy represents a spontaneous isolated chromosome translocation whereby the extra short arm of a No. 9 chromosome has replaced the short arm of a No. 14 chromosome, ie 46,XY,-14,+t(9p14q). It is probably no coincidence that these same 2 chromosomes are among those most frequently involved in various types of aberrations in humans. We believe that the translocation mutation in this case occurred during meiosis in the process of gamete formation.

Clinical features which the majority of cases show in common, and which combined together are sufficient to suggest the diagnosis, include an unusual facies with an antimongoloid slant to mildly wide-set and deep-set eyes; a downturning of the corners of the mouth; a mildly globulous nose; and protruding, slightly atypical ears. The hands show abnormalities in dermatoglyphics and finger creases and there is a single transverse palmar line. All are mentally retarded. With increased awareness of trisomy 9p as a clinical entity and wider application of the newer banding techniques for specific chromosome identification, more cases will be discovered and reported, and the nature and basis of these disorders will become better understood.

BALANCED AUTOSOMAL TRANSLOCATION t(2p-;Dq+) IN A FAMILY. *C. Clark*, Alfred I. duPont Institute, Wilmington, DE.

Chromosome No. 2 is frequently involved in chromosomal rearrangements. There are several reports involving translocations of the long arms of a No. 2 chromosome and the long arms of a D-group chromosome. These are unbalanced translocations which cause serious abnormalities and mental retardation.

I am reporting a balanced translocation in 3 members of a family involving a partial deletion of the short arms of a No. 2 chromosome translocated to the long arms of a D-group chromosome t(2p-;Dq+).

The father and a sister, who are in good health and who have no apparent clinical problems, demonstrated karyotypes 46,XY,t(2p-Dq+) and 46,XX,t(2p-;Dq+), respectively. Our patient at birth had a cleft palate, vertical talus and spine anomalies resulting in scoliosis. Chromosome analysis reveals a 46,XX,t(2p-;Dq+) karyotype. Her mother and other sib, also female, have normal female 46,XX karyotype. The mother had 3 previous pregnancies which resulted in abnormal fetuses with anencephaly, spina bifida and hydrocephalus.

LONG-TERM SURVIVAL IN TRISOMY 18. *A. P. Eaton, S. B. Kontras, A. Sommer* and *R. A. Wehe*, Birth Defects & Genetics Section, Dept. of Pediatrics, The Ohio State University and Children's Hospital, Columbus, OH.

The occurrence of trisomy 18 results in a high mortality in early infancy with only 1-2% surviving from birth to 10 years of age. Few cases are reported with long-term survival and these have shown severe physical and mental retardation. A 4 1/12-year-old who demonstrates a more favorable clinical picture is reported. *P.H.* is a white female born to a gravida 1, para 1, 19-year-old mother at 36 weeks' gestation after an uncomplicated pregnancy. Although no fetal distress was noted, the amniotic fluid was meconium-stained. Birthweight was 2.2 kg and length 46 cm. Apgar scores were recorded as 6 at 1 minute and 9 at 5 minutes. Generalized cyanosis and feeding difficulties prompted transfer to Children's Hospital at 5 days of age. Pertinent physical findings on admission included generalized cyanosis, hypotonia, prominent occiput, micrognathia, small palpebral fissures, microcorneas with the left globe appearing smaller than the right, high-arched palate, malformed and low-set ears, supernumerary left thumb, limited abduction of the hips, overlapping toes as well as a poor Moro reflex, suck and cry. Clinical impression was possibly trisomy 18. (Giemsa banding studies are in progress.) Cytogenetic studies of peripheral blood leukocytes of both parents were normal. An IVP and cardiac series were normal. Shortly after admission her condition stabilized and discharge was accomplished at 2 weeks of age. She has continued to be followed at regular intervals. Her weight has consistently followed the 3rd to 10th percentile and her height slightly below the 3rd percentile. At 47 months of age on The Gesell Developmental Evaluation, her observed behavior was approximately 45% of normal. Other pertinent physical findings, not previously described, included diastasis recti and colobomata of the iris and retina. She has had very few medical problems and is enrolled in a school for the trainable mentally retarded.

The trisomy 18 syndrome was first described in 1960 by Edwards, Smith and Patau. It has a reported frequency of 1/4500 births with a female sex preponderance. The clinical findings are widely variable, with Smith reporting at least 130 different abnormalities. This condition is highly lethal during the first year of life, with death occurring in the majority of cases by 6 months. Very few cases of trisomy 18 are reported who were still alive after 4 years of age. Those patients reported with long-term survival have demonstrated little progress in growth and development which is somewhat in contrast to the present case.

MOYA-MOYA DISEASE IN A CHILD WITH PYRUVATE KINASE DEFICIENT ERYTHROCYTES. *N. Gadoth* and *V. A. McKusick*, Dept. of Neurology and Dept. of Medicine, The Johns Hopkins Hospital, Baltimore, MD.

A 6-year-old boy with pyruvate kinase (PK) deficient hemolytic anemia developed acute left hemiplegia at 2 years of age. Two months later he became suddenly aphasic and showed signs of pseudobulbar palsy, indicating bilateral cerebral damage. Selective aortic arch, carotid and vertebral angiography demonstrated bilateral intracranial carotid occlusion, dural cortical arterial anastomosis and abnormal vascular network at the base of the brain. This clinical and radiographic picture is known as Moya-Moya disease.

The boy's family belongs to an Old Order Amish isolate from the Mifflin County, in which a severe form of PK deficient hemolytic anemia is present. No other cases of childhood cerebrovascular disease are known among the 12 sibships in this pedigree.

ALCAPTONURIA AND SUCRASE-ISOMALTASE DEFICIENCY IN 3 SIBS. *A. D. Garnica, J. L. Frias, O. M. Rennert* and *J. J. Cerda,* Depts. of Pediatrics and Medicine, University of Florida College of Medicine, Gainesville, FL.

Three sibs with proved alcaptonuria presented also with a lifelong history of watery diarrhea. This was relieved symptomatically by restriction of a dietary sucrose. Further studies, including peroral jejunal biopsy, demonstrated a deficiency of intestinal sucrase-isomaltase. Both parents and 2 other sibs exhibit no stigmata of either disorder. To our knowledge, this association has not been previously reported.

SYNDROME OF INTRAHEPATIC BILIARY DYSGENESIS (IHBD) AND CARDIOVASCULAR MALFORMATIONS (CVM). *R. D. Greenwood, K. Dooley, A. Rosenthal, A. C. Crocker* and *A. S. Nadas,* Dept. of Pediatrics, Harvard Medical School and The Children's Hospital Medical Center, Boston, MA.

The presence of peripheral pulmonic stenosis (PPS) in a number of our patients with IHBD prompted us to examine the relationship between IHBD and CVM.

Review of autopsy material between 1923 and 1973 revealed 4 patients with IHBD and CVM. PPS and patent ductus arteriosus (PDA) were present in 2, PDA in one and PPS, PDA, pulmonary atresia and ventricular septal defect (VSD) in one. Age at death was 5 weeks to 4 10/12 years. None of the necropsied patients with extrahepatic biliary dysgenesis had CVM. Cardiac disease was diagnosed in 8 additional living patients with IHBD, aged 1½-17 years. Six exhibited clinical and laboratory findings of PPS (one documented at cardiac catheterization and subsequently operated upon for associated VSD and atrial septal defect) and in 2 the auscultatory findings were compatible with the diagnosis of PPS but could not be verified.

The presence of CVM was established by autopsy, cardiac catheterization or clinical examination by a pediatric cardiologist in 10 of 12 patients with IHBD and heart disease. PPS with or without other lesions was present in 9 patients and isolated PDA in 1. Two of the patients were sibs, one of whom died and also had cystic disease of the kidneys and hemivertebras. The CVM were hemodynamically insignificant in all but 2 patients and the IHBD was of a relatively mild variety in 3 of the 12 patients. It is of interest that vascular (pulmonary arteries, ductus arteriosus) and not intracardiac structures were predominately involved.

The association of IHBD with PPS and PDA strongly suggests a common etiology for the biliary and vascular disease. Because of the uncertainty regarding the usual mechanism of the hepatic abnormalities in IHBD, its presence simultaneously with CVM is of particular interest. The possible role of intrauterine infection or neonatal hepatitis should be considered. The CVM observed resemble those of congenital rubella (CR); none of our patients, however, have other stigmata of CR. The presence of this syndrome in sibs, on the other hand, suggests possible genetic factors.

We conclude that IHBD, PPS and/or PDA constitutes a distinctive recognizable syndrome. Increased awareness by clinicians of this syndrome and further clinical, pathologic, chromosomal and viral studies will be necessary before its etiology and prognosis can be determined.

FAMILIAL ASYMMETRIC CRYING FACIES SECONDARY TO HYPOPLASIA OF ANGULI ORIS MUSCLE. *J. G. Hall* and *J. Miser*, University of Washington and Children's Orthopedic Hospital, Seattle, WA.

A mother and 2 sons by different fathers are described with asymmetric movements of the lower face. Nerve conduction and EMG studies suggest congenital hypoplasia of the depressor angularis oris. One of the boys had congenital stridor and hoarse cry but no other abnormalities were found. The family is discussed and compared with the asymmetric crying facies which has been reported to be associated with multiple congenital anomalies.

ABERRANT TISSUE BANDS AND MULTIPLE CONGENITAL DEFECTS: AN EPIDEMIOLOGIC ASSESSMENT. *J. W. Hanson* and *M. G. Freeman*, Birth Defects Section, Bureau of Epidemiology, Center for Disease Control and Dept. of Gynecology and Obstetrics, Emory University School of Medicine, Atlanta, GA.

Recent case reports of infants with multiple craniofacial and limb defects associated with aberrant intrauterine tissue bands have come from several centers. Concern expressed over a possible increased incidence of such deformities

prompted us to review cases found in the metropolitan Atlanta area.

Two sources of data were used. A review of such cases reported to the Metropolitan Atlanta Birth Defects Program since its inception in 1967 revealed 7 definite cases and 1 probable case. Review of records from the perinatal pathology unit of one large Atlanta hospital showed 8 definite cases and 2 probable cases over an 11-year period. Two other possible cases were excluded from the study because of insufficient data.

Chromosome studies done on 4 of the infants were normal. Personal interviews with 4 families of infants born since 1970 identified no common features to suggest an etiologic association. Maternal age distribution was unremarkable.

Analysis of the distribution of cases over time suggests that 1-3 such cases occur yearly in metropolitan Atlanta, an area with approximately 28,000 annual births. Our data do not support the hypothesis of a significant increase in the incidence of such defects in recent years.

Recognition and referral of such cases is probably better at large medical centers with specialized facilities, and reporting is likely improved where cases are sought actively. The significance of anatomic differences between these and other sorts of malformations in newborns may often be overlooked. A precise description of defects is invaluable in epidemiologic studies of congenital malformations and should be an essential part of the medical record of each newborn.

NAIL HYPOPLASIA WITH PSYCHOMOTOR AND GROWTH RETARDATION: A POSSIBLE CASE OF COFFIN-SIRIS SYNDROME. *J. W. Hanson*, Birth Defects Section, Bureau of Epidemiology, Center for Disease Control, Atlanta, GA.

The association of hypoplastic nails with mental retardation, poor growth, hypotonia and coarse facial features without chromosomal or specific endocrine abnormalities was first described by Coffin and Siris in 1970. Since their initial report, 3 other cases have been added to the literature under the term Coffin-Siris syndrome, which suggest that not all the features initially described are invariable parts of the syndrome. Furthermore, at least one of these patients may represent the dysmorphogenetic syndrome recently associated with maternal use of diphenylhydantoin.

A patient is discussed who has many similarities to the patients of Coffin and Siris, including poor growth, moderately severe psychomotor retardation, hypoplastic nails on 5 digits, severe hypotonia and roentgenologic abnormalities. No specific endocrinologic or chromosomal abnormality was identified. The facial features in this patient were less coarse than described in other cases. No history of maternal exposure to possible teratogens was found. No similar cases were identified in this family.

The differential diagnosis between children with this pattern of malformations and the diphenylhydantoin syndrome, nail-patella syndrome and other syndromes with nail hypoplasia or dysplasia is discussed.

SHORT-ARM DELETION OF B4 CHROMOSOME (4p-SYNDROME) WITH HYPOMAGNESEMIA. *N. Hague, V. Kantipong* and *K. Thomas*, Dept. of Metabolism, Division of Pediatrics, Oakland Medical Center & St. Joseph Mercy Hospital, Pontiac, MI.

Short-arm deletion of B4 (4p-syndrome) is an aberration with only a handful of cases reported. A review of the literature showed that life expectancy is short; only 2 cases reported beyond the age of 6½ years. Seizure disorder is a feature in a majority of these cases. The present case report appears unusual in 2 ways; 1) longer life (alive at 9 years of age) and 2) magnesium deficiency linked to seizure disorder which may either be associated with other anomalies or a concomitant secondary feature.

The present case is that of a 9-year-old female, full-term gestation of uncomplicated pregnancy and normal delivery, who was noted to have multiple congenital abnormalities at birth, and is institutionalized due to severe mental retardation. Preliminary studies at birth failed to reveal any specific cause of these multiple anomalies. Family history is noncontributory. The mother is 27 years old and healthy, and chromosomal studies on the mother and maternal grandparents are normal.

Significant history includes a small baby at birth, who presented as a failure to thrive in early infancy, developed convulsion during the first year of life and had 2 intractable seizures at 18 months and 5 years of age, which required general anesthesia for control of status epilepticus. She was on anticonvulsant agents and seizures were not well-controlled. She was evaluated once again following a third episode of status epilepticus since she was not responding to conventional seizure therapy including IV Valium. She responded immediately, however, to IV administration of magnesium sulfate within minutes. Blood magnesium level prior to magnesium sulfate injection was reported as low as 0.6 mg%. Subsequent studies confirmed evidence of hypomagnesemia and seizures remained controlled with magnesium sulfate therapy.

The birth defect consists of "small for date" baby (birthweight 100 gm with full-term gestation); microencephaly; prominent glabella; hypertelorism; low-set ears; preauricular dimple; strabismus; iris deformity; prominent appearance of pseudofacial palsy; cleft palate; minor nose deformity; hypoplastic nipples, with short manubrium sternum; congenital heart defect; hypoplastic dermal ridges; simian crease; long fingers, with biconvex nails which were long; fine texture of the skin; deformed thumb on the right with accessory digit; abnormal 2nd toe on the left; diastasis recti; and seizure disorder presently under control with magnesium (oral therapy) and a small dose of Dilantin. Chromosomal studies reveal short-arm deletion of B4 (4p-syndrome).

TOTAL LIPODYSTROPHY, TYPE 11-A HYPERLIPIDEMIA, SPONTANEOUS REGRESSION OF DIABETES MELLITUS, MULTIPLE BONY EXOSTOSIS, MENTAL RETARDATION AND IMMUNE DEFICIENCY — A POSSIBLE NEW SYNDROME. *N. Hague, V. Kantipong, K. Sorajja* and *K. Thomas*, Dept. of Metabolism, Division of Pediatrics, Oakland Medical Center and St. Joseph Mercy Hospital, Pontiac, MI.

Total lipodystrophy, as first described by Lawrence in 1946 and followed by others, is a rare clinical condition and the precise mechanism of all its clinical features remains unknown. The classic features consist of generalized absence of subcutaneous fat, insulin-resistant diabetes mellitus, hyperlipidemia, hepatic dysfunction, accelerated bone age with no pituitary abnormality, acanthosis nigricans, generalized hirsutism, bilateral nonspecific enlarged kidneys, often associated with varying grades of mental retardation. In some reported cases, an abnormal protein was isolated in the urine.

The present case is that of a 16-year-old white female, who appears to be a variant of the above syndrome, with common features such as total lipodystrophy, (generalized) hyperlipidemia, insulin-resistant diabetes in infancy (now in complete remission), mental retardation and no pituitary dysfunction (HGH). There are certain exceptions such as spontaneous regression of diabetes mellitus, no hepatic dysfunction, no hirsutism, no acanthosis nigricans, no kidney change and no accelerated bone age; and certain added features such as multiple bony exostosis, immune deficiency associated with bilateral bronchiectasis, with clubbing of fingers and toes, and cardiomegaly.

Laboratory investigation revealed, at present, a normal glucose tolerance test with normal insulin response which was grossly abnormal during early infancy; normal response of (HGH) propanalol-glucagon stimulation test; hyperlipidemia type 11-A; IgA 0 mg%, IgM 15 mg%, IgG 6 mg%; lymphocyte count in peripheral blood 1254/cm with no apparent abnormal morphology of lymphocytes, inadequate response to skin testing with SK-SD, mumps, *Trichophyton*, D-T and dermatophyton; negative Schick and tuberculin tests; and normal liver function tests (SGOT, SGPT, BSP, etc). X-ray films showed multiple bony exostosis, bilateral cylindric bronchiectasis and normal bone age. Further studies on fibroblast culture and electron microscopy on lymph glands and skin are in progress.

It appears that the combination of clinical features such as total lipodystrophy with spontaneous regression of diabetes mellitus, hyperlipidemia, multiple bony exostosis and immune deficiency with mental retardation could possibly be either a variant of what was first described by Lawrence in 1946 or a possible new syndrome complex.

A LETHAL SYNDROME IN THE NEWBORN: NATAL TEETH, PATENT DUCTUS ARTERIOSUS AND INTESTINAL PSEUDOOBSTRUCTION. *D. J. Harris, K. W. Ashcraft, E. C. Beatty, Jr., T. M. Holder* and *J. C. Leonidas*, Depts. of Pediatrics, Surgery, Pathology and Radiology, The Children's Mercy Hospital, Kansas City, MO.

We are presenting 2 male sibs with similar clinical characteristics who may exemplify an X-linked lethal syndrome. The 2 infants were born 14 months apart. The gestational ages were close to term with birthweights of 3.1 and 2.8 kg, respectively. Both infants had mandibular incisors, murmur consistent with patent ductus arteriosus and a clinical syndrome of intestinal obstruction.

The first infant was found to have midgut malrotation and a left diaphragmatic eventration, repaired on the first day. Functional intestinal obstruction related to poor GI motility persisted to his death at the age of 5 months despite several surgical procedures and total parenteral alimentation. He also had persistent heart failure which improved following ligation of the ductus.

The second infant had clinical and radiographic signs of intestinal obstruction since birth. It was decided that he should not be maintained on parenteral alimentation and he died at the age of 6 weeks.

Both infants had complete postmortem examinations. Ganglion cells were present throughout the GI tract. The small bowel was dilated, but there was no anatomic obstruction or histologic abnormality of the intestinal wall. It measured 60 cm in the second infant and responded only to large concentrations of acetylocoline (0.02 mg/ml) postmortem. Patent ductus was verified at autopsy in the second infant.

The parents are not consanguineous and come from large families. The father was age 22 at the time the first child was born and has been in good health. The mother was age 21 and when the first child was born, developed cholecystitis several weeks after the delivery. She developed intestinal obstruction after the death of the second infant and was found to have adhesions, which were lysed, but there was nothing to suggest a disorder similar to that of the 2 infants. They have one healthy girl, age 3. The most striking finding in the pedigree is the lack of males who survived infancy in the mother's and her mother's sibships (0 of 5 and 1 of 7, respectively).

Intestinal pseudoobstruction has been observed in older children and adults but not in infants either as an isolated finding or combined with other defects. It may be due to receptor unresponsiveness. The hypothesis of an X-linked lethal gene governing the syndrome of natal teeth, patent ductus arteriosus and intestinal pseudoobstruction is attractive because both infants were males and because of lack of males in the maternal ascendants.

CONGENITAL CATARACT AND SPINOCEREBELLAR ATAXIA IN FATHER AND SON. *I. Hussels-Maumenee* and *E. Maumenee*, Dept. of Medicine and Ophthalmology, The

Johns Hopkins University School of Medicine, Baltimore, MD.

Spinocerebellar ataxia accompanied by congenital cataracts and oligophrenia is a well-known syndrome carrying the eponym of Marinesco-Sjoegren. The mode of inheritance is clearly autosomal recessive with a high frequency of consanguinity among the parents as demonstrated by Sjoegren. Autosomal dominant inheritance is the most likely mode of transmission in the presented family. Also, the onset of neurologic problems is insidious and late in life.

The patient, a 58-year-old white male, first came to the attention of a neurologist because of difficult walking starting around age 50. He had been operated for congenital cataracts at age 2 years and had maintained a lifelong 20/100 visual acuity. His neurologic problems were rapidly progressive so that at age 56 he was able to walk only a few steps using 2 canes as support. Slurring of speech became noticeable around age 54-56. There was a questionable decline of cerebral function over the past years.

The family history is positive for a son with congenital cataracts and mild neurologic signs such as increased deep tendon reflexes, intermediate-to-positive Babinski sign bilaterally and general clumsiness. The patient's parents were young at his birth and unrelated. His marriage was not consanguineous.

On neurologic examination, he has an evident wide-based gait with marked scissoring of the legs. The cranial nerves were intact except for some questionable reduced abducens activity. On motor examination, the segmental strength was good in upper and lower limbs. There was no atrophy, fibrillation or tremor. The tone was increased primarily in the lower limbs, but also in the upper limbs, especially in the right arm. The deep tendon reflexes were symmetrically hyperactive. The Babinski sign was positive bilaterally. Sensory examination was normal to pin prick and touch; however, he had no sense of vibration in the lower limbs. Finger-nose and knee-shin-heel test showed marked incoordination bilaterally in the upper as well as in the lower limbs. The Rhomberg test was negative. He thus had signs of cerebellar, long tract and posterior column involvement. On pneumoencephalography the patient had borderline large ventricles.

A CASE REPORT OF 46,XX,t(4;13)(q31;q14). *E. C. Jenkins, F. M. Curcuru-Giordano and S.*

G. Krishna, New York State Institute for Research in Mental Retardation and Willowbrook State School, Staten Island, NY.

An 11½-year-old mentally retarded girl has consistently indicated the above karyotypic description. The IQ was 41. She was below the 3rd percentile in height, weight and head circumference. The face was triangular with prominent glabella, marked hypertelorism, bilateral epicanthal folds, ptosis and laterally downward-slanting palpebral fissures. The subject had bilateral cataracts, pendular nystagmus and was legally blind with small and irregular pupils. Her nose was broad, flat and depressed, while her ears were large and low-set with large conchae and scaphoid fossae. The lower jaw was large and protuberant with prominent alveolar ridges and malocclusion. The chest was shield-like with a short retracted sternum and wide-spaced nipples. A systolic murmur was present. Muscle mass was decreased but the tone was normal. Antecubital and posterior neck skin presented with dry lichenoid eczema. The hands showed clinodactyly, while the feet revealed very short 3rd and 4th toes and bilateral metatarsus adduction. A pilonidal sinus was present. There was no axillary and only sparse pubic hair. Genitalia and breasts were infantile, while the clitoris was enlarged.

A total of 259 metaphase spreads derived from short-term leukocyte and skin fibroblast cultures consistently exhibited the translocated chromosomes, 4 and 13, and a modal chromosome number of 46. Eight of 152 blastoid mitotic figures manifested random loss of chromosomes with counts of 45 (5 cells) and 44, while the same situation existed in 9 of 107 skin fibroblast-like metaphases except that all random loss effected only monosomic counts. 58 G-, Q- and R-banded karyotypes have been analyzed. There is a question as to whether or not the phenotypic presentation can be attributed to an unbalanced karyotype brought about by segregation in a reciprocal translocation heterozygote.

ADDITIONAL DATA RELATIVE TO PATERNAL AGE AND FRESH GENE MUTATION. *K. L. Jones, M. A. Harvey, L. Quan, B. D. Hall and D. W. Smith*, Dysmorphology Unit, University of Washington Medical School, Seattle, WA.

Older paternal age has been recognized as a factor in fresh gene mutations and has been documented in sporadic cases of 5 autosomal dominant conditions.

In this collaborative study, an older paternal age factor was additionally documented in sporadic cases of the basal cell nevus syndrome, the Crouzon syndrome and the Waardenburg syndrome (3 conditions in which autosomal dominant inheritance has been implied) and in sporadic cases of acrodysostosis and progeria, suggesting a fresh mutant gene etiology for these 2 conditions in which the mode of inheritance has been unknown. Paternal age data from a number of other disorders showed inconclusive or no older paternal age factor.

Recognition that older paternal age is a major factor leading to fresh gene mutation in man should be incorporated into general recommendations relative to family planning.

49,XXXXX SYNDROME IN A NEONATE. *R. L. Kaufman, G. S. Sekhon, J. E. Brazy, M. C. Sivakoff* and *G. Hatahet*, Depts. of Pediatrics and Medicine, Washington University School of Medicine, St. Louis, MO.

The patient was the 1980 gm product of a 44-week gestation in a 29-year-old gravida 1, para 0, abortus 0 white woman. The pregnancy was uncomplicated. Labor was induced because of prolonged gestation. Amniotic fluid was brownish in color. The placenta was small. One minute Apgar score was 6. Several minutes after birth the child stopped breathing and was resuscitated with oxygen. She was noted to have multiple dysmorphic features and was transferred to St. Louis Children's Hospital at age 2 days.

Each parent had had a previous marriage of 5 years and was unable to have children in those marriages. The mother's niece had Down syndrome.

At age 2 days, the child's length was 45 cm, chest circumference 25.5 cm, head circumference 32.5 cm and weight 1910 gm, all below the 3rd percentile. There were craniofacial disproportion with prominence of the parietal and occipital areas, prominent anthelix and antitragus, mongoloid slant of the palpebral fissures, hypoplastic mandible, bilateral 5th digit clinodactyly, right simian crease, left complex crease, increased arches on fingerprints and bilateral metatarsus varus. At times the 2nd and 5th fingers overlapped the 3rd and 4th fingers. There was no cardiac murmur. Buccal smear showed Barr bodies in 94% of cells

including 9% with 4 Barr bodies. Blood lymphocyte and skin fibroblast karyotypes were 49,XXXXX.

At age 2 months, a grade 2/6 murmur was noted at the left sternal border. ECG and vectorcardiogram were normal. A cardiac series showed mild cardiomegaly and slightly prominent pulmonary vascularity compatible with a small left-to-right shunt.

CONGENITAL UNILATERAL ICTHYOSIFORM ERYTHRODERMA WITH IPSILATERAL HYPOPLASIA OF UPPER AND LOWER LIMBS. *S. B. Kontras, S. Kataria, A. P. Eaton* and *F. P. Flowers*, Dept. of Pediatrics, Dept. of Medicine, Ohio State University, College of Medicine and The Children's Hospital Research Foundation, Columbus, OH.

A child with unilateral icthyosiform erythroderma with marked hypoplasia of bony structures on the same side as the skin involvement is described.

B.T. was the product of a full-term normal pregnancy and delivery. There were no illnesses and growth and development were normal. She was noted to have severe "diaper rash" present at birth. The rash was treated with Vioform, Velvachol and oral nystatin without improvement. At the age of 1 month, a difference in size of the limbs was obvious. An orthopedic consultation was obtained. The family history is significant in that both parents are in their 30s and have 2 other children who are in good health. The mother's younger sister died at 28 days of age of a heart condition and it was noted that the left side of her body was smaller than the right. The mother's cousin (maternal side) died at 3 months with a similar problem and, in addition, had skin lesions.

On physical examination, the patient was active and normally developed with shorter and smaller right upper and lower limbs. Radiographic studies revealed a 6 cm difference in length between upper limbs and a 5 cm difference in length in lower limbs. The right hand showed a simian crease. The rash in the perianal area and right suprapubic area measured 7.5 × 10 cm. A skin biopsy showed hyperkeratosis, parakeratosis, acanthosis and was consistent with an icthyosiform erythroderma.

Icthyosiform erythroderma with hypoplasia of a limb appears to be a distinct clinical entity which should be recognized because of the implications for genetic counseling. This entity was first described in a single case by Rossman in 1963. Falek in 1969 reported 2 lethal cases in sibs and suggested the possibility of either teratogenesis, genic mutation or recessive transmission. In the present case, the family history indicates 3 affected individuals in 3 generations and adds the consideration of a dominant gene with varying expression as a possibility.

THE G SYNDROME: ANALYSIS OF 2 NEW CASES. *Y. Lacassie* and *V. A. McKusick*, Division of Medical Genetics, Dept. of Medicine, The Johns Hopkins University School of Medicine, Baltimore, MD.

Two new patients presenting the typical clinical picture of the G syndrome described by Opitz et al in 1969 are described.

The first patient was examined at birth because he presented severe neuromuscular defects of the esophagus and swallowing mechanism, a peculiar face with hypertelorism, very wide open fontanel, rather low-set ears, hoarse cry and hypospadias II° (with descended testes). The specific diagnosis was evident when the maternal family (*E Family*) was examined and a first cousin (second patient) with anal atresia, rectoperineal fistula and scrotal hypospadias was found; his mother also was hyperteloric.

The first patient died before the third month as a result of his respiratory problems. Autopsy was performed revealing failure of closure of the laryngotracheal groove. The second patient was under control from 1970 until the middle of 1973, at which time he died suddenly.

FACIAL SOFT TISSUE ANTHROPOMETRY. *J. Mann* and *A. O'Keefe*, Dept. of Medical Genetics, Kaiser Foundation Hospital, Santa Clara, CA.

Birth defects literature abounds with subjective descriptions of facial features. Several of these features have become sine qua non diagnostic criteria for specific syndromes, eg palpebral slants in Down syndrome, ear shape in Potter syndrome etc.

Because of the importance of facial features in the area of birth defects, we have undertaken to define a methodology for objective criteria in describing several facial features. In this preliminary work on 257 children, we chose ear

positions and rotation, mandibular length, palpebral slants and facial shape as our experimental features.

X and Y define ear position and rotation. X and Y are obtained through calculations using measurements relating the ear to the nasion and to the occiput. G defines mandibular length. G is obtained through calculations using measurements relating the mandible and the maxilla to the occiput. P defines palpebral slants. P is obtained through calculations using measurements relating the inner and outer canthus to the glabella. F defines facial shape. F is obtained through calculations using measurements relating the nasion and mandible to the zygomas. Normal graphs are available for X, Y, G, P and F through the age groups newborn to 13 years. The group is small and we have not separated sex or ethnic groups in this preliminary study.

SKELETAL DYSPLASIA WITH SOFT TISSUE TUMORS AND OCULAR, DENTAL AND DIGITAL ANOMALIES: A NEW SYNDROME? *J. D. Miller, S. A. Temtamy, L. S. Levin* and *J. P. Dorst*, The Moore Clinic, The Johns Hopkins Hospital, Baltimore, MD.

An 11-year-old white girl presented with dwarfism, soft tissue tumors, skeletal dysplasia and ocular, dental and digital anomalies. Except for advanced parental age, pregnancy and family history were unremarkable.

The digital malformations were partial soft tissue syndactyly of some fingers and toes, which were short with broad, short and flat distal phalanges. The left thumb and great toe were particularly short. The great toes were widely separated from the other toes. The lateral 4 toes showed clinodactyly. There was inability to extend both elbows completely. The facies showed wide-set eyes; flat forehead; large, low-set, protruding ears; bulbous nose; and a slightly hypoplastic mandible. She had mild left blepharoptosis, exophoria and high myopic astigmatism. There were multiple abnormalities in the permanent dentition including congenital absence of many teeth. The upper right permanent lateral incisor was markedly elongated and conical in shape. The hard palate was of normal configuration with no submucous cleft. Supernumerary maxillary and mandibular frenula were evident. Multiple small, sessile, pink, fibroma-like lesions were found on the mucosal surface of the lips and on the buccal mucosa. Early in life soft tissue nodules, some of which were subungual, were noted on the fingers and toes. Biopsies of these tumors showed dermatofibroblastic hyperplasia. Her intelligence was normal and she had mild unilateral conductive hearing deficit. Skeletal anomalies included knock-knees and progressive thoracolumbar kyphoscoliosis which led to short-trunked dwarfism. Roentgenographic findings included serpentine scoliosis associated with increased hypoplasia of vertebral bodies along the concave aspects of the curves, localized areas of narrowing of some ribs, hypoplasia and dislocation of both radial heads and scattered radiolucencies and thinning of many bones. Digital malformations were bilateral and symmetric. In addition to syndactyly, the bones were short except for the 2nd metacarpals which were elongated and possessed 2 epiphyses. Multiple carpal and tarsal synostosis, and fusion of the bases of the 2nd and/or 3rd metacarpals or metatarsals with the corresponding carpals or tarsals were noted. Areas of bone expansion of some metacarpals, metatarsals and phalanges were also present.

The skeletal malformations and their association with soft tissue tumors suggested a diagnosis of neurofibromatosis. The absence of café-au-lait spots and histopathologic changes made such a diagnosis unlikely. The presence of symmetric digital malformations with carpal and tarsal synostosis and the orofacial anomalies are not features of neurofibromatosis. Some of the facial features, the conductive hearing deficit and the digital anomalies resemble those in the otopalatodigital (OPD) syndrome. This patient probably represents a new syndrome.

GENETIC COUNSELING IN A GROUP SETTING. *A. E. Mirkinson* and *N. K. Mirkinson*, The Cornell University Medical College, New York, NY and The Association for the Help of Retarded Children (Nassau County), Old Brookville, NY.

A group counseling technique has been evolved by the counseling section of the Genetics Laboratory at North Shore University Hospital. It is used to counsel large groups of people all having interest in the same basic genetic problem. We have counseled over 100 families in this manner including a second generation contemplating marriage. The method evolved provides expert genetic counseling information to large numbers of members of families at risk for having inherited disorders. We feel that the group setting enhances understanding, the depth of perception and the

confidence that the patient has in the information received. It provides a time setting designed to reach the largest number of potentially affected family members, and a direct link with ancillary workers for continuing care for the practical and emotional family planning problems derived in the presence of genetic inherited disease.

While our experience has been for the most part confined to families affected by Down syndrome, we feel that this technique can be profitably applied to those genetic disorders having a high incidence (relatively speaking) in the general population. It is especially applicable to those disorders in which early detection of the disorder by prenatal amniocentesis monitoring makes possible the choice of termination of the pregnancy.

A FAMILIAL CASE OF WOLF SYNDROME (4p-) (Balanced Translocation Carriers and Affected Individuals). *A. E. Mirkinson* and *F. Nataro*, The Cornell University Medical College, NY and Nassau Hospital, Mineola, NY.

The first reported incidence of a chromosomal syndrome, Wolf syndrome (4p-), is presented. This syndrome, presented in the literature as occurring sporadically, joins the long list of chromosomal abnormalities which can occur in the carrier, balanced translocation state.

RING -4 CHROMOSOME. *R. Niss* and *E. Passarge*, Institut fur Humangenetik, Universitat Hamburg, Hamburg, Germany.

A ring -4 chromosome has been identified in an 11-year-old boy with mental retardation, microcephaly, small stature, ptosis palpebrae, hypoplastic thumbs and an abnormal dermatoglyphic pattern. The behavior of the ring in interphase suggested that it was often lost in subsequent cell divisions. The G-band identification showed that loss of chromosomal material had occurred in the distal long arm.

CONGENITAL HYPOPLASIA OF THE DEPRESSOR ANGULI ORIS MUSCLE. A GENETICALLY DETERMINED CONDITION? *C. Papadatos, D. Alexiou, D. Nicolopoulos* and *E. Hadzigeorgiou*, Dept. of Pediatrics, University of Athens, Medical School, Athens, Greece.

The frequency of hypoplasia of the depressor anguli oris muscle was 37 cases among 4530 consecutive births. Diagnosis was based on clinical and electromyographic studies. Severe congenital anomalies were detected in 3 of the 37 cases while another 3 newborns had minor congenital defects. In 17 of the 37 cases there were first or second degree relatives with lower lip asymmetry. A minimum of 13 out of the 74 parents of the probands were affected. The high incidence of affection among first degree relatives of the probands is a strong evidence of hereditary factors playing a role in the etiology of this anomaly.

DOWN SYNDROME AND MATERNAL AGE IN SOUTHERN CALIFORNIA: IMPLICATIONS FOR GENETIC COUNSELING. *R. M. Peterson, H. L. Wolfinger, Jr.* and *B. K. Dixson,* San Diego Regional Center for the Developmentally Disabled, Children's Health Center, San Diego, CA.

Down syndrome has been reported in the literature to occur in approximately 1/600-1/700 births. It has clearly been shown that the frequency of Down syndrome increases with maternal age. A review of 400 cases of Down syndrome served by the San Diego Regional Center for the Developmentally Disabled from 1969-1974 revealed that 57% of the children and adults in this sample were born of mothers less than 35 years of age. Data from this study have been compared with information from previous studies in the United States and other countries.

A RARE CAUSE OF LARGE PIGMENTED CUTANEOUS MACULES AND KYPHOSCOLIOSIS. *M. Pope,* The Johns Hopkins Hospital, Baltimore, MD.

The coincidence of large pigmented cutaneous macules and thoracolumbar kyphoscoliosis strongly suggests neurofibromatosis. Naked-eye diagnosis of the pigmented cutaneous lesions is not always reliable, as illustrated by the following case report.

A 9-year-old black female was referred to exclude the diagnosis of the Marfan syndrome. Her mother was concerned about a tall slim build, failure to gain weight and a spinal curvature. She was less worried about slowly enlarging cutaneous patches over the trunk and limbs.

Examination showed a tall, slim, prepubertal female with a span slightly in excess of the height. The palate was normal and the lens undislocated. There was a slight thoracic kyphoscoliosis convex to the right. Multiple pigmented macules ranging from one-half to many centimeters were scattered over trunk and abdomen. Some were smooth-edged and others irregular. A larger lesion was noted over the left temple. System examination was otherwise normal. Neurofibromatosis was considered likely but because of the unusual scalp lesion a pigmented macule was biopsied. This showed an active junctional nevus clearly distinct from neurofibromatosis. Investigations which included Heme 7, sedimentation rate, hemoglobin electrophoresis, SMA 6 and 12, and EEG were normal. Scoliosis films showed a 26° convex lumbar scoliosis with an equal compensatory thoracic curve.

Small pigmented junctional nevi are present in all adults. They increase gradually throughout childhood and more rapidly in puberty. In general they are less than 5 mm in diameter.

Less commonly, very large lesions occur with a similar histologic appearance. They range in size up to many centimeters. Though sometimes congenital, they are most common in early and late childhood and have a particular liability to malignant melanomatous degeneration. Associated abnormalities include spina bifida, clubfeet and bony hypertrophy. Subarachnoid infiltration occurs and is sometimes complicated by hydrocephalus.

In contrast to neurofibromatosis, there is no familial aggregation so that optimistic genetic counseling should be made. To our knowledge the association of giant pigmented junctional nevi with kyphoscoliosis has not been previously reported. It can always be confidently separated from neurofibromatosis by biopsy of the pigmented areas.

CUTANEOUS SQUAMOUS CELL CARCINOMA AS A RARE COMPLICATION OF CERVICAL MENINGOCELE. *M. Pope* and *A. Todorov,* Moore Clinic, The Johns Hopkins Hospital, Baltimore, MD.

Cervical meningocele has a frequency of 1/20,000 live births. Rare complications include nerve root compression and skin ulceration. We describe the first recorded example of squamous cell carcinoma complicating such a lesion.

A 37-year-old white male was followed at our clinic with a large posterior cervical lump and severe kyphoscoliosis. The former was considered a meningomyelocele because of wasting of the small hand muscles and possible posterior column signs. A persistently non-healing ulcer developed at the tip of this mass and failed to respond to topical antibiotics. An exuberant central area with a rolled edge made surgery essential. In retrospect he remembered previous smaller ulcers at similar sites which had healed and left small depressed scars. A myelogram showed the mass to be a meningo-cele and it was easily and completely excised without complication. Histologic examination showed a squamous cell carcinoma of the ulcerated region.

Cervical meningocele is especially liable to recurrent junctional damage because of its awkward siting. Our patient remembered and showed clear evidence of recurrent ulceration and scarring of his mass. Recurrent chronic trauma can sometimes be followed by squa-mous cell carcinoma, although the mechanism is obscure. Noticeable examples include carci-noma of the lip in pipe smokers and carcinoma of the palate in "reverse" cigarette smokers. Hot tea drinking has been suspected of causing esophageal carcinoma. The particular liability of outdoor workers to facial carcinomas is well-known. Chronic leg ulcers may become carcinomatous and the frequent severe scarring of Ehlers-Danlos syndrome is occasionally fol-lowed by carcinoma. Cervical meningocele should be added to those areas in which irritation may be complicated by carcinoma.

THE RATIONAL LIMITS OF PRENATAL DIAGNOSIS. *T. M. Powledge*, Institute of Society, Ethics and the Life Sciences, Hastings-on-Hudson, NY.

Adoption of fetal visualization is a major turning point in the short history of prenatal diagnosis, both philosophically and technically. The collaborative study on amniocentesis will be published next year and will presumably reveal that technique's remarkable safety. Pre-natal diagnosis is thus beginning to move into a new expansionary phase.

It will be this paper's contention that such expansion should be curbed and that limits should be placed on the uses of these new techniques. One way this could be achieved is to divide testable conditions into categories. The first would consist of serious abnormalities about which there is wide agreement; here tests would be freely available and perhaps even encouraged, and a positive test would usually be followed by abortion. A second category would include conditions that might generally be regarded as trivial or easily correctable; tests for them should not be done even if they exist. A third — and sex choice, which is already being done, falls into this group — would include conditions where large-scale abortion for this reason alone might have disruptive social consequences.

The last category would be the most fluid, a grey area where individual parental desires should probably have the greatest influence on the decision to test. Diseases in this category would be expected, in time, to move into one of the other groups — for instance, as tests became more specific or treatment improved.

The need for such controls will be defended on both philosophic and practical grounds.

A SYNDROME OF SYNDACTYLY, CRANIO-FACIAL AND SKELETAL ANOMALIES. *M. E. Rios, R. L. Kaufman, W. H. McAlister* and *V. V. Weldon*, Depts. of Pediatrics, Medicine and Radiology, Washington University School of Medicine, St. Louis, MO.

A white male, the second child of 25-year-old parents, was noted to have several dys-morphic features at birth. These included downward-slanted palpebral fissures; hyper-telorism; epicanthal folds; beaked nose with a prominent soft tissue nasal bridge; low-set ears; high-arched palate; cryptorchidism; bifid thumb and syndactyly of the 3rd, 4th and 5th fingers bilaterally; broad 1st toes; partial syndactyly between 2nd and 3rd toes; and complete syndactly between the 3rd and 4th toes bi-laterally. Several surgical procedures were per-formed between 1-2 years of age to correct the hand anomalies, epicanthal folds and cryptor-chidism. A testicular biopsy showed structures consistent with infantile seminiferous tubules. In 1972 Perthes disease of his right femoral epiphysis was diagnosed and treated. At age 13 years, his weight and height were in the 3rd percentile and his head circumference between the 50th-98th percentile. Besides the anomalies noted above, he had posteriorly rotated ears with prominent anthelix and dimples on the lobes; micrognathia; bronze pigmentation with prominent venous marking of the upper chest;

pectus excavatum; scars in both inguinal regions; no palpable testes; multiple scars in both hands; and short thumb, 3rd, 4th and 5th fingers bilaterally.

Radiographic findings included diffuse osteopenia; thick diploid space of the skull, especially in the frontal region; hypoplastic mandible and maxilla; hypertelorism; loss of the normal nasofrontal junction depression; and increased basal angle. The clavicles were short and bowed and the 1st ribs hypoplastic. There was spina bifida occulta of L5 and S1 and the 2nd and 3rd cervical vertebras were fused. The neural arch of L1 on the right was hypoplastic. The hands showed flexion contractures. The 1st metacarpals were hypoplastic. The remaining distal 1st phalanx was cleft. There were hypoplastic distal phalanges and a middle 5th phalanx, underdevelopment of the distal radius, a broad distal ulna and a decreased carpal angle, but no carpal fusion. The radii were distally hypoplastic and both proximal radial heads were dislocated. The forearms were shortened. There were coxa valga, broad proximal femoral necks, flattened proximal femoral heads with subluxation and secondary degenerative changes on the right, and broad proximal fibular metaphyses. The distal phalanges in the feet were shortened, especially the first.

Our patient has some resemblance to the *F* form of acropectorovertebral dysplasia described by Grosse et al.* However, he had more striking craniofacial anomalies, different digits involved in syndactyly, less involvement of the feet and lacked the carpal and tarsal synostosis prominent in their patients.

A NEW PHENOTYPE OF THE CEREBRO-HEPATORENAL SYNDROME OF ZELL-WEGER IN SIBS. *M. Robinow, R. Bobo, W. Schubert* and *A. Klein*, The Children's Medical Center, Dayton and the Children's Hospital, Cincinnati, OH.

Two male infants in a sibship of 3 showed strikingly similar clinical and laboratory findings. Both children had marked scaphocephaly, an unusual facies and poor muscle tone. Soon after birth they developed failure to thrive, developmental retardation and seizures. Laboratory studies revealed very severe hypoproteinemia and some evidence of parenchymal liver disease. Radiography showed severe bone

*(Part III. *Limb Malformations*, Birth Defects: Orig. Art. Ser. V(3):48-63, 1969.)

dystrophy. Pneumoencephalography demonstrated cerebral atrophy and ventricular enlargement.

The first child died at the age of 6 months after progressive mental and physical deterioration. The second boy started on a similar downhill course soon after birth. A massive pericardial effusion occurred at 3 months and required pericardiotomy. Soon afterwards the hypoproteinemia began to improve spontaneously. Now, at 11 months, he seems somewhat improved clinically, though his liver function continues to deteriorate.

Tissues obtained from the first child at autopsy and from the second at biopsies of brain, liver, kidney and bone marrow have shown the characteristic findings of the Zellweger syndrome.

A PERICENTRIC INVERSION OF A NO. 4 CHROMOSOME WITH A t(4q-10p-) AND A FAMILIAL t(DqDq) IN A MENTALLY RETARDED GIRL. *M. Robinow, S. M. Soukup* and *W. A. Yarema*, Children's Medical Center, Dayton, The Children's Hospital Research Foundation, Cincinnati and St. Elizabeth Hospital Medical Center, Dayton, OH.

A complex chromosome abnormality, consisting of a pericentric inversion of a chromosome No. 4, a t(4q-10p-) and a familial t(13q14q), was found in a 12-year-old girl showing various minor dysmorphic stigmata, moderate mental retardation and an expressive aphasia. The structural chromosome rearrangements were analyzed by Giemsa, quinacrine fluorescence and terminal acridine orange banding techniques. No loss of chromosome material could be demonstrated to account for the patient's defects.

SOMATOMETRY OF THE FACE IN PRESCHOOL CHILDREN. *I. Rostenberg, M. Jiménez, M. Daltabuit* and *S. Armendares*, Sección de Genética, Departamento de Investigación Científica, I.M.S.S., México, D.F., México.

Face somatometry was performed in 278 normal mestizo children of both sexes from Mexico City. The measurements studied were the following: bizygomatic diameter, bigonial diameter, morphologic face height, upper face height, nasal length, nasal breadth, outer bipalpebral distance and inner bipalpebral distance. The following indexes were calculated: morphologic facial index, upper facial index, nasal index and interpupillary distance. Also, for comparative purposes 5 children with face dysmorphology as a manifestation of the Marfan, Hurler, Sanfilippo, Morquio and Scheie syndromes were studied. It was observed that in them some of the normal values were deviated, which suggests that face somatometry can be a good diagnostic aid.

HIGH VERTEBRAL ANOMALIES, WEBBED NECK, HETEROCHROMIA OF THE IRIS AND CLEFT PALATE. *M. Saadat, M. Tafozoli* and *M. Ziai*, Aharis Children Medical Center, Tehran, Iran.

Association of heterochromia of the iris and cleft palate with high vertebral anomalies, although conceivable, has not been reported previously. On the other hand, manifestations of first arch syndromes including cases of Waardenburg syndrome are not associated with high vertebral anomalies. However, according to Waardenburg, under the title of status dyspraphicus many combinations of spinal anomalies with manifestations of first brachial arch syndrome could be seen.

A 2½-month-old white girl was born to a 25-year-old mother, gravida 2, para 1. Birthweight was 3 kg. There was no history of exposure to radiation, contagious diseases, etc during pregnancy. The parents were not blood related.

Physical examination on admission revealed an acutely sick infant. Weight was 2.5 kg, length 48 cm and head circumference 36 cm. Her head was normocephalic, but mild asymmetry of the face was noted. The right iris was blue and the left one was brown. Pupils were equal and reacted to light. Fundi were normal. The ears were low-set and there was a small preauricular skin tag on the left side. A midline cleft palate was present. Mandible was somewhat small. The neck was short and webbing was prominent. The shoulders were asymmetric. Wet rales were audible bilaterally; no heart murmur. Liver edge was palpated below right costal margin. The tip of the spleen was also palpable. Her external genitalia and limbs were normal. Except for a moderate degree of diaper rash, her skin was normal. There was no webbing around the joints. Her buccal smear showed normal female pattern. Chest x-ray film of the spine demonstrated spina bifida, hypo-

plasia of the vertebras of the cervical and upper thoracic regions, besides Sprengle deformity on the right with the omovertebral bar.

This case presents an unusual combination of anomalies previously not reported all in one patient.

ACROMELIC ANOMALIES SUGGESTIVE OF A NEW SYNDROME. *G. F. Smith* and *D. W. Day*, Section of Genetics and Human Development, Rush Presbyterian St. Luke's Medical Center, Chicago, IL.

A 31-week-old white male was referred for genetic evaluation of acromelic anomalies, obstipation and gross motor development delay. The patient's mother (gravida 2, para 2, age 31 years) and father (age 31 years) were both healthy and of normal appearance and intelligence. There was a normal 2-year-old female sib. The mother ingested 50 mg of clomiphene citrate (Clomid) to help induce this conception. The normal gestation spontaneously terminated in labor at 38 weeks. Subsequent course was uneventful.

Physical examination revealed weight to be 6.7 kg (3rd%), length 60 cm (10th%) and head circumference 43 cm (10th%) (Boston Children's Growth Curves). There was normal cephalic configuration with prominent forehead; the anterior fontanel (8 × 5.5 cm), parietal foramen and all cranial sutures were open. Hair pattern showed normal right occipital whorl with a preauricular downward sweep and low posterior hairline. The face showed prominent epicanthal folds, broad nasal bridge, mild antimongoloid slant, right esotropia, minimally low-set ears with poorly formed and folded helix without lobule and a small-appearing mouth with a longer, thin upper lip. The mouth frequently assumed a "puckered appearance," with a high-arched palate. The nose was unremarkable. Cardiac examination showed a grade 3/6 systolic murmur and decreased femoral pulses, suggesting mild coarctation. Fecal masses were palpable in abdomen and bilateral cryptorchidism was present. Acromelic anomalies were present bilaterally. Hands showed 1) marked radial clinodactyly of 1st, 2nd and 5th fingers; 2) camptodactyly of 3rd and 4th fingers; 3) broad distal phalanges and nails of 1st and 2nd fingers; 4) duplication of distal osseous portion of 2nd phalanges; and 5) osseous hypoplasia of midphalanx of 2nd finger. The feet were symmetric, with broad great toes and clinodactyly of the 4th toe.

Laboratory data: EEG, endocrine, urine amino acid and general laboratory screening exams were all normal. EMI computerized cephalic scan showed mild dilatation of lateral and third ventricles. Radiograms showed shallow acetabula, premature osteosynostosis of third and fourth ossification center of sternum and bone age delayed below the "slow" 10th percentile. Patient and parental chromosome studies were normal. Denver Development Screening Test proved abnormal (only 2 test items of greater than 5 months age level were passed: "bears some weight on legs" and "turns to voice").

Dermatoglyphics of the hands showed concentric whorls on fingers 2-5 bilaterally; thumbs — ulnar loops; bilateral simian lines; and left thenar area — ulnar directed loop. The feet demonstrated a long deep axis.

This case presentation bears some signs in common with the Rubinstein-Taybi syndrome. However, it does not show that syndrome's typical facial gestalt. The hand and foot anomalies of our case appear more extensive than those seen in the Rubinstein-Taybi syndrome. We raise the question of this infant being a variant or a new syndrome.

POLYDACTYLY OF TRIPHALANGEAL THUMBS WITH UPPER LIMB AND PECTORAL DYSPLASIA. *S. A. Temtamy* and *J. P. Dorst*, The Johns Hopkins Hospital, Baltimore, MD.

A 22-year-old white female was referred for genetic counseling. She was the result of her mother's second pregnancy which was 8 months and uneventful. Family history was unremarkable. The father was 36 years old and the mother 34 years old when the patient was born. At birth, the patient was noted to have bilateral preaxial polydactyly. The 2nd digit on both hands was triphalangeal and was removed at the age of 18 months. Since her early childhood, she was noted to have a left parasternal, grade 1-2/6 systolic ejection murmur. Because of easy fatigability, complete cardiac evaluation at the age of 21½ years, including right cardiac catheterization was done and showed normal findings. Other laboratory investigations, including CBC, were normal. On examination, the patient was of average build. She had malformations of both hands, inability to supinate both forearms, a slightly shortened right humerus, prominent clavicles, bilateral

hypoplasia of the sternal head of the pectoralis major muscle, slight winging of the scapulas, pectus excavatum and multiple pigmented nevi. The hands showed scars of removed triphalangeal thumbs. The remaining right thumb was thin, elongated, digitalized, inflexible and non-opposable. The left thumb was also thin and elongated but was partially flexible and opposable. Both thenar eminences were hypoplastic, particularly on the right. The lower limbs were normal.

Roentgenograms showed a triphalangeal thumb on the right, with an elongated 1st metacarpal, and a left biphalangeal thumb with a short 1st metacarpal. Partial scaphoid lunate fusion, an os centrale, a small capitate and a large pisiform bone were noted bilaterally, as was shortening of the middle phalanges of the 2nd and 5th fingers. Both medial epicondyles were prominent and the carrying angles were increased especially on the right. Both scapulas had flat inferior angles and were rotated outward, and there were coracoclavicular joints. The medial ends of both clavicles were broad.

Except for polydactyly of the triphalangeal thumbs, the clinical and roentgenologic changes in the upper limbs of this patient are those generally considered specific for the Holt-Oram syndrome. Unilateral polydactyly of a biphalangeal thumb was noted by Schonenberg (1968) in a patient with the Holt-Oram syndrome.

Triphalangeal thumb with or without polydactyly of the thumb but without cardiac disease is inherited as an autosomal dominant trait in certain families. It will be interesting to obtain shoulder, upper limb and wrist roentgenograms in such families to know whether the changes described above may be present. If so, it would mean that these limb and shoulder abnormalities are not specific for the Holt-Oram syndrome.

THE PARTIAL TRISOMY 3q SYNDROME. *J. Herrmann, T. Ruffle, L. F. Meisner, C. Viseskul* and *E. F. Gilbert*, Depts. of Pediatrics, Pathology and Preventive Medicine, University of Wisconsin, Madison, WI.

A family included several phenotypically normal members with a 46,XX or XY,t(3q-;12q+) karyotype and a severely malformed infant with a 46,XY,12q+ karyotype. He represents trisomy for at least the distal two thirds of the long-arm chromosome 3. A previous male sib probably was also affected.

ACROFACIAL DYSOSTOSIS TYPE NAGER. *J. Herrmann, P. D. Pallister, E. G. Kaveggia and J. M. Opitz*, Depts. of Pediatrics and Medical Genetics, University of Wisconsin, Madison, Boulder River School and Hospital, Boulder, MT and Central Wisconsin Colony and Training School, Madison, WI.

We report 4 personal cases and summarize information from 11 previously reported cases of a particular form of mandibulofacial dysostosis which is referred to as acrofacial dysostosis type Nager (AFD Nager). This condition frequently affects at least 2 developmental field complexes, one involving the craniofacial skeleton and one the radial ray. The Treacher Collins syndrome and AFD Nager can be distinguished clinically and appear to be etiologically distinct. While no single clinical finding is diagnostic and precise differentiation may not be possible in some instances, the general pattern of manifestations is different in both conditions. This is summarized in the following table:

Manifestation	*AFD Nager*	*Treacher Collins*
Hypoplastic zygoma	mild-moderate	often severe
"Antimongoloid" palp. fissures	frequently mild	often severe
Lower lid coloboma	rare	frequent
Hypoplastic maxilla	mild-moderate	often severe
Hypoplastic mandible	often severe	rarely severe
Cleft palate, uvula	frequent	rare
Dysplastic auricles	lower portion	entire portion
Abnormal forearms	frequent	rare
Abnormal hands	frequent	rare
Further skeletal findings	frequent	rare
Etiology	unknown (?autosomal recessive)	autosomal dominant

FAMILIAL CYSTIC KIDNEYS AND PANCREAS, WITH FIBROSIS OF LIVER IN A PATIENT WITH PROGERIC FEATURES. *E. T. Heuser, R. Koch and B. H. Landing*, Depts. of Pediatrics and Pathology, University of Southern California and Childrens Hospital of Los Angeles, Los Angeles, CA.

This child was the product of a normal pregnancy, labor and delivery. At age 8 weeks, he had persistent jaundice, hepatosplenomegaly, diarrhea, failure to thrive and anemia. A tentative diagnosis of hepatitis was made. Thereafter, jaundice and liver size diminished but elevated bilirubin persisted. At 1 year of age, he had an episode of sepsis and urinary tract infection; ureteropelvic obstruction and "microcystic disease" of the kidneys were diagnosed. At age 4½, he was anicteric, but at age 5, hepatomegaly was noted. At age 9, icterus, pruritus, hepatosplenomegaly and easy bruising were present and he was 104 cm tall. Baldness appeared at age 10. At this time, a 3-week-old male sib died with fibrosis of the liver and cystic kidneys. By age 13, the patient had progressive renal failure and portal hypertension. At 14, his height was 135 cm. He had alopecia, deeply wrinkled external ears and was not pubertal. There were scaling and upward spooning of the fingernails. Calcific masses were present in the right axilla and over both shoulders. There were resorbtion of ungual tufts in the hands, demineralization of bones, and femoral and iliac arterial calcification. Fundi were normal. Death occurred at age 16 in hepatic and renal failure.

Autopsy revealed a habitus and facies resembling progeria. Massive medial calcinosis of atria, aorta and large muscular arteries was present. The liver was fibrous. Kidneys showed structural malformation, with collecting tubular and nephronal cysts. There were cysts in the head of the pancreas. Other findings were tumoral soft tissue calcinosis, ectopic pancreas in small bowel, accessory spleens, bilaterally bilobed lungs, esophageal varices, secondary parathyroid hypertrophy, generalized osteoporosis and malacia. The liver and kidney pathoarchitectonics were the same as in his infant brother.

FAMILIAL HEPATIC CIRRHOSIS AND ENDOCARDIOPATHY. *R. M. Holland-Moritz and A. M. Stern*, Dept. of Pediatrics, University of Michigan Medical Center, Ann Arbor, MI.

Three children of a sibship of 4 presented with persistent jaundice and left-sided heart failure. The jaundice was detected shortly after birth whereas symptoms of heart disease were delayed until after the second year. The 2 youngest, identical twin girls, and their sister, the oldest child, were afflicted whereas their parents and intermediate brother were not. The clinical picture of the 3 girls was essentially the same, consisting of gross hepatosplenomegaly, ascites, esophageal varices, osteoporosis, cooing apical and harsher aortic systolic murmurs and exacerbations of chronic pulmonary congestion. Though cardiac decompensation was present, their hearts were only slightly enlarged. Their body weights were below the 3rd percentile except when ascites was present. Developmental milestones were mildly delayed.

Their serum bilirubin levels, alkaline phosphatase, bromsulphalein retention, SGOT and SGPT were persistently elevated. The chest x-ray films showed Kerley B lines and pulmonary edema as the heart disease progressed. ECG showed left ventricular hypertrophy in the older child and surviving twin. Liver biopsy revealed portal fibrosis but no evidence of neonatal hepatitis, hepatocyte necrosis or biliary obstruction. The karyotype of one twin was 46,XX.

Because of massive esophageal bleeding on 5 occasions, the older twin had a mesocaval shunt on 1/19/73. She died on 1/29/73 following several episodes of gross hematemesis. The oldest sister had replacement of her mitral valve with a porcine prosthesis on 3/9/73. She had a very stormy postoperative course and died on 5/25/73 of hepatic insufficiency and cardiac failure. Their autopsies showed hepatic cirrhosis, fibrocongestive splenomegaly, esophageal varices, cardiomegaly, membranous subaortic stenosis and, in the younger child, shortened and thickened chordae tendineae. The older child's mitral valve and attachments showed identical changes. The extrahepatic biliary systems were normal.

The mode of transmission appears to be recessive. The authors have not been able to find a report of similar cases in the literature.

C9/D13-TRANSLOCATION RESULTING IN DUPLICATION/DEFICIENCY. *P. N. Howard, K. M. Yarbrough* and *G. R. Stoddard*, Institute of Genetics, University of Southern Mississippi, Hattiesburg, MS and Medical Laboratory, Ellisville State School, Ellisville, MS.

Several recent reports have discussed a duplication or trisomic condition for part or all of a No. 9 chromosome. We have been studying a familial translocation involving a reciprocal exchange between 9q and 13q.

The 12-year-old, profoundly retarded white proband suffers from multiple anomalies and is a patient at a state mental institution. Routine chromosome analysis revealed an abnormal karyotype — 46 chromosomes with a missing D-group chromosome and an extra C-group chromosome. G-banded cells revealed a trisomic condition for most of chromosome 9 and monosomy for part of chromosome 13. Thus, the proband has a chromosome complement of 46,XX,-13,+der(9),t(9;13)(q22;q12)mat as the result of adjacent-2 segregation during gamete formation in the mother.

MICROSTOMIA, LINGUA SCROTALIS AND MICROPHALLUS — A NEW SYNDROME. *I. Hussels-Maumenee*, Dept. of Medicine and Ophthalmology, The Johns Hopkins University School of Medicine, Baltimore, MD.

A 13-year-old boy was referred with unilateral glaucoma secondary to uveitis. On physical examination he was found to be above the 97th percentile for height and weight. He had microstomia and lingua scrotalis; his ears were big and fleshy. There was no thyroid enlargement. Thoracic and abdominal examination were unremarkable. On urogenital examination, he had normal descended testicles and had early pubertal signs. His phallus, however, measured only 1 cm. He had normal range of motion in his joints; his hands were flat and somewhat poorly differentiated. He had postaxial brachydactyly of his feet and mild hallux valgus bilaterally. On neurologic examination, his intelligence was low-normal. The cranial nerves were intact; so was sensation, tonus and motor strength. The deep tendon reflexes were present in all limbs and there were no pathologic reflexes. The family history was negative for lingua scrotalis, microstomia and microphallus. He is the eighth of 9 sibs. His father was 35 and his mother 31 years old at the time of his birth. On laboratory examinations, he had a slightly elevated IgG for age; all other tests were unremarkable. This patient is presented as a new syndrome of unknown etiology.

SEVERE MOHR SYNDROME OR MILD MAJEWSKI SYNDROME? *S. A. Temtamy, L.*

S. Levin, J. D. Miller, K. McClanine and W. Goldie, The Moore Clinic and Dept. of Pediatrics, The Johns Hopkins Hospital, Baltimore, MD.

We studied a newborn Philippino female with features of the Mohr syndrome, who had severe micrognathia, glossoptosis and rudimentary epiglottis. The infant was the result of her mother's third pregnancy, which was full-term but complicated by a gross polyhydramnios. The first pregnancy ended by miscarriage. Both parents were normal, 29 years old and unrelated. A 1½-year-old brother was normal. Family history was unremarkable. At birth the Apgar score, the placenta and cord were normal. Her birthweight was at the 60th percentile, length 50th percentile and head circumference 80th percentile. Orofacial malformations were hypertelorism, bilateral epicanthic folds, flat nasal bridge, median pseudocleft of the upper lip which was accentuated by a heavy maxillary labial frenum and severe micrognathia with short ramus of the mandible and a relatively wide body. The tongue was normal in size and was not lobulated; however, there was significant glossoptosis. A soft, yellow, sessile nodule, 4 mm in diameter, was noted on each lateral border of the tongue. The hard palate was V-shaped and no cleft was evident. She had heptadactyly of the right hand and both feet with preaxial and postaxial polydactyly and syndactyly of some fingers and toes. The infant had decreased muscle tone and poor head control. An excretory urogram was normal. During her 15-day stay in the nursery she had no respiratory distress. Her main problems were feeding and a stridorous breathing when lying in the supine position. She was initially fed by gavage but was gradually shifted to a special feeder. At age 7½ weeks, she was readmitted to the hospital because of feeding problems, failure to thrive and aspiration pneumonia. A rudimentary epiglottis with absent cartilage and collapsible oropharynx were detected by tracheolaryngoscopy. A tracheostomy and an elective gastrostomy were lifesaving.

The gross polyhydramnios and the hypoplastic epiglottis noted in our patient are features of the Majewski syndrome, not previously noted in cases of the Mohr syndrome. Our patient, however, did not have other features of the Majewski syndrome, ie thoracic dystrophy with short ribs and respiratory distress, short limbs with rounded tibias or urogenital anomalies. Similar orofacial and digital anomalies occur in both syndromes. The phenotypic overlap between Majewski and Mohr syndromes, as illustrated by our patient, and the early neonatal deaths and stillbirths in previously born affected sibs of reported cases of the Mohr syndrome suggest that Mohr and Majewski syndromes may be mild and severe expressions of the same disorder. This question may be answered by the study of lethal cases of the Mohr syndrome.

MACRODACTYLY, HEMIHYPERTROPHY AND CONNECTIVE TISSUE NEVUS: A NEW SYNDROME?

S. A. Temtamy and J. G. Rogers, The Moore Clinic, The Johns Hopkins Hospital, Baltimore, MD.

Macrodactyly, like other digital anomalies, is either an isolated malformation or occurs as a part of syndromes, such as congenital partial gigantism, neurofibromatosis, Ollier disease, Maffucci syndrome, Klippel-Trenaunay-Weber syndrome and congenital lymphedema.

We studied a 7-year-old white male with macrodactyly and hemihypertrophy who did not clearly fit into any of the above entities. Abnormal enlargement of the fingers was first noted at 4 months of age; the index finger continued to grow rapidly and was amputated at 2½ years. At this stage hypertrophy of the left middle finger and thumb, and the right index and middle finger was noted. Digital enlargements occurred in both length and circumference and were slowly progressive. At age 3½ years, mild scoliosis and disparity in leg length were noted. On examination at age 7 years the child had obvious macrodactyly and hemihypertrophy. He approximated the 50th percentile in both height and weight, had mild pectus excavatum, flaring of the lower ribs, winging of the scapulas and mild scoliosis. There were slightly dilated veins over the left anterior chest and 4 depigmented areas over the trunk. The skin over the dorsum of both hands, the left foot, the back of the elbow and in the axilla was thick, coarse and depigmented. The right upper limb was 1 cm longer than the left and the right lower limb 2 cm longer; the right foot was larger than the left. The 2nd toe showed mild enlargement.

IVP was normal and the kidneys equal in size. Radiographs of the spine showed some shortening of the sacrum and structural abnormality of L5. His intelligence was normal. Skin biopsy from the dorsum of the right foot showed a well-defined but nonencapsulated area in the middermis where collagen appeared coarse, fragmented and stained more deeply than the surrounding normal collagen. There was a suggestion of thickening and clumping of elastic tissue. This was interpreted as connective tissue nevus.

The family history revealed no similarly affected individuals. He was the fourth offspring of a 35-year-old mother and a 40-year-old father, who were unrelated. Examination of the mother showed coarse facial skin with excessive freckling and some pedunculated pigmented lesions, which on biopsy proved to be a common dermal nevus. Other members of this family were not available for examination.

The association of progressive macrodactyly with hemihypertrophy and connective tissue nevus may represent a new syndrome exhibiting some features in common with neurofibromatosis. One other case with the same anomalies has previously been reported by Werthemann (1952).

A NEW POSTAXIAL POLYDACTYLY SYNDROME? *S. A. Temtamy* and *J. G. Rogers*, The Moore Clinic, The Johns Hopkins Hospital, Baltimore, MD.

A 5 10/12-year-old Turkish boy, the offspring of normal first cousins, was referred to us because of multiple malformations. The mother was 33½ and the father 39½ years old at the time of his birth. He was born at term following the mother's eighth pregnancy. This had been complicated during the first month by a 10-day febrile illness, presumptively viral. There were 3 older male sibs, one who died of a hypoplastic left heart at 2 days of age. The remaining pregnancies had ended in abortion, 1 spontaneous and 3 induced. At birth, the proband was noted to have a single umbilical artery and multiple malformations. The malformations were bilateral hydrocele, phimosis, craniofacial asymmetry, congenital torticollis, bilateral ear malformations and hemivertebras with agenesis of 11th and 12th ribs, right facial nerve paresis, ureteropelvic junction obstruction, congenital heart disease and digital malformations. The cardiovascular anomalies were a retroesophageal right subclavian artery, hypoplastic left ventricle, truncus arteriosus with pulmonary atresia and blood supply to the lungs from the aorta.

On examination his height and weight were below the 3rd percentile. There were plagiocephaly, a high forehead, narrow palpebral fissures, an elongated nose and a small mouth. The uvula was bifid and there was a submucous cleft of the palate; the lower medial and lateral incisors were fused bilaterally. The neck was short and webbed with low hairline and right torticollis; both ears were malformed and posteriorly rotated. The nipples were widely spaced, low-set and hypoplastic. His hands showed postaxial polydactyly and mild webbing, with clinodactyly (radial) of the 5th digit and of the 2nd digit (ulnar), due to short middle phalanges, with a bilateral single flexion crease on the 5th digits. The 5th digits possessed nails and like all the other nails, they were clubbed and cyanosed but not dysplastic. He had short 2nd toes and bilateral partial soft tissue syndactyly of the 2nd and 3rd toes. An extra rudimentary postaxial digit on the right foot had been removed shortly after birth.

The right testis was undescended and the left testis was in the inguinal canal. IVP showed left hydronephrosis. Skeletal roentgenograms showed an asymmetric skull with no evidence of craniosynostosis or increased intracranial pressure. He had incomplete fusion and hemivertebras at T12 and L1 and a butterfly vertebra at T4. The ribs were quite narrowed posteriorly and widened anteriorly. The IQ was 71; this may have been depressed by immaturity and deprivation. Biochemical, metabolic and chromosome studies showed no abnormalities. A maternal uncle was said to have postaxial polydactyly of one foot.

THE DUANE/RADIAL DYSPLASIA SYNDROME: AN AUTOSOMAL DOMINANT DISORDER. *S. A. Temtamy, A. S. Shoukry, I. Ghaly, R. El-Meligy* and *S. Y. Boulos*, National Research Centre and the Cairo University Children Hospital, Cairo, Egypt.

The Duane anomaly, an unusual congenital form of strabismus, was noted in an Egyptian man who also had radial dysplasia. Two of his 3 children had radial dysplasia. The first-born child, a female, was said to have had congenital club hands and short upper limbs, and died at the age of 5 days of congenital anuria. The proband, the second affected child, had bilateral radial dysplasia, malrotation of the left kidney with some pyelocaliceal dilatation and absence of the right kidney. He had no associated Duane anomaly. The lower limbs were normal. Both father and son had malformed ears and the father had associated bilateral facial nerve weakness and right congenital hearing deficit, mostly sensorineural. Pectoral and upper limb muscle hypoplasia were noted in the son. Pregnancy and family history were unremarkable and chromosomes were normal. The association of the Duane anomaly with radial dysplasia as seen in the present family is the second example of autosomal dominant inheritance of this association with variable expressivity. In the presently reported family, the associated anomalies were malformed pinnas, pectoral and upper limb muscle hypoplasia, congenital deafness and facial nerve weakness with renal anomalies; congenital heart disease was noted in the previously reported family by Ferrell et al (1966), where a father and 3 out of his 5 children had radial defects. While the father had radial defects and the Duane anomaly without associated congenital heart disease, the proposita had radial defects and the ASD but did not have the Duane anomaly; a sister, similar to the father, had radial defects and the Duane anomaly; and a brother had radial defects only. All associated malformations noted in these 2 families were previously noted in sporadic cases of the Duane anomaly. The presence of such associated malformations indicates a developmental correlation which is genetically determined in the familial cases. Absence of the Duane anomaly in all previously reported cases of the Holt-Oram syndrome, in familial cases of radial defects as isolated malformations and in other radial dysplasia syndromes suggests that the association of radial dysplasia with the Duane anomaly in these 2 families may represent a distinct genetic entity which, similar to other radial dysplasia syndromes, may have a high incidence of other mesodermal defects, including congenital heart disease and renal malformations. The definition of the variety of anomalies which may be associated with the Duane/radial dysplasia syndrome must await reports of additional cases.

ANTIMONGOLISM OR MONOSOMY 21: 46,XY,-21,+ SMALL METACENTRIC. *M. S. Tenbrinck*, Child Evaluation Center, Dept. of Mental Retardation, Phoenix, AZ.

F.B. (2/12/70) was born after 25 weeks' gestation. During the first trimester, the mother had experimented with "uppers and downers," LSD, took "a lot of" Doriden® for sleep and repeatedly smoked cannabis to "highs." She spotted from the third month on and before delivery had early toxemia and one episode of syncope.

At birth the child weighed 1109 gm. He was exchange transfused, had RDS and was kept in the hospital for 3½ months. His developmental milestones have been delayed, such as walking at 26 months, talking at 36 months.

He is below the 3rd percentile in height and weight. He has poor muscle mass and sparse subcutaneous fat. His head is narrow. The eyes have an antimongoloid slant and epicanthus. There is slight left lid ptosis. The bridge of his nose is rather prominent. The palate is high-arched but without tooth crowding. The ears are large and low-set. There is a blowing systolic murmur at the left sternal border. The hands have slender tapering fingers and transverse palmar creases (not true simian lines). The testicles were palpated in the inguinal canals. The IQ was 55 at 3 7/12 years. Hypertonia, micrognathia, hypospadias and seizures were absent.

The cytogenetic report was 46,XY,-21,+ small metacentric. Cytogenetic study of the family showed normal karyotypes of mother (46,XX), father (46,XY) and older sister (46,XX). The mother denied drug experimentation during her first pregnancy. Cytogenetic studies were performed at Children's Hospital, Los Angeles, CA.

DOWN SYNDROME: TRISOMY AND TRANSLOCATION 47,XX,18q-,t(18q21)+. *M. S. Tenbrinck*, Child Evaluation Center, Dept. of Mental Retardation, Phoenix, AZ.

A.C.G. (7/8/69) was recognized as having Down syndrome at birth. Cytogenetic studies performed on 6/16/71 and 8/31/71 were reported as 47,XX,18q-,t(18q21)+. Analysis of the cells revealed 47 chromosomes. In addition to an extra chromosome in the G group, consistent with Down syndrome, there is also a deletion of the large arm of an 18 chromosome which is translocated to one of the G group.

The girl demonstrated classic Down syndrome stigmata. At 3 10/12 years her IQ was 54.

A cytogenetic study of the available family members was made. The maternal grandmother, a maternal aunt and uncle, as well as the mother, demonstrated the translocation. (The mother had spontaneous first trimester abortions before and after the birth of *A.C.G.*) The maternal grandfather and one maternal uncle showed 46,XY karyotypes. The father's karyotype was 46,XY.

Cytogenetic studies were performed at Children's Hospital, Los Angeles, CA.

A RARE FORM OF ARTHROGRYPOSIS. *D. D. Weaver* and *J. G. Hall*, Depts. of Medicine and Pediatrics, University of Washington Medical School, Seattle, WA.

An 18-year-old male is reported with arthrogryposis involving his arms and hands, apparently caused by congenital hypogenesis of the flexor muscles of the upper arms and forearms, and scapular muscles. His monozygotic twin was unaffected. At birth, he had fixed extension and rotation of arms with flexion contractures of the wrist and fingers. At the time of transplantations of the pectoralis muscles to the ulnas, no flexor muscles were found, but some fibrous bands appeared to have replaced some missing muscles. These changes apparently represent a rare form of arthrogryposis involving the arms. The case is discussed with emphasis on possible etiology.

OCULAR MANIFESTATIONS OF DE LANGE SYNDROME. *R. Weleber* and *F. Hecht*, Dept. of Ophthalmology and Dept. of Pediatrics (Clinical Genetics), University of Oregon Medical School, Portland, OR.

That the ocular manifestations of de Lange syndrome can be helpful in differential diagnosis is not widely known. Most people are aware that bushy eyebrows, synophrys, antimongoloid slant, long lashes and telecanthus are present. However, most are unaware of the other ocular findings such as blepharophimosis, ptosis, mongoloid slant, esotropia, exotropia, nystagmus, microcornia, blue scleras, high myopia, pupillary anomalies, orbicularis oculi paresis and pallor of the optic disk. We have intensely studied a 20-year-old girl who presented with features of de Lange and bilateral posterior subcapsular cataracts. Chromosome studies were normal. As far as we can ascertain, posterior subcapsular cataracts have not been reported with de Lange patients. Patients with cataracts should receive additional biochemical investigation to attempt to detect enzyme deficiencies which might predispose to or cause cataract formation. Diagnosis of de Lange in adult patients is difficult. Heterogeneity of the syndrome probably exists. We strongly recommend the reporting in detail of atypical cases of de Lange syndrome.

Contributors

O. S. Alfi
Associate Professor of Pediatrics
Division of Medical Genetics
University of Southern California
Los Angeles, CA 90033

J. F. Annegers
Department of Medical Statistics
and Epidemiology
Mayo Clinic and Mayo Foundation
Rochester, MN 55901

F. Antillón
Departamento de Oftalmología
Hospital de Pediatría
Centro Médico Nacional
Instituto Mexicano del Seguro Social
Apartado Postal 73-032
México 73, D. F., México

R. M. Antley
Assistant Professor of Medical Genetics
Indiana-Purdue University
Indianapolis, IN 46202

V. Apgar*
Lecturer in Medicine
Division of Medical Genetics
Department of Medicine
The Johns Hopkins University School
of Medicine
Baltimore, MD 21205

S. Armendares
Jefe de la Sección de Genética
Departamento de Investigación Científica
Instituto Mexicano del Seguro Social
Apartado Postal 73-032
México 73, D. F., México

K. W. Ashcraft
Department of Surgery
The Children's Mercy Hospital
Kansas City, MO 64108

R. S. Baum
Director of Neonatology
Methodist Hospital
Indianapolis, IN 46202

M. Bernal
Pediatra
Departamento de Pediatría
Hospital de Gineco-Obstetricia
Centro Médico Nacional

Instituto Mexicano del Seguro Social
Apartado Postal 73-032
México 73, D. F., México

D. Bixler
Chairman
Department of Oral-Facial Genetics
Indiana University Medical Center
Indianapolis, IN 40202

W. Blankenship
Associate Professor of Pediatrics
University of California
Davis, CA 95616

D. S. Borgaonkar
Associate Professor of Medicine and Head
Chromosome Laboratory
Division of Medical Genetics
The Johns Hopkins University School of
Medicine
Baltimore, MD 21205

J. B. Brayton
Assistant Professor of Pediatrics and
Laboratory Animal Medicine
The Johns Hopkins University School of
Medicine
Baltimore, MD 21205

N. J. Burzynski
Professor of Oral Medicine
University of Louisville
Health Sciences Center
Louisville, KY 40208

L. L. Bushkell
Resident
Department of Dermatology
School of Medicine
University of Minnesota
Minneapolis, MN 55455

J.-M. Cantú
Investigador Asociado
Sección de Genética
Division de Biología de la Reproducción
Departamento de Investigación Científica
Centro Médico Nacional
Instituto Mexicano del Seguro Social
Apartado Postal 73-032
México 73, D. F., México

R. J. Cantwell
Assistant Clinical Professor
Mailman Center for Child Development
Department of Pediatrics

---

*Deceased

347

University of Miami
Miami, FL 33124

J. Červenka
Associate Professor
Division of Oral Pathology
School of Dentistry
University of Minnesota
Minneapolis, MN 55455

F. Char
Associate Professor of Pediatrics
University of Arkansas
School of Medicine
Little Rock, AR 72233

D. E. Comings
Director
Department of Medical Genetics
City of Hope National Medical Center
Duarte, CA 91010

F. A. Conte
Assistant Professor of Pediatrics
University of California
San Francisco, CA 94122

V. del Castillo
Residente de la Sección de Genética
Departamento de Investigación Científica
Instituto Mexicano del Seguro Social
Apartado Postal 73-032
México 73, D. F., México

B. K. Dixson
Genetic Counselor Coordinator
San Diego Regional Center
Children's Health Center
San Diego, CA 92123

G. N. Donnell
Professor of Pediatrics
University of Southern California
Los Angeles, CA 90007

J. E. Douglas
Assistant Professor of Medicine
University of Arkansas
School of Medicine
Little Rock, AR 72233

K. W. Dumars
Associate Professor and Director
Division of Developmental Disabilities
    and Clinical Genetics
Department of Pediatrics
University of California
Irvine, California College of Medicine
Irvine, CA 92664

W. T. Dungan
Professor of Pediatrics
University of Arkansas School of Medicine
Little Rock, AR 72233

A. J. Ebbin
Associate Professor
Genetics Division
Department of Pediatrics

University of Southern California School
    of Medicine
Los Angeles, CA 90033

L. R. Elveback
Department of Medical Statistic and
    Epidemiology
Mayo Clinic and Mayo Foundation
Rochester, MN 55901

M. Epstein
Program in Surgery
University of Texas Medical School at
    Houston
Houston, TX 77025

F. H. Farrington
Associate Professor
College of Dental Medicine
Department of Pediatric Dentistry
Medical University of South Carolina
Charleston, SC 29401

W. A. Fawcett
Department of Pediatrics and the
    Clinical Investigation Center
Naval Regional Medical Center
San Diego, CA 92134

M. Feingold
Director
Center for Genetic Counseling and
    Birth Defects Evaluation
New England Medical Center
Boston, MA 02111

U. Francke
Assistant Professor of Pediatrics
Division of Medical Genetics
University of California, San Diego
School of Medicine
La Jolla, CA 92037

S. Franco-Vázquez
Cardiólogo pediatra
Hospital de Enfermedades del Tórax
Centro Médico Nacional
Instituto Mexicano del Seguro Social
Apartado Postal 73-032
México 73, D. F., México

F. C. Fraser
Director
Department of Medical Genetics
The Montreal Children's Hospital
Montreal 108, Quebec H3H 1P3

R. J. Gorlin
Professor and Chairman
Division of Oral Pathology
School of Dentistry
University of Minnesota
Minneapolis, MN 55455

A. Grix
Resident
Department of Pediatrics
University of California
Davis, CA 95616

B. D. Hall
Assistant Professor of Pediatrics
University of California
San Francisco, CA 94122

S. D. Handmaker
Fellow in Medical Genetics
Department of Pediatrics
University of California
San Francisco, CA 94122

Present Address
Department of Pediatrics
Charles R. Drew Postgraduate Medical
  School
Los Angeles, CA 90059

S. Harami
Senior Data Analyst
Image Processing Laboratory
Jet Propulsion Laboratory
California Institute of Technology
Pasadena, CA 91109

D. J. Harris
Department of Pediatrics
The Children's Mercy Hospital
Kansas City, MO 64108

W. A. Hauser
Department of Neurology
St. Paul-Ramsey Hospital and Medical Center
St. Paul, MN 55101

A. Hernández
Residente
Sección de Genética
División de Biología de la Reproducción
Departamento de Investigación Científica
Centro Médico Nacional
Instituto Mexicano del Seguro Social
Apartado 73-032
México 73, D. F., México

J. Herrman
Assistant Professor of Pediatrics
University of Wisconsin Center for Health
  Sciences and Medical School
Madison, WI 53706

E. T. Heuser
Assistant Professor of Pathology
University of Southern California
Los Angeles, CA 90007

L. S. Hillman
Instructor
Division of Neonatology
Department of Pediatrics
Washington University School of Medicine
St. Louis, MO 63110

J. Himebaugh
Senior Laboratory Technologist
University of Michigan Medical Center
Ann Arbor, MI 48104

T. M. Holder
Department of Surgery

The Children's Mercy Hospital
Kansas City, MO 64108

G. Jensen
Resident
Division of Oral Surgery
School of Dentistry
University of Minnesota
Minneapolis, MN 55455

M. Jiménez
Residente de la Sección de Genética
Departamento de Investigación Científica
Instituto Mexicano del Seguro Social
Apartado 73-032
México 73, D. F., México

O. W. Jones
Head
Division of Medical Genetics
University of California, San Diego
School of Medicine
La Jolla, CA 92037

R. J. Jorgenson
Assistant Professor
College of Dental Medicine
Department of Pediatric Dentistry
Medical University of South Carolina
Charleston, SC 29401

R. L. Kaufman
Director
Medical Genetics Clinic
St. Louis Children's Hospital
St. Louis, MO 63110

L. T. Kurland
Department of Medical Statistics and
  Epidemiology
Mayo Clinic and Mayo Foundation
Rochester, MN 55901

B. H. Landing
Professor of Pathology and Pediatrics
University of Southern California
Los Angeles, CA 90007

H. J. Lawce
Cytogenetics Laboratory
City of Hope National Medical Center
Duarte, CA 91010

S. G. Lazoff
Resident
Department of Pediatrics
Stanford University Medical Center
Stanford, CA 94305

L. Luzzatti
Professor of Pediatrics
Department of Pediatrics
Stanford University Medical Center
Stanford, CA 94305

G. M. Mahan
Consultant Pediatrician
San Diego Regional Center

Children's Health Center
San Diego, CA 92123

P. Malvaux
Visiting Professor in Pediatrics
The Johns Hopkins Hospital
Baltimore, MD 21205

S. J. Marsh
1409 Brnwell Street
Columbia, SC 29201

P. R. Martens
Senior Research Assistant
Department of Pediatrics
University of Tennessee Center for the
    Health Sciences
Memphis, TN 38103

W. K. McCord
Department of Pediatrics and the Clinical
    Investigation Center
Naval Regional Medical Center
San Diego, CA 92134

V. A. McKusick
Chairman
Department of Medicine
The Johns Hopkins Hospital
Baltimore, MD 21205

M. Melnick
Postdoctoral Fellow
Departments of Medical Genetics and
    Oral-Facial Genetics
Indiana University Medical Center
Indianapolis, IN 46202

J. Melnyk
Director
Department of Developmental Cytogenetics
City of Hope National Medical Center
Duarte, CA 91010

J. D. Miller
Fellow in Medicine
The Johns Hopkins Hospital
Baltimore, MD 21205

A. E. Mirkinson
Physician in Charge
The Genetics Laboratory
North Shore University Hospital
Manhasset, NY 11030

N. Mirkinson
Association for the Help of Retarded Children
189 Wheatley Road
Brookville, NY 11545

H. Muller
Research Specialist
Department of Psychiatry
UCLA School of Medicine
Los Angeles, CA 90027

S. Nadler
Resident in Pathology
Children's Hospital of Los Angeles
Los Angeles, CA 90027

W. E. Nance
Professor of Medical Genetics and
    Medicine
Indiana University Medical Center
Indianapolis, IN 46202

J. Opitz
Professor of Pediatrics and Medical
    Genetics and Director
Wisconsin Clinical Genetics Center
University of Wisconsin Center for Health
    Sciences and Medical School
Madison, WI 53706

P. D. Pallister
Clinical Director
Boulder River School and Hospital
Boulder, MT 59632

E. G. Panizales
Fellow in Pediatrics
Mailman Center for Child Development
Department of Pediatrics
University of Miami
Miami, FL 33124

B. R. Parker
Clinical Assistant Professor of
    Radiology
Stanford University Medical Center
Stanford, CA 94305

H. M. Pashayan
Associate Professor of Pediatrics
Tufts University Medical School
Boston, MA 02111

K. Patau
Professor of Medical Genetics
University of Wisconsin Center for
    Health Sciences and Medical School
Madison, WI 53706

B. Paul
Research Scientist
Birth Defects Institute
New York State Department of Health
Albany, NY 12202

G. Persinger
Research Associate
Department of Developmental Cytogenetics
City of Hope National Medical Center
Duarte, CA 91010

R. Peterson
Resident
Department of Pediatrics
University of California
Davis, CA 95616

I. H. Porter
Professor and Chairman
Department of Pediatrics
Albany Medical College
Albany, NY 12208

W. Porter
Manager
Biomechanical Research and Development

Section
Department of Electronic Instrumentation
City of Hope National Medical Center
Duarte, CA 91010

A. Poznanski
Professor of Radiology and Co-Director
of Pediatric Radiology
Univ. of Michigan Medical Center
Ann Arbor, MI 48104

M. Preus
Research Assistant
Department of Medical Genetics
The Montreal Children's Hospital
Montreal 108, Quebec, Canada H3H 1P3

S. Pruzansky
Director
Center for Craniofacial Anomalies
University of Illinois
Chicago, IL 60612

M. Raafat
Post Doctoral Fellow in Medicine
Division of Medical Genetics
Department of Medicine
The Johns Hopkins University School of
Medicine
Baltimore, MD 21205

Present Address
Assistant Professor
Department of Pathology and Head
Tissue Culture Unit
The Cancer Institute
Cairo University
Cairo, Egypt

J. Ramírez
Patólogo
Departamento de Patología
Hospital de Gineco-Obstetricia
Centro Médico Nacional
Instituto Mexicano del Seguro Social
Apartado 73-032
México 73, D. F., México

P. Reed
Geneticist's Associate
Division of Developmental Disabilities
and Clinical Genetics
Department of Pediatrics
University of California, Irvine
California College of Medicine
Irvine, CA 92664

W. A. Reynolds
Associate Physician
Department of Radiology
Henry Ford Hospital
Detroit, MI 48202

F. D. Riggs
Staff Pediatrician
San Joaquin General Hospital
Stockton, CA 95201

K. P. Robertson
Genetics Laboratory Supervisor
Louisiana Heritable Disease Center
Department of Pediatrics
Louisiana State University School of
Medicine
New Orleans, LA 70112

M. Robinow
Director
Birth Defects Clinic
The Children's Medical Center
Dayton, OH 45419

R. E. Robinson
Resident in Pediatrics
Children's Hospital of Los Angeles
Los Angeles, CA 90027

G. Rubio
Jefe
Departamento de Patología
Hospital de Gineco-Obstetricia
Centro Médico Nacional
Instituto Mexicano del Seguro Social
Apartado 73-032
México 73, D. F., México

J. J Rybak
Resident
Department of Radiology
Stanford University Medical Center
Stanford, CA 94305

C. Salinas
Fellow in Medicine
The Johns Hopkins Hospital
Baltimore, MD 21205

R. G. Sanger
Assistant Professor of Pediatric Dentistry
University of Southern California
Los Angeles, CA 90027

R. Schmickel
Associate Professor of Pediatrics and
Communicable Diseases
University of Michigan Medical Center
Ann Arbor, MI 48104

C. I. Scott, Jr.
Associate Professor of Pediatrics
University of Texas Medical School at
Houston
Houston, TX 77025

G. S. Sekhon
Director
Cytogenetics Laboratory
St. Louis Children's Hospital
St. Louis, MO 63110

Y. Setoguchi
Medical Director
Child Amputee Prosthetics Project
Institute for Rehabilitation and
Chronic Diseases
University of California
Los Angeles, CA 90024

N. W. Shinno
Instructor
Genetics Division
Department of Pediatrics
University of Southern California School of
   Medicine
Los Angeles, CA 90033

K. Silk
Resident
Department of Otorhinolaryngology
Indiana University Medical Center
Indianapolis, IN 46202

T. J. Sorauf
The Children's Medical Center
Dayton, OH 45419

R. Sparkes
Associate Professor
Departments of Medicine and Pediatrics
UCLA School of Medicine
Los Angeles, CA 90024

M. Steigner
Resident in Pediatric Dentistry
Department of Dentistry
Harbor General Hospital
Torrance, CA 91309

R. E. Stevenson
Director
Greenwood Genetics Center
Greenwood, SC 29646

R. E. Stewart
Assistant Professor and Chief
Pediatric Dentistry
Harbor General Hospital
Torrance, CA 91309

A. N. Stroud
Senior Biologist
Image Processing Laboratory
Jet Propulsion Laboratory
California Institute of Technology
Pasadena, CA 91109

R. L. Summitt
Professor of Pediatrics
Anatomy and Child Development
University of Tennessee Center for the
   Health Sciences
Memphis, TN 38103

R. T. Szymanowski
Staff Physician
Department of Otolaryngology
Henry Ford Hospital
Detroit, MI 48202.

S. A. Temtamy
Fellow in Medicine
The Johns Hopkins Hospital
Baltimore, MD 21205
Present Address
1 Amman Square
El-Dokki, Cairo, U.A.R.

H. Thompson
Associate Professor of Pediatrics
West Virginia University School of
   Medicine
Morgantown, WV 26505

T. F. Thurmon
Associate Professor and Director
Louisiana Heritable Disease Center
Department of Pediatrics
Louisiana State University School of
   Medicine
New Orleans, LA 70112

W. Tiddy
Director of Dental Services
Boulder River School and Hospital
Boulder, MT 59632

J. W. Towner
Assistant Professor
Genetics Division
Department of Pediatrics
University of Southern California
School of Medicine
Los Angeles, CA 90033

M. C. Tracy
Cytogenetics Technologist
Louisiana Heritable Disease Center
Department of Pathology
Louisiana State University School of
   Medicine
New Orleans, LA 70112

N. Uga
Fellow in Medical Genetics
Indiana-Purdue University
Indianapolis, IN 46202

J. Urrusti
Jefe
Departamento de Pediatría
Hospital de Gineco-Obstetricia
Centro Médico Nacional
Instituto Mexicano del Seguro Social
Apartado 73-032
México 73, D. F., México

R. J. Warren
Director
Genetics Associates
8686 Coral Way
Miami, FL 33155

F. Weber
Assistant Clinical Professor of Pediatrics
Department of Pediatrics
UCLA School of Medicine
Los Angeles, CA 90024

L. Weiss
Director
Cytogenetics Laboratory and Genetic Counseling
   Clinic
Department of Pediatrics
Henry Ford Hospital
Detroit, MI 48202

O. Welsh
Associate Professor of Dermatology
University Hospital
Universidad Autónoma de Nuevo León
Monterrey, México

R. S. Wilroy, Jr.
Associate Professor Pediatrics and
  Child Development
University of Tennessee Center for the
  Health Sciences
Memphis, TN 38103

M. G. Wilson
Professor of Pediatrics and Chief
Genetics Division
University of Southern California School
  of Medicine
Los Angeles, CA 90033

H. Yune
Professor of Radiology
Indiana University Medical Center
Indianapolis, IN 46202

Author Index

Subject Index